KARL JASPERS

VIBS

Volume 250

a volume in
Studies in Existentialism
SE
Mark Letteri, Editor

KARL JASPERS

From Selfhood to Being

Ronny Miron

Rodopi

Amsterdam - New York, NY 2012

Cover Design: Studio Pollmann

The paper on which this book is printed meets the requirements of "ISO 9706:1994, Information and documentation - Paper for documents - Requirements for permanence".

ISBN: 978-90-420-3531-7
E-Book ISBN: 978-94-012-0806-2

Printed in the Netherlands

CONTENTS

EDITORIAL FOREWORD

I am pleased to inaugurate Studies in Existentialism (SE), a special series within the Value Inquiry Book Series. I am grateful to Editions Rodopi for the opportunity to develop this body of work on the theme of existentialism, and to the members of the Society for Existential Analysis for their kind sponsorship of the series. Editions Rodopi offers the following statement of purpose, upon which I cannot improve: "Studies in Existentialism publishes works on the thinking of individual existentialists, such as Kierkegaard, Nietzsche, Sartre, Beauvoir, and Arendt, and books on topics of human existence such as freedom, values, anguish, and interpersonal relationships." I invite all prospective authors who are interested in "existentialism," however construed, to contact me with ideas for projects.

Ronny Miron's *Karl Jaspers: From Selfhood to Being*, the first book in this series, gives us a comprehensive and masterful analysis of the thought of Jaspers. I am happy to begin Studies in Existentialism with her eminently worthy undertaking (published originally in Hebrew). Despite his importance to the Continental tradition, Jaspers often receives insufficient attention, at least in English. Herewith, a remedy.

Mark Letteri
Studies in Existentialism Series Editor

GUEST FOREWORD

Interest in the philosophy of Karl Jaspers has been increasing in recent decades. Many books and articles examine various aspects of his thought, which was until recently overshadowed by the philosophy of Martin Heidegger. Ronny Miron's book about Karl Jaspers is another contribution to this trend. At the same time, the importance of this book should not be underestimated. In many ways, it opens a new era in research into Jaspers's thought.

Thanks to its research horizon, this book offers a comprehensive analysis of the entire oeuvre of Jaspers, both psychiatric and philosophical, and does not focus only on his philosophical writings. This is no small matter; through analyzing Jaspers's complete works, Ronny Miron succeeds in showing the deep structures of Jaspers's thought. This comprehensive approach is examined using a sophisticated research method, combining the diachronic aspect and the synchronic aspect. Accordingly, Ronny Miron follows the development of Jaspers's ideas, and her work in this channel involves the chronological mapping and analysis of the sequence of the ideas. The synchronic aspect focuses on the consistent, systematic analysis of the sequence of ideas. The diachronic, developmental perspective uncovers the fundamental changes that gradually led Jaspers from his original interest in mental pathology to his philosophical interest in Being and transcendence. The synchronic viewpoint indicates the perpetual elements constituting Jaspers's philosophy into one whole, inseparably combining the human effort to obtain meaning and self-understanding with the search for Being and transcendence as a space and horizon of existentialist search.

In contrast with the common approaches sketching a picture of development and change in this philosophy, from interest in questions of existence to interest in questions of Being and transcendence, Ronny Miron offers a profound and original reading of Jaspers's thought. Her approach is unique in offering her new reading from dialog with the wide-ranging interpretations of his work, in both the Continental and the English-speaking research traditions. Ronny Miron is not a critic, denying the range of interpretations written before her; instead, she views these interpretations as part of an ongoing conversation enabling profound insights into Jaspers's philosophy. She sees this philosophy as based on two themes: selfhood and Being. Jaspers's thought is a constant attempt to decipher the interrelations between these two elements, rather than a transition from one element to the other.

The questions of selfhood and its relation to transcendence, and to Being, have always been fundamental questions in human culture and in philosophy. Ronny Miron's interpretative work enables us to read Karl Jaspers's thought as a constant attempt to answer these questions. The precise and systematic tracing of the changing interrelations between selfhood and Being in the work of Karl Jaspers reveal to us a rich, original, and dynamic philosophy, worthy of a central position in the current philosophical and theological discussion. Ronny Miron's important achievement in this book is embodied in her ability to reposition a philosophy that had, for many years, been on the margins of the discussion, and for this we owe her a debt of gratitude.

Avi Sagi
Chair, Program for Hermeneutics
General Philosophy Department
Bar–Ilan University, Israel

ACKNOWLEDGMENTS

This book was originally written in Hebrew. The English version is published with the assistance of the Center for Continental Philosophy and Culture at Bar-Ilan University. I would like to extend my deepest gratitude to the Center's head, Avi Sagi, who supported the translation of the book into English and provided good advice and encouragement. I would also like to thank Avidov Lipsker of the Department of Hebrew Literature at Bar-Ilan University, and Aner Govrin, of the Program for Hermeneutics Studies at Bar-Ilan University.

The book was translated into English by Ruth Ludlam. I am grateful to her for her serious approach and dedication in creating the English version of a book whose origins are in Hebrew and German.

I also wish to thank my good friend Orit Klapisch for her support and encouragement over many years.

This book is dedicated with love to my children Shira, Noa, Itamar, and Neta, for their patience and love.

INTRODUCTION

1. Opening

In one of his lectures on philosophical intuition, Henri Bergson claimed that every great philosopher ultimately aimed to express in his writings one simple intuition, a point where there "is something simple, infinitely simple, so extraordinarily simple, that the philosopher has never succeeded in saying it. And that is why he went on talking all his life."[1] That this statement of Bergson's also appears to be true of the philosophy of Karl Jaspers. This philosophy, that was formulated against the background of the *fin de siecle*, and that dealt with such a wide range of issues—metaphysics, ethics, politics, education, religion, history, art, and more—wished to contend with one fundamental problem: the ability of modern human beings to establish a metaphysical consciousness.[2] The heart of this book will clarify the formation of metaphysical consciousness in Jaspers's writings between 1910 and 1947.

The basis of metaphysical consciousness in Jaspers's thought is the human search for the meaning of life and existence (*Dasein*). This search is grounded in the discontent that accompanies people and in the intuition that there exists some entity beyond the immediate reality in which people live and act. This intuition becomes an evident awareness in Jaspers's thought. On the one hand, it expresses people's endeavor to elucidate the discontent they experience within being.

On the other hand, it reflects people's position in the face of the possibility of the existence of a transcendental entity whose boundaries exceed the realm in which human existence operates. Jaspers's thought is rooted in the Kantian ethos according to which people act as autonomous entities and create in their consciousness the reality in which they live, but at the same time it challenges Immanuel Kant's approach that human consciousness has no access to "the thing-in-itself."

Understanding that metaphysics is embedded in the human condition does not enable people to escape their basic tasks in existence for another reality, which in their distress they can envisage as satisfying and perfect.The hold of metaphysical consciousness over immanence entails the possibility in principle that the feeling of discontent, or more precisely the objective aspects of this feeling, will be accessible to the instrument of formal consciousness. This datum creates what I call throughout this study the "epistemological viewpoint," portraying Jaspers's attempt to encompass what can be known about his topics of discussion, even only partially. For instance, as part of his perception of the field of psychopathology, Jaspers attributed great importance to knowing the physical symptoms of a mental disorder; in his book *Psychology of Worldviews* he attempted to ground his arguments on selfhood in the general and structural features of the phenomenon of multiple worldviews; and in his later philosophical writings he dealt consistently with illuminating the contribution of the objective worldview of the consciousness to the clarification of the issues under discussion: Existenz, the world, and Being.

The epistemological viewpoint does not contradict the fundamental intuition accompanying Jaspers's searches, and we should not view it as an attempt to present a substitute for intuition, which as such needs no establishment in the tools of consciousness. Jaspers's definition that philosophy "rejects the mythos that gave it birth" and presents an argued and rational understanding in contrast to the dreams and deceptions of the history books[3] may explain the nature of the epistemological viewpoint in his thought. It uses rational tools to clarify the irrational source of philosophy, whether myth or intuition.

However, Jaspers did not view the experience of discontent as a final state of human existence. His primary aim was to escape this discontent and to formulate, on the basis of the primary intuition regarding the existence of a transcendental entity, an explicit philosophical consciousness of this entity. The understanding that the very experience of discontent indicates the reality of the thing whose absence a person senses served as a basis for what I call throughout the book "the ontological viewpoint." This viewpoint portrays the intention of the consciousness to explicate the existence of the thing at the center of the discussion. At the same time, this consciousness is accompanied by the awareness of the limitations of rational thought in relation to this entity, which Jaspers believed contained transcendent aspects, such that by their very definition they cannot be accessible to people's perception and understanding. For instance, Jaspers argued that the unique personality of each mental patient is not revealed through the physical manifestations of his or her condition, and in his philosophical writing he discussed the limitations of consciousness and its inability to provide complete understanding of Existenz and of transcendence.

Unlike the epistemological viewpoint, which seeks to expose the general and objective aspects of the object and to turn them into a conscious element of the discussion, the ontological viewpoint appeals to its object's particular aspects, and has intuitive certainty of its reality. The transcendental aspects of this entity were perceived as inexplicable using the instruments of consciousness or even those of philosophy, and this obliges the ontological viewpoint to maintain the inexplicable element on which metaphysical consciousness is based. While the presence of the epistemological viewpoint in Jaspers's thought helped clarify the boundaries of the accessibility of human consciousness to the "thing-in-itself," the ontological viewpoint reflected the philosophical position regarding the gap between the particular nature of a human being's search for experience and the perfection of experience as the "thing-in-itself."

Jasper's statement that philosophy "also rejects theology" due to its connection to revelation[4] may illuminate a crucial facet of the ontological viewpoint. Philosophy cannot accept the presence of the transcendental experience on which theological thought is based as a datum that is taken for granted. In particular, it cannot accept the attempt to characterize this experience in a concrete way that could be perceived as formal knowledge about transcendence. It is true that, like theology, metaphysical philosophical consciousness recognizes the existence of a transcendental being. However, metaphysical consciousness is not grounded in an approach according to which recognition of a transcendental entity is detached from the unique character of the person establishing a relation toward Being. Jaspers's philosophical effort to regard revelation as "a historic form of phenomenal transcendence,"[5] grounding it in the immanent starting point of the person relating to it, may cause the loss of revelation's universal character, a character that theology sometimes aims to prove. The concept of historicity will be discussed in Chapter Six. However, only in this way may revelation be a significant component in the framework of philosophical consciousness aimed at explicating the entity of an experience beyond the boundaries of immanence.

Just as mythology, theology, and philosophy were for Jaspers three spheres that together form metaphysics and that exist in constant tension, so, too, we must recognize the inseparability of the two viewpoints, epistemological and ontological, presented in this book as founding elements of the metaphysical consciousness that develops in his thinking. As Jasper says:

> Philosophical metaphysics tried by pondering transcendence in existence, by thoughts that reach the ultimate origins and limits of existence, turn somersaults, and require present fulfillment by a historic Existenz. *In philosophical metaphysics we adopt mythical reality from everywhere and seek to understand what is alien to us in mythology and revelation* [emphasis mine].[6]

Metaphysics in Jaspers's thought is not presented as based on objective foundations that may enable communications between people (Jaspers's perception of communications will be discussed in Chapter Five), but as an experience where people meets themselves each time while clarifying their disposition vis-à-vis transcendence.[7] This process can serve as a basis for an illusion, since neither transcendence nor self can be fully philosophically explicated. However, Jaspers claimed that the effort entailed in fulfilling this double task and the insights formulated as a result may cause a person to "abysmally delude himself, but as a thinker he can also find there his most profound self-assurance".[8]

This process of forming the metaphysical consciousness in Jaspers's thought ultimately reflects the human attempt to find meaning in existence primarily by relying on the intuition about the existence of a transcendental being. At the same time, the reality of this entity is not perceived in Jaspers's thought as being limited to the relations of people toward it, but instead it exists in its own right, as the "thing-in-itself."

2. Periodization of Jaspers's Works

Metaphysical consciousness in Jaspers's works originates in two basic drives: to elucidate selfhood and to explicate being. Jaspers's dealing with these two drives was expressed in the works published in the two periods of his life discussed in this book: the medical-psychological period (1910–1919) and the philosophical period (1932–1947), during which his main philosophical works were written. His writings from the third period, the socio-political period, not discussed in this book, include publications written after the Second World War.[9] In this period, Jaspers showed, both in the theoretical issues he discussed and in his participation in official committees, a public awareness that was not typical of his earlier periods, and this had a deep impact on the nature and contents of his writings.

The criterion for distinguishing the periods is mainly thematic. It relies on the continuity or centrality of the topic under discussion. The writings from the first period, dealing with selfhood, will be discussed in the first part of this book, Explication of Selfhood. The second period, characterized by philosophical writing, displayed a displacement of selfhood from the heart of the discussion, in favor of the explication of Being. This period will be discussed in the third and final part of the book, Explication of Being. A discussion of the thematic and methodological aspects of the transition from the first to the second period will appear in the second part of this book, Transition Mechanisms.

A. The Medical-Psychological Period

During the first period of his writings, Jaspers wrote articles about psychiatry (1910–1913), and the books *General Psychopathology* (1913) and *Psychology of World Views* (1919). Along with his practice and academic study of medical issues related to mental illness, and against the background of positivistic approaches in science in general and in contrast to them, in this period Jaspers tended to examine different aspects related to the patient's self and private world.

The book *Psychology of World Views*, which Jaspers wrote after leaving the field of psychopathology, expressed his wish to obtain a wider view of human beings, beyond the boundaries of mental psychopathology. The choice to examine the subjective experience of the individual from a point of view of normality opened new horizons for Jaspers, enabling him to examine more abstract aspects of this experience. At the same time, Jaspers consistently avoided exploring aspects related to the concrete reality in which the subjective entity under discussion lived and operated. These features of the discussion of selfhood in this book testify to the development that occurred in Jaspers's approach compared with his earlier writings. His turning to the abstract aspects of selfhood indicated the philosophical direction he was about to adopt in the coming years. Jaspers himself described this book with hindsight as "my unconscious way to philosophy."[10] However, the separation of the discussion of selfhood from the discussion of concrete reality and the absence of additional aspects that Jaspers saw as essential for philosophical discussion do not enable us to include this book in the second period, when his philosophical writings were developed.

Relatively little research literature exists about Jaspers's writings from the medical-psychological period, and it usually does not deal with the challenge of linking them to his philosophical thought. We may assume that the research literature perceived these early writings as irrelevant to understanding Jaspers's philosophy. Unlike the common approach, the interpretation I offer in this book to these writings deals with the challenge of revealing the complex relation between them and his later thought, and focuses on the perception of selfhood (*Selbstsein*) developed in them.

B. The Philosophical Period

The second period of Jaspers's writings began in the early nineteen thirties, with the publication of *Philosophy* (1932), and it includes his main writings up to the end of the Second World War: *Reason and Existenz* (1935), *Philosophy of Existence* (1938), and *Out of Truth* (1946). In this period, Jaspers, appointed in 1920 as Professor of Philosophy at Heidelberg University, strengthened his position as a philosopher dealing with classic philosophical issues such as consciousness, human beings, the world, and Being. In his writings from this period, Jaspers continued to discuss the issue of selfhood that had interested him already in his early work, and he even dealt with it in greater depth compared with the first period. However, the main issue that interested him during the second period was clarifying Being and transcendence.

Both these periods are at the center of this study, which will show their continuity and development.

C. The Socio-Political Period

In the third period, encompassing the works written after the Second World War—mainly essays and political books—Jaspers became a thinker familiar to the general public.[11] Even when consciously addressing a wide audience of readers, using a simple and flowing style, and trying to participate in the formation of the new social and cultural reality, Jaspers never stopped viewing himself as a philosopher, and in this period he even wrote *Philosophical faith in the face of Revelation.* Jaspers redefined his thinking and changed its name from "philosophy of existence" to "philosophy of reason"—a name he believed expressed the "age old essence" (*uralte Wesen*) of philosophy.[12] However, this book is the exception that proves the rule of this period, when Jaspers discussed mainly social issues that interested Germany after the war: educating the youth; the idea of academia; the question of German guilt; the conditions and possibilities of humanism in the new political and social situation; and especially the question of the role and essence of reason and philosophy in the new reality.[13] In this period Jaspers was prominent among German thinkers seeking to establish a new identity and to found a "different Germany" on the basis of cosmopolitan values and universal ideals.[14] The new Humanism to whose development he wished to contribute, presented human freedom and its decisions regarding the truth and necessity of values as the corner stone supporting everything. In his introduction to the periodical *Die Wandlung*, reflecting his personal experiences and value decisions, Jaspers formulated the principles of this approach:

> *By no means can we say that we have already lost everything.* As long as we have not wasted in desperate anger everything we could have had as something that cannot be lost: the element of history—for us [this element is] first and foremost a thousand years of German history, and then the history of the West and finally the history of the whole of humanity... We will gain contact with everything human beings have experienced all over the world in the most extreme form. A German outcast in his homeland can find his support in the wide spaces of this humanity [emphasis mine].[15]

In his work written after the war, Jaspers sought to express the profound political and cultural changes Germany experienced after the war. Although there exists significant influence of his early work on the writings of this period, these works should be examined first and foremost against the background of the challenges of the period when they were written.[16] This sort of study requires a different methodology and poses different questions than those on which this book focuses, and this book will concentrate only on the works from the first two periods.

3. Philosophizing Framework

Jaspers opened the three-volume work *Philosophy* with the question "What is Being?," and stated that this question arose from the basic situation of people in the world.[17] This is not just one of many questions people ask about existence, but a fundamental question (*Grundfrage*) relating to what philosophy has discussed since its inception.[18] Jaspers listed three aims derived from the question of Being: philosophical world orientation, self-fulfillment and the openness toward transcendence[19], and devoted to each of these aims a separate volume: (1) *Philosophical World Orientation*; (2) *Existential Elucidation*; (3) *Metaphysics*. The three volumes, discussing the three classic issues of philosophy—world, humanity and God—include all the issues Jaspers's thought discussed in its different periods. The fact that he chose to present the framework of his discussion in *Philosophy* (1932) is no accident. This book, written after *Psychology of World Views* (1919), was undoubtedly Jaspers's "visiting card," through which he wished to distance himself from the fields of psychiatry and psychology, and turn to the professional study of philosophy. *Philosophy* is in many ways the most mature and systematic of Jaspers's works, and he himself defined it as "closest to my heart".[20]

Alongside the three areas of philosophy, Jaspers presented three types of existence that were destined to become the basic distinctions on which his philosophy was based: "objective Being," "subjective Being" and "Being-in-itself." Objective Being (*Objektsein*) expressed everything accessible to human consciousness and everything that can become "known being" (*Gewußtsein*) through science. Subjective being (*Ichsein*) is separate from the object being and expresses the unmediated layer of individual human existence.

When people think about their existence in the abstract, they see it as an object, they become in their eyes Being-in-itself (*Ansichsein*) and see all other beings as subject to it.[21] Just as the three areas of philosophy are not separate from each other, but constitute one whole, so also the three forms of existence are not separate from each other, but together portray the complex where human life occurs. So the question of Being is a sort of *organon* of Jaspers's whole philosophy, meaning that it defines the objects about which he philosophizes, and their combination forms the whole of his thought.

Jaspers apparently based this basic division of fields of philosophy on Kant's division into the three transcendental ideas of pure reason: the idea of the knowledge of the world, which is the absolute idea of all the conditions of the phenomena; the idea of the study of the soul, which is the idea of humanity as the final subject of all philosophy; and the idea for knowing God, which is the total unity of the conditions of all objects.

The transcendentalism through which Kant defined the three ideas shows that unlike the categories, they cannot be derived from the mind, and they do not refer directly to the objects of the mind as such.[22] In addition, I argue that the relation between Kant's ideas of reason and categories of mind is similar in principle to that between Jaspers's three areas of philosophy and the disciplines that deal with them formally. Just as Kant's philosophy perceived the ideas as complementing for reason what was missing in the categories of mind, which apply only to experience, so Jaspers perceived "philosophical world orientation," "existential elucidation," and "metaphysics" as complementing the three disciplines of their background: science, whose object is the world; psychology, whose object is the spiritual life; and theology, whose object is religion. While Jaspers never indicated his attitude toward Kant's distinctions, the use he made of them goes beyond the adoption of an efficient method of organization, and expresses the anchor he found in this philosophy that continued to guide him when he wrote his different works.[23]

4. Philosophical Method

Alongside the obvious relation of Jaspers's philosophical framework to Kant's basic concepts, we can also observe a certain proximity between these two thinkers in their philosophical method. According to Kant's transcendental method, people cannot achieve knowledge of any state of affairs without revealing the general and a-priori system of rules on which it relies.[24] Like Kant's transcendental method, Jaspers's method of transcending (*Transzendieren*) also aims to clarify the fundamental premises or a-priori certain logic on which philosophizing is based. This method enabled Jaspers not to see the philosophical framework set out in *Philosophy* as a starting point, but already as the result or the implementation of his method of transcending. In this respect, the three areas included in this framework: (1) Philosophical World Orientation, (2) Existential Elucidation, and (3) Metaphysics, should be seen as an objective framework within which the fields of science, psychology, and religion are rooted.

(1) In *Philosophical World Orientation*, the method of transcending is applied to everything that can be scientifically objectified. The German word *Wissenschaft*, meaning science, has a much wider range of meaning than the English word "science," which is usually used to mean the exact sciences. The German term indicates a process of methodical investigation both of human existence with all its theoretical and practical aspects, whose results are universal knowledge that can be phrased using accurate definitions. Sometimes this term appears as "science in general" (*Wissenschaft überhaupt*), in contrast to science whose object is single and more limited (*Einzelnwissenschaft*).[25] The transcendence from this framework should have applied to specific contents of human existence in the world. However, Jaspers clarified that it is based on the understanding that the Kantian perception sees the world as a disintegrating "phenomenon."[26]

The transcendence in philosophical world orientation is primary and limited in the horizons it aims at, compared with the two following transcendences, but it serves as an introduction and a condition for them. This transcendence is essential in philosophy aimed at explicating "Being" and "transcendence," as is demonstrated in the following passage:

> We search for coming to the limits that we expect, for the world, *as appearance, does not rest on its laurels, does not have a self-subsistent existence*... These boundaries, in their concrete form, do not allow us to ignore them. *I do not recognize them from general knowledge but I become aware of them only through empirical reality itself.* The more world experience [*Welterfahrung*] is fulfilled in theoretical and practical terms the more lucid is the manner of transcending the world. Without world there exists no transcendence [emphasis mine].[27]

(2) Within *Existential Elucidation*, the method of transcending is applied to the perception of the individual as a Being existing in a concrete reality in order to expose its selfhood in its peculiar specificity.[28] Jaspers presented the experience of Existenz that was shaped in this framework as what exists beyond objectivity but within the boundaries of immanent reality.[29] In this respect, the concept of Existenz combines the perception of the individual as a unique being that cannot be generalized, and the understanding that this individual can transcend the level of objectivity and even consolidate a relation toward transcendence.

Jaspers's argument that Existenz itself cannot be understood, but instead reveals to philosophy the incomprehensible (*Unverstehbare*)[30], encompasses the basic difference separating the two philosophical frameworks. While in *Philosophical World Orientation* reality and the action of the individual's mind are two sides of the same coin, in *Existential Elucidation* reality and thought are separate, so that what is considered universal in *Philosophical World Orientation* is no longer perceived as such. In *Existential Elucidation,* the one-time uniqueness of individuals is perceived as a basis that enables them to transcend the boundaries of empirical reality. Existenz, as the name for this uniqueness, becomes possible only in this boundary, where it is an experience that is not an individual case of generality. So it is perceived as inaccessible to the tools of objective reason.

(3) In *Metaphysics*, the method of transcending serves as an instrument to breach the other philosophical frameworks, *Philosophical World Orientation* and *Existential Elucidation*, in order to achieve a certainty that does not depend on existence and to form a relation toward transcendence. However, the act of transcending in *Metaphysics* is only possible by Existenz that has achieved philosophical world orientation and whose selfhood is clear to itself.[31] The implementation of the method of transcending in the two philosophical frameworks presented above should be seen as a basis and a preparation for its implementation in *Metaphysics*. The concept of "transcendence" (*Transzendenz*), whose elucidation is at the heart of the philosophical framework of *Metaphysics*, indicates the existence of a Being that is not existence (*Dasein*), consciousness (*Bewusstsein*), or Existenz. Transcendence, transcending all of these, represents what will never become an object, the complete contrast to finality and the expectation and openness to everything that formal consciousness cannot access.[32]

The three forms of transcending presented above are anchored in the idea of the "whole" (*Ganze*).[33] This idea has two faces: the subjective face is based on the origin of the "whole" being in the individual's drive to reveal the meaning of Being, and we must understand it as being beyond all forms of objectivity. The objective face of the "whole" is based on serving as an object for the person's desire. This desire does not enable people to be satisfied with their boundaries and directs them to things beyond themselves. The "whole" is perceived in Jaspers's thought as a substrate in which philosophy is anchored, and that motivates it, and at the same time as a horizon that it constantly aims to approach in order to become an explicit element in people's consciousness.

The anchoring of the method of transcending in the idea of the "whole" supports the understanding of the three contexts of philosophizing as not only derivatives of different disciplines but as parts of a comprehensive whole that exists beyond them. This shows another similarity between Jaspers and Kant, who deduced from his transcendental dialectic the following:

> We easily see that pure reason has no other aim than the absolute totality of synthesis on the side of conditions, and that reason has nothing to do with absolute completeness from the side of the conditioned. For it needs only the former series in order to presuppose the whole series of conditions and thereby give it to the understanding a priori.
> ...Finally we also come to be aware that a *certain connection and unity* showing itself among the transcendental ideas themselves and that pure reason by means of it brings all its cognitions into a system. To progress from the cognition of oneself (of the soul) to cognition of the world, and, by means of this, to the original being, is so natural that this progression appears similar to the logical advance of reason from premises to conclusion [emphasis mine].[34]

Although Jaspers's thought reflects the aim to make the "thing-in-itself" explicit, he avoids presenting his method of transcending as an instrument whose use guarantees the solution of the question of Being. The definition of the method of transcending as "only an act, not a result"[35] strengthens the understanding that this method served mainly as an instrument to reveal the three facets of the human being: the wish to make the world familiar, the drive to consolidate selfhood, and the search for God.[36] The focus on these aspects indicates that Jaspers's thought did not concentrate on consolidating the contents to fill metaphysical consciousness, but with revealing the conditions of consciousness or even the state of mind (*Stimmung*) that could facilitate the achieving of this consciousness. Jaspers aims to explicate the ways a person could imagine (*Vergenenwärtingen*) the very possibility of the existence of an absolute being. He also stressed that even within the act of transcending implemented in the realm of metaphysics, the philosopher remains in dialectic that leaves him in a constant contradiction whose solution, were it possible, would empty transcendence of meaning.[37] In this respect, the method of transcending serves as a means for marking new targets for philosophy, which ensures that metaphysical consciousness is subject to a constant process of development. Because it remains unanswered, the question of Being serves as a motivation and as an urge for a mode of being where philosophizing accompanies experience of reality.

5. Philosophical Experience of Boundary

Jaspers's method of transcending relies on the experience of boundary that is one of the primary insights that characterize his thought throughout the different periods. This experience has two aspects: first and foremost it expresses the need of individuals to constantly evaluate the entirety of insights and experiences they have accumulated so far, and to formulate them as assets at their disposal in the future. But what is perceived as an asset is not translated into an experience of self satisfaction or what Jaspers defined as "calmness" (*Gelassenheit*) regarding people's achievements. The basic drive motivating people to appraise their achievements and to focus on what has not yet been achieved reflects the condition of philosophizing that aims to create an approach that unifies all the different philosophical insights.[38] Without this drive, what has already been achieved could become fossilized and lose its creative power. The other aspect of the boundary experience was aimed at marking new targets for philosophizing and presenting them to the individual as a demand for perfection, since even if this perfection cannot be achieved, it drives people and does not let them stand still. The very search for perfection and the explication of the experience in its absence are what formulate, in Jaspers's thought, the way for creating a metaphysical consciousness.

In addition, philosophical experience of the boundary reflected the target at which philosophizing was aimed in each of the stages of the development of Jaspers's thought: In *General Psychopathology* this experience served as a basis for determining the boundaries of the science of psychiatry and for distinguishing them from what was known as "the person in his individuality and wholeness."[39] In *Psychology of World Views* this experience was at the basis of the aim "to determine the boundaries of our mental life."[40] In *Philosophical World Orientation* it served as a means for determining the relation between science and philosophy. In *Existential Elucidation* it served to redraw the boundaries between the world and the ways of knowing the particular experience of Existenz. In *Metaphysics* this experience helped clarify the awareness of the limitations of the consciousness grounded in the selfhood of Existenz alone, an awareness that led it to create a relation toward transcendence that exists beyond it. Finally, in *Out of Truth* the boundary experience, which was at the basis of the perception of the "encompassing," helped discern the relation between the immanent and transcendent aspects of Being.

The duality typical of the different expressions of the boundary experience, namely between what philosophizing has already achieved and what is perceived as a perfection not yet achieved, is at the basis of the distinction Jaspers presented between contextual boundaries (*jeweilige Grenzen*) and boundaries in principle (*prinzipielle Grenzen*). The contextual boundaries can be crossed, and they present a challenge for scholars and philosophers, even if they cannot serve as starting points for philosophy. The boundaries in principle, however, dispute the world view as a phenomenon, and scientific research reaches the limit of its ability. But although the boundaries in principle denote the end of the area that can be studied using formal tools of consciousness, they open for people the option of philosophical transcending. According to Jaspers, "every boundary immediately raises the question what is beyond it."[41] Following the relation to the philosophical framework established by Kant, Jaspers's distinction between "contextual boundaries" and "boundaries in principle" is apparently parallel to two boundary concepts in Kant: the barrier or limit (*Schranke*) and the boundary (*Grenz*). Kant states:

> Boundaries (*Grenzen*) (in external things) always presuppose a space that is found outside a certain fixed location, and that encloses that location; limits (*Schranken*) require nothing of that kind, but are mere negations that affect a magnitude insofar as it does not posses absolute completeness. Our reason, however, sees around itself as it were a space for the cognition of things in themselves, although it can never have determined concepts of those things and is limited to appearance alone.[42]

The "limit" is a sort of "stop sign" indicating the point up to which a person can reach, and no further. The "boundary," in contrast, turns the discussion to what happens within its framework, perceived as a sign of the end of the realm of experience at a person's disposal. Like the concept of "limit," the concept of "boundary" also reflects the end of the area of human experience. From an ontological point of view, we apparently cannot go beyond the "boundary," just as we cannot break through the "limit." However, standing at the edge of the "boundary" does not indicate the end of our possible experiences, since from that boundary point are visible the wide horizons surrounding our existence that are not included within our experiential consciousness. In Kant's terms, we cannot cross the boundaries with our reason, but unlike the "limit," in the "boundary" people have an idea about the existence of a space beyond us, a space where in Kant's opinion human consciousness locates the "thing-in-itself." Ultimately the concept of the "limit" is built by elimination, while the positive concept of "boundary" originates in a sort of intuition that sees it as a sign of the area of internal and external space.[43]

Jaspers used the idea of the "boundary" in order to determine the limits of philosophy from which the method of transcending would be implemented was not alien to the usage Kant made of his two boundary terms. Kant used the negative "limit" term to distinguish between the borders of mathematical and natural sciences knowledge and the borders of metaphysics: in the first, the meaning of the restriction is that the knowledge existing in these areas has not yet reached completion, although it is in a constant state of accretion. In these borders there exists movement from one conditioned thing to another. Kant called the concepts determined in these areas dogmatic, in the sense that they cannot be transcended by possible experience,[44] since he saw their borders as reflecting the limitations of the phenomenon and the way it is represented in our consciousness.[45] In contrast to the restriction existing in empirical areas of knowledge, in metaphysics the boundary is mainly positive, and as such it creates an insurmountable gap between what is known and what is not known, and must limit itself. In this context the essence of reason is exhausted in the relation to what is beyond it. This relation reflects the effort of reason to extend its boundaries in order to approach what is beyond the "boundary"—although this experience is itself accompanied by the awareness of reason that it cannot cross the boundary between itself and the experience beyond it.

Kant's philosophy was for Jaspers not only a great source of inspiration, from which and against which he philosophized, but it also provided him with instruments to formulate his own philosophy. Kant's influence on Jaspers is significantly greater in depth and breadth to the influences he absorbed from other philosophers.[46] However, Jaspers did not remain committed to the borders set by Kant's philosophy, and often Kant's ideas served as vessels into which he poured new and even contrasting contents than those where they first appeared. Jaspers apparently wished to transcend Kant's philosophy in one step, or alternately to withdraw from it by one step: unlike Kant, who placed at the center of his work the discussion of consciousness and revealing its boundaries, Jaspers's thought focused on the person bearing this consciousness. This approach helped Jaspers reveal additional forms of human experience in existence, which he thought reflected the human tendency to transcend itself.

The boundary experience and the method of transcending it show us that at the basis of Jaspers's attempt to form a metaphysical consciousness were the philosophical goals he set himself but had not yet achieved. The very experience of the absence of perfection and its role in determining the targets of philosophy was, for Jaspers, evidence of the reality of perfection itself. In this respect the method of transcending served not only as a "limit" to remaining in what had already been achieved, but also as a means that could lead the philosophers each time to new districts beyond the "boundary" where they were standing.

6. Methodological Approach

In his retrospective essay "About My Philosophy," Jaspers described the two elements to which philosophical practice is directed: the "being" and the "self." As he writes:

> The philosophical mediation is an execution (*Vollzug*) where I reach the *experience* and *myself.* This is no calm thought where I deal with an object without involvement. Philosophizing is the praxis of my own thinking source in which the full essence of the human is realized in individual people. The peak of the praxis is the internal action (*inneres Handeln*) through which I become what I am. [This action] is *making the experience discoverable (Offerbarwerden), it is the activity of the selfhood (Selbstein) which is at the same time experienced as passivity in the turning into the given to yourself* (*Sichgeschenktwerden*) [emphasis mine].[47]

These two components of philosophical practice appear in this book as central axes around which Jaspers's intellectual biography developed, and as establishing elements of the metaphysical consciousness he expounded. During the earlier stages, Jaspers dealt with the element of "self" from different points of view. This element reached its climax in Jaspers's philosophical writings with the establishment of the philosophy of existence. The discussion of "Being" took place alongside the discussion of selfhood. However, difficulties that arose in this framework pushed aside the selfhood from the center of the philosophical discussion, and Jaspers formulated a new philosophical framework, at whose center were the concepts of "Being" and "transcendence." In truth, the selfhood never ceased to interest Jaspers. But its philosophical explication showed him that behind the person's original drive to reach self-understanding pulsated another drive, deeper and more basic, leading people to search for meaning and intent beyond the boundaries of their self-being. This book aims to show that the two basic philosophical urges—the urge to explicate selfhood and the urge to form a relation toward Being and transcendence—were interlinked and simultaneously influenced the development of Jaspers's thought in its entirety. The division of Jaspers's work into periods should be seen mainly as playing a methodical role.

The order of issues discussed in the book's chapters is determined largely on a chronological basis. By ordering the material in this way, the development of Jaspers's ideas is examined from a genealogical point of view—what preceded what, which ideas served as a basis for later and more mature ideas, and what the different contexts added to explicating the philosophical questions under discussion. This approach, viewing the order of the ideas' appearance as critical for their understanding, aims to deal with the difficulty raised by Jaspers's thought—a thought that does not present its themes in a complete and systematic way, and necessitates picking out the arguments that appeared in different contexts while clarifying these contexts. The genealogical point of view aims to reveal the dynamic of the development of Jaspers's philosophy from the writings that appeared in the psychiatric period up to those written in the philosophical period.

This approach is not sufficient, since a purely genealogical study would limit the research to "the history of Jaspers's philosophy" without discussing the original issues developed in his thought. Alongside the genealogical issue, sometimes in parallel and sometimes using it as a starting point, the different philosophical issues will be examined from a thematic point of view. One crucial aspect that the thematic examination will deal with throughout the book is the dependence of the understanding of ideas that appeared in the early writings on those that appeared in later writings. However, this dependence is not a disadvantage in the context of a discussion that conducts an immanent phenomenological explication of the philosophical text. The understanding that occurs in this sort of discussion is always "temporary," and reflects the discussion at the stage when it appeared, but will later be formulated differently, more accurately, in the more advanced stages of explication.

The presence of the two viewpoints, genealogical and thematic, inevitably creates tension not only between the different parts of the book, but also within each of the chapters. This tension originates in the basic fact of the hermeneutical circle that for describing the stages of development requires the writer to have already a thematic understanding of the issues discussed, but this understanding only becomes clear to the reader after completing the entire move, at the end of the book. We should aim to understand the study as one whole, like the way Jaspers wished his book *Philosophy* to be read:

> The meaning of philosophizing is a single thought, ineffable as such: the *consciousness of being* [*Seinsbewusstsein*]. In this work it ought to be approachable from every chapter; each should be the *whole in detail*, though leaving dark what will first illuminate itself through the rest [emphasis in the original].[48]

The book focuses then on clarifying Jaspers's wide-ranging work, first and foremost from within itself and from studying the complex mutual relations between its parts. The choice to conduct a critical phenomenological explication of the philosophical text makes the writings of the philosopher himself the focus and main sources for the study. The research seeks to illuminate the different facets of Jaspers's thought and its dynamic motion through an immanent penetration of Jaspers's thought as reflected in his writings, without requiring an external justification and without proposing a critical judgment of the validity of his arguments. This understanding of the role of the interpreter is at the basis of the decision not to deal in this book with questions about the range of influences on Jaspers's thought, and not to try to discover the similarities and differences between him and other thinkers of the existentialist tradition, or to locate his work within the historical context of his time.

The scholarly literature about Jaspers focuses mainly on his philosophical writings, and places special emphasis on the three-part work *Philosophy*—the first and most systematic of them. This literature, a large part of which was written during Jaspers's lifetime, contains two main trends: one aims at a particular issue and presents an immanent interpretation of the sources dealing with it directly. Among the authors belonging to this trend we can list leading scholars of Jaspers's work: Richard Wisser, who discussed the concept of truth; Leonard Ehrlich and Aloys Klein, who dealt with perceptions of faith and religion; Sebastian Samay, who discussed questions of objectivity and science; Hans Kunz and Alan M. Olson, who focused on transcendence; and Kurt Salamun, who illuminated the ethical aspect. The other trend is an attempt to formulate a general impression of Jaspers's thought, often without grounding in a systematic explication of his writings. The second trend can be exemplified by the work of Fritz Heinemann, Otto Friedrich Bollnow, Heinrich Knittermyer, and others.[49] The literature included in these two trends does not address philosophically Jaspers's early works, dealing with psychiatry, and the ideas developed in *Psychology of World Views* are hardly mentioned.[50] Apart from the clear break with these early works, characteristic of most interpretations in both trends, they lack an integrative view of Jaspers's work grounded in an analysis of his entire corpus.

However, despite the large scope of scholarly literature in the two trends presented above, indicating the interest and challenge Jaspers presented to those who dealt with his work, it would be difficult to remain unaware that Jaspers's thought remained to a large extent on the margins of the philosophical discourse of the past few decades. This phenomenon may be explained in several ways. The first explanation involves the character and great influence of Martin Heidegger. Jaspers was Heidegger's contemporary, and they were both perceived as representing the German existentialist current. The dominance achieved by Heidegger with the publication of his book *Being and Time* in 1927, five years before the appearance of Jaspers's *Philosophy* in 1932, made gaining their place and status quite difficult for Jaspers and other contemporary philosophers. Even the thought of Husserl, Heidegger's teacher, was gradually pushed aside from the philosophical discourse, while Heidegger's gained a status and importance that was already indisputable, and even today is at the center of philosophical activity. While Jaspers had to deal with the ban on publishing his writings in Nazi Germany, Heidegger, who joined the Nazi party, continued to publish and establish his status in Germany during the Nazi regime's years in power. It was during the nineteen thirties and forties, when Jaspers's philosophical writing reached its maturity that his way to the contemporary philosophical discourse was barred, even before his thought became available for public criticism.

Alongside this historical-biographical explanation, we can suggest another explanation for the relatively marginal status of Jaspers's philosophy. This explanation involves his style of writing and the premises on which his thought was based. Jaspers deliberately avoided coining distinct philosophical terms, and in practice allowed his ideas and concepts to draw their meaning from the general context in which they appeared. This approach contributed to the unsystematic nature of his thought, and made expressing his already complex and vague ideas difficult, which often left his readers with the impression that they were not accessible to rational analysis.[51] In this respect we can argue that Jaspers's philosophy gave its readers a task that he himself did not achieve: exposing the basic structures and formulating the fundamental concepts in which it was grounded. Jaspers largely missed one of the central challenges facing any philosopher: presenting efficient thought patterns or instruments to help deal with philosophical problems even outside the boundaries of his thought.[52] Readers undertaking the challenge of Jaspers's complex philosophy are required to follow the development of Jaspers's ideas and concepts throughout his writings and formulate for themselves their overall meaning.

The interpretation I propose in this book attempts to deal with the challenge of revealing the unity of the world from which Jaspers wrote—from his beginnings as a young psychiatrist and up to his late maturity as a philosopher with his own original approach. The analysis wishes to complete what is missing in existing research literature about Jaspers, to conduct an immanent phenomenological explication of his writings, and at the same time to crystallize an integrative interpretation of the range of issues they discuss. Yet, this will not take place in a vacuum. The different approaches and interpretations in the secondary literature are perceived in this framework as part of Jaspers's text. In the interpretation offered in this book, and in the illumination of the different facets of Jaspers's thought, I will not argue with them and where possible will build upon them in offering an original interpretation of this philosophy. The current research literature about Jaspers largely focuses on different issues about his thought and activity in what was earlier called the "third period," and so it will not be discussed in this book. As explained, the research literature dealing with Jaspers's philosophical thought in the two first periods of his thought, mainly in the second period, was mostly written during his lifetime and so can be seen as part of the contemporary discourse. The discussion of the different interpretations of Jaspers's thought will be an integral part within the process of developing the interpretation offered in this study to Jaspers's thinking. The critique of these interpretations does not presume to offer the "correct method" of studying Jaspers's work, and does not claim exclusivity.[53]

7. Structure

After the Introduction, this book is divided into three parts comprising eleven chapters: Part One, containing four chapters (One to Four), deals with the explication of selfhood. This part discusses the writings of the first period and some of those from the second period that deal with selfhood. The perception of selfhood presented in this part relies on the concepts "self" (*Selbst*), "mental" (*Seelische*), and "subjectivity" (*Subjektivität*) that typified Jaspers's early writings. From the book *Philosophy* onwards, these terms made way for the concept of "Existenz." This study seeks to illuminate the development of Jaspers's thought by following his use of these concepts. It also studies the process of widening the philosophical framework from the pathological-psychological viewpoint in the early writings to the philosophical viewpoint typical of his writings in the second period, when Jaspers established his philosophy of existence. Jaspers, like other philosophers of the philosophical trend called Existentialism, preferred to remove this definition from his thought. The term "philosophy of existence" (*Existenzphilosophie*) was first coined by Friz Heinemann, considered one of the important German scholars of this trend already while it was in formation, in his book *New Way of Philosophy* (*Neu Weg der Philosophie*) (1929). In his later, more mature work, Heinemann discussed the characteristics that could include Jaspers's philosophy in this trend, and its uniqueness compared with other thinkers of this trend.[54]

My main argument in this part is that the philosophical effort to explicate selfhood is influenced by its solipsistic image, but at the same time contains several attempts to deal with this image. The first stages of his work, mainly in the psychiatric period and to a large degree also in *Psychology of World Views*, were characterized by an almost complete dominance of the solipsistic understanding of selfhood that led largely to a subjugation of the different issues under discussion to the question of their relevance to the understanding of selfhood. However, the discussion in Chapter Three and Four suggests a process of the formation of Jaspers's critical awareness of his early approaches and an understanding of the difficulties arising from them. This awareness enabled Jaspers to abandon some of the insights of his early work and prepared the ground for the inclusion of new philosophical concepts, through which Jaspers aimed to ground Existenz in a wider context. This book examines the influence of the new issues discussed in his philosophical writings on his perception of selfhood.

Part Two includes an introductory methodological chapter, three chapters (Five to Seven), and a chapter of conclusions. This part discusses three of Jaspers's central and most original ideas—"communication," "historicity," and "boundary situations." These ideas, which I define as "transitional mechanisms," are presented as central instruments that helped Jaspers rescue the perception of selfhood from the influence of the solipsistic image that had accompanied its discussion up to the appearance of these ideas. These three ideas, discussed mainly in the *Existential Elucidation*, helped expand and deepen the perception of selfhood. These ideas also opened new horizons for Jaspers that served as a foundation for the establishment of a new philosophical axis in his work, aimed at explicating Being.

Part Three contains four chapters (Eight to Eleven), and deals with the explication of Being based entirely on writings included in the philosophical period. Even in this framework Jaspers continued to discuss selfhood, but the developments typical of it, first and foremost the distancing from solipsism, diverted it from the center in favor of the concepts of "Being" (*Sein*) and "transcendence" (*Transzendenz*). The primary motive for discussing the question of Being and for seeking transcendence was presented as belonging to Existenz; however, it ceased to function as a touchstone of the different issues that arose in Jaspers's philosophy.

Finally, a note about the style of writing. The choice of a phenomenological method conducting an immanent explication of the original texts leads, almost inevitably, to a style that humanizes the different concepts under discussion, abstract though they otherwise are.

PART ONE

THE EXPLICATION OF SELFHOOD

One

SELFHOOD THROUGH MENTAL ILLNESS

1. Note on the Framework

The discussion of Karl Jaspers's early writings, *General Psychopathology* (1913)[1] and his articles on mental illness published in neurology and psychiatry journals, based mainly on experimental investigations, is quite different from the speculative and abstract philosophical discourse. The book *General Psychopathology* was published in several editions. The first edition is the shortest. In the second and third editions there were few changes. The fourth edition (1942) incorporates his main philosophical approaches, developed from the nineteen thirties onwards, and therefore it is critical to the discussion of Jaspers's philosophy. After this edition, five more editions appeared in the same format as the fourth, the latest appearing in 1973. Most scholars of Jaspers's thought did not attribute to these writings any real significance in understanding his philosophy, whose starting point they dated to *Psychology of World Views* (1919), and in many cases even to *Philosophy* (1932). When these early works did receive attention in scholarship, the focus of the discussion was the influence of other philosophical approaches, such as those of Edmund Husserl, Max Weber, Immanuel Kant, and Wilhelm Dilthey on forming Jaspers's methodical view of the science of psychiatry.[2] Jaspers's experts saw these scientific writings as irrelevant to the understanding of his philosophical work, and so did not examine their connection to his philosophical writings.

The following discussion is based on the premise that Jaspers's scientific work relied, as meta-science, on a fundamental understanding of human nature. This understanding reflects the early roots of ideas developed and expanded much later in the perception of Existenz in Jaspers's philosophical writings. While Jaspers sometimes presented them as axioms instead of as part of a critical debate, their clarification has great importance in the philosophical explication offered in research aiming to reveal the primordial insights that comprised the focus of the world of Jaspers the person—the same world in which he worked as a psychiatrist and later as a philosopher. The central argument in this chapter is that Jaspers's perception of psychopathology, where he expressed what he viewed as a guiding "ideal" of "correct science," reflected his first steps in establishing the perception of selfhood—an issue that became explicit and conscious in his philosophical writings. In this respect, we can view the perception of psychopathology as a sort of introduction to the explication of selfhood, since it constitutes one of the points of view from which he examined human beings. Obviously, the perception of psychopathology turns out to be part of the framework of Jaspers's explication of selfhood only in light of the philosophy of Existenz, which developed later. Without the philosophy of Existenz, the discussion of his early writings would be restricted to their uniqueness and innovation in relation to the perception of science current at the time. However, since the discussion of selfhood is one of the two components of metaphysical consciousness developed in his philosophical writings, one can see Jaspers's perception of mental illness as evidence of the philosophical impulse that drove him already early in his development.

2. Mental Illness as an Expression of the Individual's World

In the opening passage of the first edition of *General Psychopathology*, Jaspers introduced a distinction between the psychiatrist and the psychopathologist—a distinction fundamental to his perception of the field of psychiatry:

> *In the practical psychiatric occupations (Berufe) the interest is always in man in his individuality and wholeness*; whether he is referred to a psychiatrist [for] observation, treatment, or therapy, or whether [the psychiatrist] gives an opinion of his [the person's] personality to the court, to other authorities, to the science of history, or whether the patient approaches him for consultation during visiting hours. While his work here deals completely with the individual case the psychiatrist searches... being a psychopathologist for general concepts and rules. In contrast with the psychiatrist, who in the practical profession is a living personality for whom science is only an instrument, for the psychopathologist science is its own goal. He wants to identify and recognize, characterize and analyze, but not only the individual person, but the general... [emphasis mine].[3]

The choice of the word *Beruf* in this context and the perception of science presented in this chapter testify to the clear influence of the sociologist Max Weber, which Jaspers himself admitted explicitly. In his Protestant ethical approach, Weber explained the German word *Beruf* as a religious term denoting a life task determined by God, and in Calvinism a person's occupation was also understood as a calling that leads the person to redemption in this life and salvation in the afterlife.[4]

The difference in principle between psychiatrists functioning as scientists, psychopathologists, and psychiatrists practicing mental healthcare, depends on their attitude toward the science in which they are involved. Scientists see science as an aim in itself, and are interested in learning the general features of mental illnesses in isolation from the individual patient who suffers from them. In contrast, for practicing clinical psychiatrists, science serves as a means compared to which their personal intuition has a more important function. Jaspers's perception that the meeting of the patient's personality and that of the psychiatrist is a context where different aspects of the character of each are revealed was fundamental to the requirement that the psychiatrist be aware of different aspects related to the patient's entire life.[5] This approach was well reflected in the definition of psychiatry as an expertise (*Kennerschaft*)—a definition that added another aspect to its perception as a science (*Wissenschaft*).[6] This means that psychiatry cannot be fully defined by general concepts, but represents a whole range of relationships between two people that becomes more sophisticated and deeper by means of continuous awareness of the foundations on which it is based in an attempt to realize them in practice.

From this distinction between psychopathologists and the psychiatrists we may deduce their different views regarding the mental patient: while psychopathologists focus on the pathological discoveries in patients' behavior and on their physiological condition and determine the appropriate treatment, psychiatrists see their patients as whole and unique people. They treat each patient as an individual case. Therefore, their attention is focused first and foremost on the patient's personality and world, and only as a result of this is the relevance of scientific definitions to the patients' needs and condition examined. Their different views of the patient served Jaspers as a basis for the definition of the different types of restrictions under which they operate. Psychopathologists are viewed as always working within "restrictions" (*Beschränkungen*) resulting from the system of rules and concepts of the science of psychiatry, although these change along with the development of the science in general and the area of psychopathology in particular. Psychiatrists, on the other hand, encounter a more thorough "border" (*Grenze*), because a person as an individual can never be fully understood using concepts amenable to recognition and contemplation.[7] Since this "border" is finite in nature, it cannot be removed or overcome. This concept is linked in Jaspers's writings of this period to the quality of the person's "individuality" (*Einzelnheit*), which does not enable scientific and comprehensive arguments to be made regarding a person. This quality necessitates giving precedence to the mental patient as a human being over the scientific need to reach a pathological diagnosis.[8] These distinctions of Jaspers's show that the inseparable cohesion of physical and psychic forces, characteristic of mental patients as individuals, does not enable their treatment to be limited to the point of view of illness on which science focuses, and we must add a wider understanding of mental patients, centering on their unique personalities.

Jaspers's tendency to base his approach to the mental health field on the patient's humanity extended to psychopathology as a field of knowledge and practice. It also goes beyond the differences between the different types of interest the psychopathologist and the psychiatrist take in the mental patient under their care. As Jaspers wrote:

> For him as a *psychopathologist*, it is sufficient that he knows about the *infinitude* of each individual that he cannot fully understand; as a *human being* he can, without any connection to this, see even more; or when others see this same more (*Mehr*) that cannot be compared to anything else, he must avoid trying to convince them using psychopathology [emphases in the original].[9]

In these words, Jaspers gave deeper expression to his approach that placed the person's humanity in the center of the psychiatric approach—an attitude that turns out to be necessary not only for a better understanding of the patient, but also for establishing the psychiatrist's professionalism. In this context, Jaspers aimed for psychopathologists to use in their professional work not only the achievements of the scientific socialization that they absorbed during the years of their training, but also the entirety of their personality, whose boundaries extend much farther. In this respect, Jaspers's understanding both sides of the therapeutic situation—that of the therapist and that of the patient—reflects his attempt to protect the person's individuality. This protection is essential not only for patients, so that they will not be viewed solely through the generalizing categories of the scientist, but also for psychiatrists, who do not cease functioning as complete individuals during their work as physicians.

In this approach of Jaspers's, we can see the influence of Dilthey's basic approach, connecting "experience" (*Erlebnis*), "understanding" (*Verstehen*), and "expression" (*Ausdruck*). Dilthey stated that any experience belongs a-priori to the concrete context, and only in this context can it be understood and can it become possible at all. In his opinion, the understanding of the experience, the subject aiming to achieve it and the thing or object to which the subject's consciousness is directed are communally linked. He determined that the understanding aimed at objects is at the same time an understanding of the subject experiencing the action of understanding. Dilthey discussed this issue in the context of what is known as the "methods dispute" (*Methodenstreit*), dealing with the issue of the method desirable for the humanities and the differences between it and the method required for life sciences.[10] In this spirit, we can note that unlike the approach on which the science of psychopathology was based at that time, Jaspers wished to soften the sharp distinction between the experiencing subject, in this context the psychiatrist, and the object on which the experience focuses, namely the patient seeking therapy, in order to reveal the connection the two share and establish a therapeutic approach grounded in a broad understanding of this connection. He aimed to prevent the identification of the science of psychopathology with reality in order to enable a wider viewpoint aimed beyond the mental reality reflected in the science of psychiatry, providing the contents of this science with depth, and contributing to a wider understanding of human reality.

Understanding mental illness as a mirror of the individual's world, as arises from the basic distinctions presented above, enfolds two facets: on the negative side, it reflects Jaspers's criticism of the positivistic tendency in science, and especially in psychopathology, which had led to the reduction of patients to their illness, and of scientists to their scientific knowledge. On the positive side, the subjective individuality of the patient is placed at the focus of psychiatric practice. But beyond the contribution of these two facets to achieving a fuller understanding of Jaspers's psychiatric approach, their discussion is critical in this study due to their relevance to the clarification of the early basic principles in the background of the development of his philosophy of Existenz.

3. Criticism of the Science of Psychiatry

Already in the title of the first section of *General Psychopathology*, "The restriction and the task of general psychopathology,"[11] Jaspers expressed his aversion to the positivistic approach common in his period that saw the study of the physiological and neurological aspects as a sufficient expression of what could be known about mental illnesses.[12] While this criticism did not involve detracting from the importance of the conceptual framework of psychopathology, which phrases in objective language the symptoms typical of different mental illnesses, Jaspers himself developed an "objective psychopathology."[13] His main criticism was aimed at the medical training (*medizinische Bildung*),[14] which did not direct those destined to psychiatric practice to have a wide view of human beings, and especially did not present this view as the first tool a psychiatrist needed when meeting a patient.[15] In his basic approach that psychiatry was not merely a science,[16] Jaspers wished to propose a new understanding of the mental attitude the psychiatrist should adopt when meeting the patient. At the center of this attitude was the awareness of the boundary between people as individuals—an awareness that Jaspers considered the key to the full understanding of the human soul and of the forces that operate within it.

Against the background of the positivistic approaches current in science of this period, Jaspers saw fit to discuss the question of whether a mutual influence existed between the physiological and mental aspects of mental illness, or whether they operate in parallel channels. In this context, he stated that the issue is a subject for empirical research beyond the realm of his interest in psychiatry. However, he argued that what should be decisive in the approach toward mental illness is the basic fact that the physical and mental manifestations appear together, and that it is impossible to separate them, since the physical and mental study are conducted differently.[17] The enigmatic "continuity" that Jaspers believed connected the physical symptoms of the illness and its mental manifestations is not reflected in the science of psychopathology. On the one hand, as the objective study of the physiological aspects of mental illness progresses, the related mental element eludes it. On the other hand, the study of the mental phenomena reaches a border where it can no longer find the presence of the physical element.[18] Jaspers developed in the fourth edition of *General Psychopathology*, in the chapter "Concept of health and illness," the general principle that there is no clear distinction between health and sickness. Scholars consider this approach as a milestone in the introduction of the phenomenological method into the area of mental health.[19] From these general statements it seems that not only can the precise border apparently separating the physical and mental aspects of mental illness not be marked, but also that we cannot always find a physical expression of mental phenomena. The absence of a unified concept of sickness, resulting from the difficulty in separating the physical aspects of a mental illness from its mental aspects, was at the basis of Jaspers's far-reaching claim that the starting point of psychopathology is factually within the area of normality.[20] Since individual differences exist even among normal people, Jaspers believed that psychology was as essential for psychopathology as physiology. In some cases, psychology could not serve the psychiatrist in working with mental patients, and this should encourage psychopathology to develop its psychology.[21] In any case, Jaspers wished to emphasize that the decision regarding the normality or pathology that should be attributed to a certain mental phenomenon was always based on an assessment that was inaccurate. If the assessment is based solely on the physical aspects it could detract from the possibility of understanding the unified nature of the individual personality, and, as a result, prevent a correct perception of the patient's condition.[22]

So, Jaspers did not oppose the contribution of science in the study of the soul, but instead the positivistic pretension of a comprehensive scientific representation of the soul. The book *Psychology of World Views*, written after *General Psychopathology*, shows that he directed his criticism mainly at making science into a "world view" that served as "something whole and something universal,"[23] instead of being what it should—part of a comprehensive understanding of the person as an individual being. Psychiatrists, who aim to understand the mental patient's soul, should use science as a tool in their work, but should absolutely not view science as the sole source of their complete understanding of a person suffering from a particular illness.

Jaspers's perception of the area of psychopathology was not limited to his criticism of the positivistic tendencies current in science at the time. Understanding the alternative presented in his approach may not only explain and clarify his critical position, but also illuminate the first crystallization of philosophical aspects that later became corner stones of his thought. The connecting point linking his perception of psychopathology at this stage and the philosophy of Existenz he developed later is his understanding of the human being, which was really a decisive element in his perception of these two fields: just as the science of psychopathology cannot provide a complete understanding of mental illness, let alone provide a comprehensive grasp of the person who suffers from such an illness, so also philosophy itself bound by the limitations of the representation of our consciousness cannot expose the full being of a person.[24] Just as while he was a psychiatrist and a researcher Jaspers tried to form a different viewpoint of the person, so later, as a philosopher, he constantly aimed to liberate the attitude toward people from the restrictive viewpoints and even the wide contexts surrounding it. This attempt led, as will be clarified later, to his understanding of selfhood as a solipsistic Being.

Unlike his critical approach toward the solipsistic tendencies in the science of psychopathology in his day, Jaspers showed a positive attitude toward phenomenology, whose influence started to penetrate the area of mental health at that time. The basis for the legitimacy Jaspers granted phenomenology in his psychiatric approach stemmed from the contribution of the central concepts of "intentionality" and "phenomenon" to reaching the "things in themselves" to the blurring of the traditional distinction between "normal" and "abnormal."[25] In his article, "The Phenomenological Research Direction in Psychopathology" (1912),[26] Jaspers presented the role he intended for phenomenology in the study of mental illnesses: to delimit, describe, and name some types of experiences and the facts that appear in them in an unmediated manner. The advantage of phenomenologists for the science of psychopathology is that they can observe pathological phenomena without the theoretical burden, the premises, and the conceptual framework that accompanies them in the research literature. This approach enables them to devote themselves to the phenomena they investigate in order to achieve a tangible representation of the physical and concrete aspects of mental illness while being liberated from the knowledge we apparently have about these phenomena.[27] The sensory differentiation and the ability to think rationally, with which phenomenologists are equipped, will help them provide the science of psychopathology with what Jaspers called the "experience of being" (*Vorhandensein*) of the mental illness[28]—an understanding that encompasses the scientific viewpoint regarding the mental illness and focuses on the individual personality of the person suffering from it.

Jaspers understood phenomenology as a theoretical method, as an instrument through which the psychiatrist could detail the real expressions of the concrete mental phenomenon and give them a general aspect. He defined phenomenology as a source of static understanding (*statisches Verstehen*) of individual situations and qualities.[29] Since according to his approach the phenomenological method reveals mainly "fragments" from the mental element present intermittently in every real and concrete experience, Jaspers believed that we should not expect it to provide a wide and general view of the pathological state of the soul.[30] However, this was apparently the advantage of phenomenology and the reason for incorporating it into his approach, since as a theoretical method it lacked the pretension to propose causal or general explanations for the phenomena it described,[31] leaving room for additional viewpoints to complement it.

As Jaspers's discussion expanded, it became apparent that the static understanding, partial by nature, cannot enable psychiatrists to deal with the endless variety existing in the individual case, nor can it provide them with a general aspect. Jaspers stated that even after a certain phenomenon is distinguished from other phenomena, we encounter "a new chaos of an infinity of named phenomena that still do not satisfy at all our scientific need."[32] In light of the singularity and uniqueness of the individual cases, phenomenologists, who remained within the boundaries of static understanding, were not helped by the guidelines of organization and generalization they achieved by focusing on the external expressions of the phenomenon. Jaspers's argument in this context was that unlike the natural sciences, where the organization of phenomena according to a particular law can suffice, in psychopathology the "genesis" of the phenomenon has significance, and tracking it can familiarize us with a range of mental qualities. The genetic understanding (*genetisches Verstehen*) of phenomena, an essential addition to the descriptive approach, aims to offer an analysis of a wide range of mental phenomena "at the level of the final components," and to enable renewed recognition of their uniqueness.[33] The expression "phenomenological chasms," indicating the uniqueness of the mental phenomenon revealed in the individual case, defines to a large extent the type of consciousness in which the genetic viewpoint is anchored. In this spirit, Jaspers noted that awareness of the chasms between human beings as individuals presenting symptoms that seem apparently related to a mental illness enables at most proposing a limited form of organization of these symptoms.[34]

Against this background, we can state that the principle according to which different mental phenomena were distinguished from each other did not depend, as far as Jaspers was concerned, on their differences or similarities. Characteristics related mainly to the direct and relatively immediate expressions of mental phenomena do not show us much about the individual personality at the focus of Jaspers's interest. Since the particular subjective Being of the person serves as a framework from which the different expressions of the illness develop, he believed that generalizations about any mental phenomena were valid mainly regarding the concrete individual afflicted with a mental disorder. Unlike the static understanding that delimits mental phenomena and distinguishes them from other accompanying phenomena, the genetic point of view enables a broader view of the mental illness appearing in a certain patient—since the illness in itself is only part of the wide totality of this patient's personality as a human being. Observation grounded in the genetic viewpoint reflects Jaspers's basic attempt to understand the origin of the different phenomena that appear in each person as an individual case, instead of the attempt to reveal the unified nature of the mental phenomenon expressed in different people.

The attempt to formulate out of two viewpoints, the static and the genetic, a general approach to the understanding of mental illness was termed by Jaspers "real phenomenology." This approach enhances not only the differences between different mental phenomena, but also emphasizes the particular influence of mental phenomena on different patients for whom science has presented a uniform definition. In Jaspers's opinion, the non-generalizable uniqueness of human beings is the origin of the unbridgeable gap between people as infinite beings. Since people deal with their illness in a unique way, the therapeutic approach cannot rely only on the presence of symptoms common to several patients. Jaspers's approach, which set itself a goal of preserving awareness of the unique relation of the mental phenomenon to the particular personality where it is expressed, reflects the insight that the main part of the mental illness is not revealed through the classification of the phenomena by their objective features, but instead through observation of the mental patient as an individual.

The importance of the discussion of Jaspers's criticism of the science of psychopathology in his day for this study, dealing with the development of his metaphysical approach, which is mainly philosophical, stems from this criticism revealing some features of the method of transcending (*Transzendieren*), on which he based his later thinking. This method, which in this context would be better defined as a "transcending viewpoint" and not as a method that is implemented systematically and consciously, guided his general approach, which recoiled from definitions and distinguished concepts that he saw as restricting the possibility of achieving full understanding of the person experiencing a mental disorder. The transcending viewpoint was reflected concretely in Jaspers's consistent attempt to reveal the limits of the scientific approach, especially the one influenced by the positivistic approach that examined the patient's condition in light of the physiological symptoms capable of objective examination. His positive attitude to the contribution of the science of psychiatry to a certain understanding of mental disorders enables us to argue that transcending from the physiological viewpoint in itself does not reflect an anti-systematic approach by any means. Jaspers saw fit to examine individual cases of illness in light of general principles, indicating that the transcending viewpoint did not require a complete negation of the approach being criticized, but instead reflected an effort to rescue from it the aspects relevant to a more complete understanding. This revealed the most important principle on which the method of transcending in Jaspers's later work was based. This method cannot be implemented without clarifying the attitudes that serve it as a base from which it can transcend. In this respect, the meeting between Jaspers's position and other approaches, and the discourse with them, not only helped clarify and sharpen Jaspers's arguments, but were even an integral part of the mental position where the transcending viewpoint is anchored. However, from the perspective of his entire thinking, we can say that the transcending viewpoint not only guided the meeting of Jaspers's approach with other approaches, but also applied later to his approach. For instance, the perception of subjectivity, which in the context of the discussion of psychopathology reflected the viewpoint that transcends the scientific understanding of mental illness, was itself in *Psychology of World Views* a datum from which Jaspers developed a deeper understanding of subjectivity. This means that an insight that at an early stage was the result of the transcending viewpoint later served itself as a basis for transcending, a method that helped Jaspers's thinking constantly break into more distant realms.

In some respects, we have difficulty determining whether Jaspers's later perceptions of the self were the result of the method of transcending, or whether this method itself adapted to the basic intuitions that guided him. The difficulty in deciding this question stems first and foremost from Jaspers himself not indicating at that time any method that was guiding him. He based his perception of mental illnesses and their sufferers on his objection in principle to the formation of a fixed and defined method that would guide the practice of the psychiatrist or scientific research. This claim also explains the choice to describe Jaspers's approach as a "transcending viewpoint" and its preference over the term "method of transcendence," which is more relevant to his later writings. Also, the frequent use of the term "viewpoint" demonstrates Jaspers's consistent effort to avoid forming over-defined structures that could restrict the openness he considered essential to the discussion of phenomena in which people's involvement grants them an infinite character.

4. The Primacy and Centrality of Subjectivity

The essence of Jaspers's interest in psychopathology becomes clear when he addresses the question of the borders of science and his wish to focus psychiatry within the borders of the person's individuality. What he called "the mental in its real reality" served for him as a starting point for clarifying the mental experience the patient undergoes as a human being. As he says:

> We want to feel, conceive, and think what happens in the human soul, to catch the thing and think about it. The general drive to reality means in psychopathology the drive to *the real mental life* that we wish to know later in contexts *partially capable of sensory understanding,* like *the objects* of the natural sciences [emphases in the original].[35]

Jaspers's use of terms such as "reality," "person," and "mental life" instead of "patient" or "mental illness" demonstrates the basic interest he showed in the humanity of the patient and the priority he granted it over the aspects that the science of psychopathology studied. The need to indicate explicitly the "translation" of this drive in terms of a general foundation for the field of psychopathology—as if this were not the explicit subject of the discussion—also strengthens the distinction that the scientific explanation presenting the reasons and conditions for illness cannot fully express the interest the psychiatrist has in the complete personality in psychopathology and in the patient. As he says, "In the absence of the ability and the will to observe the mental and to compare it before our eyes in its fullness, the [physician] has no option of practicing psychopathology."[36]

In any case, Jaspers's attempt to expand the viewpoint of subjectivity in the framework of his perception of psychiatry reveals two facets: restrictive and expansive. The restrictive facet of subjectivity arises already from Jaspers's criticism of the science of psychopathology, a criticism resulting from his understanding of the human soul as only partially accessible to the scientific research instruments and to observation in general. However, when Jaspers discusses subjectivity more directly, this restriction of science is presented as a mirror of the mental element itself "experienced really… as foam floating on the depths of the ocean"[37] and as a reflection of the "atmosphere" or "mood" (*Stimmung*) surrounding the wide context in which mental reality exists.[38] These vague phrasings, through which Jaspers chose to express his ideas, demonstrated the loose and clouded way the mental element is sometimes revealed to the observer. The difficulty in fully exposing subjectivity served as a basis for Jaspers's requirement that the psychiatrist be aware that the individual cannot be fully explained using the normal tools of consciousness, which no matter how far they go will always encounter a remnant that is impermeable to them. This facet, which appears as a theme throughout his works of this period, first expresses the influence of Kant's two concepts of boundary discussed in the Introduction. Against this background, the psychiatrist can be presented as facing the "border" of the person as an individual, and the psychopathologist as facing the "barrier" presented by the conceptual framework of the science of psychopathology.

One of the critical implications of the understanding that locates subjectivity within the boundary of human consciousness is that no complete theory or uniform system regarding the character of mental patients as people, regarding their illnesses, can control psychopathology.[39] As part of his criticism of the science of psychopathology, Jaspers also criticized the comprehensive theories of psychiatry, which he presented as aiming to achieve control of people in the same way they treat objects. This approach, apparent in the different efforts to organize the knowledge about the patient into predetermined patterns, reflected in his opinion their distance from the patient's real reality and their helplessness in the face of the changing expressions of the mental illness that appear uniquely in each case. Jaspers called these theories "prejudices" (*Vorurteile*) of psychiatry, and in the same spirit defined the approaches based on the premise prevalent at that time, seeing mental illness as a brain disease, "the brain mythologies."[40]

There can be no doubt that the basic difficulty Jaspers had with the methods that tried to direct observation of mental life from control resulted from his fear that they would influence the perception of the mental element as part of the person's physicality or as an expression of it. For him, such an approach not only distorts the inexhaustible aspect of the person. It could also lead gradually to a focus on some components of the mental life and give them a total meaning within the person's whole life, while at the same time neglecting other components that did not force their way into the heart of the system and ejecting them from the framework of understanding the mental phenomenon. However, Jaspers's criticism of the science of psychopathology, which was linked to recognition of his contribution to a particular understanding of pathological mental phenomena, did not enable him to present the focus on subjectivity as a comprehensive response to the faults of positivistic psychopathology. He proposed settling for a methodical organization of our viewpoint on limited aspects of the "mental."[41] As he said:

> Instead of pushing ahead the last components, mechanisms, and laws, from which *all* the mental will is perceived or will necessarily be perceived in the future, we follow only *special* ways, use *special* methods that present for us *individual* sides of the mental life [emphases in the original].[42]

A method perceived as depicting a certain viewpoint can bear fruit precisely in the place where the methods suited mainly to the natural sciences cannot penetrate. The psychiatrist cannot even rely on a single viewpoint, but needs multiple viewpoints in order to achieve full understanding of human mental illnesses.[43] As he says:

> Only psychopathology whose starting point is the borderless search, the infinite variety of reality, the wealth of subjective approaches and of objective facts, the multiplicity of methods and the uniqueness of each, does justice to its task as a scientific discipline.[44]

Viewing the human soul as an endless space of behaviors and external expressions is what requires psychiatrists to provide a more minimalistic definition of their viewpoint and a continuous consciousness of the "border" between themselves and the person as an individual. The distinction between the system and the method along with the requirement for multiple viewpoints to guide the scientific practice of psychiatry join the effort to establish awareness of the boundaries of the representation of subjectivity in the instruments of scientific consciousness and of consciousness in general. For Jaspers, only this consciousness grants us reason to assume that awareness of the potential contribution of science to the understanding of the mental phenomenon will not develop into flawed and harmful understanding.

The expansive facet of subjectivity deals with the understanding of the human experience as reflected in everyday reality in different and sometimes surprising ways.[45] The genetic viewpoint of mental illness, mainly directed at what Jaspers defined as a "chasm" between people as individuals, transpires as essential for clarifying this facet of subjectivity. In light of the emphasis on the difficulty in defining the subjective aspects of illness, at this point Jaspers's effort to make positive claims about it is especially noticeable. However, while the dealing with the limited accessibility of the mental aspect in its totality relied mainly on awareness of the boundaries of science and also of the elusive character of the soul, Jaspers wished to establish the expansive understanding of subjectivity on real means originating in the personality of the psychiatrists themselves.

The psychiatrists' personality skills, especially empathy, present vividly the alternative Jaspers wished to offer the conceptual system of science, an alternative that emphasized the need for processing the mental-emotional experiences the psychiatrist undergoes during the meeting with the mental patient. Jaspers defined several skills in this context, such as empathy (*Einfühlen*), internalization (*Hineinverstehen*), participation (*Miterleben*) and internal priorities (*innerliche Vorgänge*).[46] Unlike those requiring the study of the objective symptoms based mainly on rationality, the skills that help the psychiatrist become acquainted with the wide and varied aspects of subjectivity relate to the psychiatrist's personality. These skills are not simple to define accurately and completely, just as what they are aimed at exposing is not definable. The non-verbal aspect, so central in these skills, served as a basis for Jaspers's perception of them as anchored in "something outside consciousness"[47] that served to decipher the particular character where the mental illness in each individual case is revealed, and where it affects the entire life of the person suffering from it.[48] The genetic viewpoint of mental illnesses, which turns out to be a main instrument for obtaining an expansive view of subjectivity, serves as a basis for the psychiatrist-patient relationship. In this framework, psychiatrists can get close to their patients free of principles defining the "correct" boundaries of the relationship between them and their "final" purpose. Jaspers called the framework of the psychiatrists' relationship with their patients "understanding in the participatory experience" (*miterlebendes Verstehen*), and "subjective approach," and argued that it could lead to "unmediated, informal, and personal" understanding of the patients' mental condition, and even indicated the possibility that this understanding would remain with the psychiatrists as a pure experience, without being processed using defined conceptual tools. Jaspers went even further when he claimed that the ability to develop such an approach should be the "ultimate aim of the profession," and an infinite ideal within the framework of a science that perceives mental phenomena as an infinite multiplicity of forces where we can never exhaustively understand the connections between them.[49] We may understand the rationale on which he based his approach in this context from the following passage:

> We cannot "portray" (*abbilden*) mental phenomena, nor compare them before our eyes using anything sensory and distinguishable. We can only direct (*hinleiten*) *ourselves and others* from all directions to actualize the particular (*Bestimmte*) to ourselves. The genesis, the conditions, and the constellations in whose framework these phenomena tend to appear, the objective contents that may exist... *must be illuminated from outside the mental phenomenon considered real* [emphases mine].[50]

Jaspers also criticized "objective psychology," based on identifying the objective symptoms through rational thinking and sensory observation, and called it "psychology without the psyche." In contrast, what he termed "subjective psychology," grounded in the psychiatrist's subjectivity and aiming at the patient's subjectivity, stressed the uniqueness of the mental experience that for Jaspers was perceived as having weight and value for its understanding even in the absence of an objective anchor that defined it.[51] The definition of the mental element in the person as "an unreducable remnant"[52] is a quite important basis for the formation of a wide view of subjectivity as a one-time, total experience. Subjectivity is actually a primary core from which the different mental phenomena develop. Jaspers compared "the last, smallest possible components" that act in phenomenology to the role of atoms in chemistry.[53] He placed at the forefront of the aims of psychopathology the achieving of the ability to represent them in our consciousness. As he said:

> While the ideal of phenomenology is actually an infinity of unreducable mental qualities, organized covertly, there exists another ideal, contrary to us, *the ideal of the last, smallest possible components*, as there exists for instance in chemistry. From the combination [of these two ideals] should be derived all the most complex mental phenomena. An analysis of these components is supposed to describe satisfactorily all the mental phenomena. After all *such an approach cannot reject in its result the sufficing of one single and last mental atom from which all the mental is constructed in its different combinations, rejecting its as illogical* [emphases mine].[54]

These words, continuing Jaspers's criticism of phenomenology and of the science of psychopathology, indicate that subjectivity, which Jaspers viewed as a key to understanding mental illness, does not reflect his ruling in favor of one of the sides on any imaginary spectrum—a spectrum between general physiological symptoms adding up to a syndrome that serves as an indicator of a particular mental illness at one end, and individual, perhaps exceptional, cases of real patients expressing some symptoms at the other end. The subjectivity glimpsed from Jaspers's writings in this period appears as a primary element relating to the understanding of the person as such, and its representation in our consciousness appears as a source for understanding the range of phenomena of health and illness. Jaspers discussed extensively the difference between two facets of the personality: "development" and "process." The diagnosis of the first requires empathy from the therapist to a range of aspects of the mental patient's world including his unconscious aspects, while the diagnosis of the second requires the ability to recognize logical connections and is based mainly on the typical objective features of various mental illnesses. However, Jaspers believed that subjectivity serves as a unifying element for these two aspects.[55] Against this background we can understand the basic idea behind Jaspers's programmatic statement that the starting point of the study of mental illness is in human experience defined as normal.[56]

Apart from the implications for psychiatrists' attitude toward their patients and their self-perception, the expansive view of subjectivity is also connected to the definition of the sources of the knowledge field of psychopathology. Jaspers argued in this context that besides the areas of neurology and psychology, considered a natural part of it, psychopathology also needs to rely on the other fields of human consciousness. In practice, this implies the need for multiplying and varying the viewpoints that guide research conducted in psychopathology. Already in the first edition of his book, Jaspers allocated a central role to philosophy in designing the methodological tools for psychopathology, through which we could examine and criticize the premises on which it was based.[57] While philosophy does not touch directly upon the field of psychopathology, a variety of Jaspers's statements show that he saw it at that time mainly as a general source of inspiration. Evidence of this is found in the general statements in the context of his comments on philosophy in the first edition of his book, such as that the very fact that the individual was infinite was not sufficient for him as a person;[58] that apart from psychiatry, and independently of it, there arise metaphysical, aesthetical, and ethical evaluations;[59] and that we must avoid relying on organized structures of thought and turn to what he called "spirit-rich thoughts" [quotation marks in the original].[60]

Although these statements were detached from the context Jaspers discussed in the first edition of *General Psychopathology*, they made a certain contribution to establishing the general trend aiming at a wider view of the human being as an essential basis for the practice of psychopathology. In this context, Jaspers's criticism of Freud's psychoanalysis apparently reflects his search for a wider view of a human being that he perceived as an urgent need of psychopathology. In his opinion, the root of psychoanalysis's mistake is the attempt to offer absolute knowledge about the person and in its isolation from the history of ideas that represented for Jaspers a wider and non-dogmatic view of human beings. He argued that "the pretend liberation of the person [psychoanalysis wished to present] is as false as the humanity on which it sought to reflect." In his opinion, any conception of a human being that detaches the scientific modes of thought from the methods of philosophical thinking misses the essence of a person and will end up deteriorating into fanaticism or mythology.[61]

In the fourth edition of *General Psychopathology*, expanded and permeated by his philosophical ideas that had already reached maturity, Jaspers destined philosophy a positive and much wider role. At that time he stated that "not only does empiricism not tied to prejudice lead us to the real boundaries set by philosophizing, but to the contrary, only philosophical awareness facilitates an empirical research approach".[62] Henceforth philosophy is perceived as contributing more directly to the human quality of psychopathologists, through which they can clarify to themselves their motivation in practicing this profession.[63] Jaspers, who was already a philosopher with an independent approach when this edition was published in 1942, presented philosophy as a tool that enables contact with the fullness of human life that finds its full expression compared to its limited appearance in the scientific realm.[64]

In the end, the two facets of subjectivity, the restrictive and the expansive, are two sides of the same coin. On the one hand, restricting what can be argued about the human soul is motivated by the awareness that subjectivity is a wider and more extensive experience than can be represented using scientific tools. On the other hand, the demand to expand psychopathology's frame of reference to enable access to the humanity of the person suffering from a mental illness, portraying the alternative to the scientific viewpoint of mental illness, contains criticism of approaches that did not recognize the existence of an experience that cannot be represented using the instruments of science. We can see these two facets of subjectivity as a continuation of Jaspers's striving to undermine the general foundation on which science's approach to reality and to human beings was based. While in his criticism of the science of psychopathology Jaspers wished to remove mainly what he saw as the source of distortion, in his perception of subjectivity he tried to fill the vacuum left by his critical position. The deep individualistic element in Jaspers's writings in this period did not allow him to decide whether to focus on the psychiatrist's character or on explicating the desirable viewpoint of the patient, and his words remained aimed at the subjectivity shared by the patient and the physician due to them both being human beings. Against this background, Jaspers's point of view appears to aim to liberate patients, and no less the physicians treating them, from the burden of general definitions that miss the particular nature of the interpersonal relations and the human contact with reality. By redefining the boundaries in principle of the realm of psychiatry, the perception of subjectivity—relating to both the patient and the psychiatrist—expresses the outcome of the transcending viewpoint as an instrument that helped Jaspers formulate positive arguments regarding selfhood, which was present in the background of his approach to the science of psychopathology.

In a way, the criticism of the science of psychopathology and the perception of subjectivity presented above expresses the basic tension between two points of view that would accompany Jaspers's philosophical thinking later. While the criticism of science reflects the presence of the *epistemological viewpoint*, focusing on the question of what can be known about the issue under discussion, the perception of subjectivity represents the presence of the *ontological viewpoint*, searching for the tools by which we can imagine the Being of the object at which our thought is directed. These two viewpoints are distinct in their philosophical intention, but they cannot be completely separated. This is because what we can know about subjectivity expresses only one facet or part of this Being, which does not in itself exist for us except within some boundaries, some of which are dictated by our conscious ability. Perhaps it is the taken-for-granted importance of the epistemological viewpoint for the scientific discussion of psychopathology that led to the special emphasis Jaspers granted to the aspects related to subjectivity, what concerned the ontological viewpoint aimed at the Being of the mental patient and the physician as subjects. As we will see below, the aim to express the Being of subjectivity, and later the Being of Existenz, accompanies the entire explication of selfhood. In this respect, the prominent presence of the ontological viewpoint in the perception of the science of psychiatry indicates the start of a trend that would become more dominant as this philosophy developed, and would start expressing itself using philosophical tools.

We should note that this emphasis does not imply Jaspers's complete detachment from the epistemological viewpoint. The presence of this viewpoint is maintained throughout the explication of selfhood—especially through the continued criticism of positivism in science, but also in the discussion of different aspects of objectivity related to Existenz. However, since the epistemological viewpoint remains in the background during this discussion while the ontological viewpoint receives greater emphasis, the tension between them remains implicit. Only during the explication of Being, where both viewpoints are granted importance, does the tension between them ripen, and its clarification become an inherent part of the explication of Being. The full meaning of Jaspers's early statements about selfhood, like the one related to other issues raised from this discussion, will only be clarified later, when Jaspers develops philosophical perceptions of Existenz and of Being.

5. The Idea of the Person as a Whole

The emphasis on the individualistic aspect of mental illness, aimed at protecting mental patients and the psychiatrists who treat them from the absorbing power of the general definitions of the science of psychopathology, was presented in the first edition of *General Psychopathology* as based on "the whole of the mental."[65] This statement accorded with Jaspers's basic approach that indicated the limits of research dealing with the human soul, but apart from that it was not developed further. In the expanded edition of *General Psychopathology*, published after Jaspers's main philosophical works, he added a chapter called "The Person as a Whole." In this chapter, he tried to fill his view of human wholeness with real contents, and grounded it in the philosophy of Existenz and the metaphysical ideas developed in his philosophical writings.[66] This broad framework of discussion enabled Jaspers to present a more mature perception of the subjective Being that had interested him already early in his career, and at the same time to give this Being a significance and context far beyond the boundaries of the discussion of mental illness.

The perception of the person as whole is based on an intuition regarding the existence of a real Being not accessible to the experimental consciousness aimed at empirical existences, but capable of being experienced in a total manner in the unmediated experience.[67] Using this approach, which is anchored in the awareness of the gap between what people experience and what can be represented using the instruments of research, Jaspers wished to reject two approaches: both the positivistic that sees the whole as a sum of is parts, and the idealistic (or mystical) that sees the whole as a supreme essence separate from the details comprising it.[68] The perception of the person as a whole offers an alternative to these approaches, according to which the whole is informed by the parts, but it transcends them and exists beyond them. Jaspers aimed at establishing this general perception, whose implications went far beyond the realm of psychopathology, as a regulative idea that would help understand the multiple facets of the human soul as establishing an infinite Being. In his opinion, the inability to reach a synthesis between the different approaches regarding the relationship between the whole and its parts[69] should testify to the relative and restricted nature of the knowledge obtained in psychopathology, and in any case should cast doubt over any existing knowledge about the human soul.[70]

The general trend characterizing the expanded edition of *General Psychopathology*, to anchor the science of psychopathology in a wider perception of people using ideas developed in his philosophical writings, is clear in his use of the concept of the "encompassing" (*Umgreifende*) in this context.[71] The general principle behind this approach is that philosophizing is always directed at a Being beyond the immanent components it deals with and beyond the philosopher, who cannot exhaust it using the instruments of formal consciousness. This principle may explain the central role granted in the perception of the "encompassing" to transcendence, one of its seven components, defined as the "encompassing of all encompassings."[72] Transcendence, as the horizon furthest from human consciousness, was presented in this context as the origin of the urge people have to form a relationship with what is beyond the boundaries of their existence, and as a primary motivation for philosophizing. Naturally, Jaspers was unable to include in his discussion in *General Psychopathology* all the aspects of the "encompassing."

However, he distilled from it the general principle he saw as relevant to understanding the human soul. As he wrote:

> The question what is man leads in psychopathology to wholes. However, like any whole we encounter so also personality is measured in light of the encompassing of human Being, as a phenomenon about which we can speak with a typical comprehensible quality. *All the patterns of human Being existing before our eyes that we can analyze scientifically are not the encompassing itself, but are contained within it* [emphasis mine].[73]

The "wholenesses" Jaspers refers to in this passage probably reflects the different viewpoints on human experience represented in the different components of the "encompassing." In this context, each of them portrayed one facet or aspect of the person (such as environment, personality, physiology) whose understanding could contribute to a fuller understanding of mental pathology.[74] In the philosophical context, Jaspers did not see any of the components of the perception of the "encompassing" as false in itself, but argued that when they were given total meaning, both the particular truth contained in them and the surrounding truth beyond them were missed. Jaspers's position reflects the influence of Hegel's perception of truth according to which the real is only the whole. This perception constitutes a central motif in Hegel's *The Phenomenology of Spirit.*[75] In this spirit, he did not propose, in this context, rejecting approaches differing from his, even when he believed they provided a limited understanding of the human soul and incorrectly claimed totality.[76] Just as the perception of the "encompassing" served as a framework containing a variety of terms clarified in different contexts, so, in this context, the perception of a person as a whole was proposed as a wide framework to provide meaning and context to the range of expressions of the mental element.[77] As he says:

> We do not know the whole of the mental life nor the whole of the individual personality, but we direct our intentions toward this whole through invented totalities: [through] the whole life story, [through] the varied character of the person, [through] the unity of the illness, *through totalities that are not in themselves the whole*, but only final criteria, the results of an analysis *that shows us the ways for possible perceptions of the whole* without ourselves owning this approach. [emphases mine][78]

The perception of the wholeness of the soul as a possibility not yet realized did not express in this context a skeptical or relativistic position such as the one derived from the scientific viewpoint that Jaspers criticized. The perception of subjectivity, in which his attitude toward psychiatric medicine was anchored, was aimed not only against a positivistic understanding of the soul but also as preparation for opposing or even contradictory expressions of the mental element encountered by psychiatrists in their work with mental patients and psychopathologists studying the soul. Jaspers gave vivid expression to the way a person faces the idea of the human being as a whole when he wrote:

> Knowing a person is likened to sailing on the infinite ocean in order to discover continents. Any anchorage... shows some facts, but when we claim to be in the center of things, this [anchoring] increases the other awareness so that the theories are no more than a sand bar we have reached without achieving real landfall.[79]

Jaspers anticipated that along with the maturation of the awareness of the existence of an imperceptible and perhaps enigmatic layer of the human soul, so would deepen the awareness that an exhaustive perception of the human soul was beyond what can be formulated by scientific tools, and beyond human ability altogether.

The discussion of the imperceptible aspects of the human soul within the perception of a person as a whole complements the perception of subjectivity as formulated in his writings on psychopathology, and gives it a more general significance. However, the expanded edition of the book was written when Jaspers was already a philosopher with a personal, independent approach, and this inevitably raises another puzzling question: what point did Jaspers see in making the effort to rewrite, sometimes superficially and fragmentarily, ideas that he had already presented in his philosophical books in a much more mature and profound manner? The expanded version of the book omitted the subtitle of the first edition, defining the book as a "guide for students, physicians, and psychologists." However, using the book's original name in the expanded version, and maintaining the chapters dealing with the physiological aspects of illness almost in full left no doubt that, from Jaspers's point of view, the book was perceived as aimed mainly for mental health professionals instead of philosophers, especially since from a philosophical point of view this book contains no innovations.

The importance of discussing this question in this study, seeking to offer a genealogical insight into Jaspers's thinking, is almost obvious. On the first level, we could argue that Jaspers the philosopher believed a connection existed between the fields, and also between the chapters of his biography as a psychiatrist and as a philosopher, and so the positions Jaspers expressed in the fourth edition of *General Psychopathology* cannot be detached from his intensive philosophical activity in the many years between the editions. However, for the purpose of our discussion of his early writings, more important is the fact that when he was a philosopher he chose to integrate in a mainly non-philosophical book the aspects of his philosophy of Existenz. Jaspers was usually careful to insert references to his philosophy books, meaning that it was clear to him that the whole philosophical framework was necessary to complete the picture.[80] This distinction supports the basic argument of this chapter that, already in his early writings, subjectivity expressed Jaspers's main interest in the science of psychopathology. Not only does this enable a new reading of Jaspers's writings from this period, it also makes them relevant to the philosophical discussion of his later writings, whose center is a more systematic analysis of selfhood. This argument is demonstrated in Jaspers's words that "the practice of the physician is concrete philosophy," spoken at the opening of "Centenary conference of the German society of natural sciences scholars and physicians," held in Wiesbaden in 1958.[81]

On the basis of the argument that Jaspers's perception of psychopathology indicated the beginning of his attempt to achieve explication of selfhood, we can state that the philosophy of Existenz presented in the following chapters is to a large degree a continuation and development of the two basic trends discussed in this chapter: the focus on subjectivity and the search for a more encompassing whole. The first trend led to placing selfhood as the central issue already in *Psychology of World Views* (1919). The second trend was developed later, when the framework of explicating selfhood had been exhausted, or more precisely, reached a dead end, and the focus of the discussion was diverted to explicating Being and Transcendence. Within the discussion of these concepts Jaspers was able, as we will see below, to achieve a more complex understanding of the self Being, and to base upon it in his thinking a new ideal of wholeness.

Two

SELFHOOD IN WORLD VIEWS

1. From Pathology to Normality

The main contribution of the transcending viewpoint to the discussion of mental illness and the essential role of the psychiatrist and psychopathologist was that it helped Karl Jaspers present a wider view of the phenomenon of mental pathology—a view that not only included an analysis of its physiological aspects, but also referred to the mental patient's subjective personality. However, the discussion of Jaspers's perception of selfhood based on his psychiatric writings encounters difficulties. The main difficulty is related to his being unable, within this framework, to develop tools suitable for characterizing subjectivity as a particular experience or clarifying the ways of approaching it. From Jaspers's general statements a description arises indirectly of the inspiration that should accompany the treatment of people suffering from mental illness. However, the subjective being of the patient remains enigmatic and concealed so that its discussion deviates from the framework of scientific discourse. Jaspers's attempt to make the particular features of the individuals' subjective being into part of the range of considerations in treating mental illness relied mainly on the critical image he had formulated regarding the science of psychopathology. But the more dealing with the scientific world view helped him clarify his position regarding the correct treatment of mental illness and the worthy character of the psychiatrist, the more it showed him the way out of psychopathology and science in general.[1]

These insights may to some extent create the impression that the attempt to find in Jaspers's psychiatric writings his approach toward selfhood is forced, due to the dependence of this presentation on an explication of his later philosophical writings. However, this dependence, expressed throughout this book, is no disadvantage in the framework of a phenomenological discussion, where the understanding achieved is always "temporary," reflecting the stage of the discussion when it was revealed, but destined to be formulated differently, more accurately, at later stages of the explication. Although the perception of subjectivity formulated in the early writings was limited in terms of the ability to grant it meaning, it served as a basis for a more structured and systematic discussion already in *Psychology of World Views* (1919)[2]—the first book Jaspers wrote after leaving his practical and scientific work in psychiatry (hereafter: *Psychology*). The subjective being discussed in this book, the focus of discussion in this chapter, was no different than the one that occupied Jaspers in his early writings, since even while he was a psychiatrist Jaspers did not exhaust his discussion with the pathological viewpoint. But after he no longer saw himself as committed to formulating an approach that would provide an immediate response to the distress of patients, distress that sometimes included physical problems, Jaspers was able to place subjectivity at the focus of a discussion that would treat it from a wider perspective. However, as we will see below, the psychological viewpoint of selfhood did not liberate Jaspers from the basic questions that had interested him as a psychiatrist. Quite the opposite, since it apparently granted a central role to the aspects that had been implicit in his psychiatric writings, and perhaps had been no more than a cover for his statements as a scientist, it now exposed him to a greater extent to the fundamental difficulties involved in its clarification.

The interpretation presented below will not deal with the explication of the different perceptions of selfhood presented in *Psychology*—constituting the main part of the book[3]—but instead will focus on the explication of the implicit and explicit premises behind Jaspers's perception of selfhood in this work.

2. "World View"

The title *Psychology of World Views* might mislead the reader into thinking that the book deals with a psychological subject or that it was written by a psychologist. The basic perceptions it presents and the nature of the discussion leave no doubt that in this book Jaspers took his first steps as a philosopher. Jaspers clarified that the choice of this title had political and instrumental reasons originating in his relations with the academic staff of Heidelberg University at that time. He hinted in the preface to the book (1954) about the struggles he had experienced, among others with Heinrich Rickert and Wilhelm Windelband, who "at this period became enemies independently from scientific correctness," as he put it. Jaspers's perception of *Psychology* as an unconscious expression of his path toward philosophy was expressed in his statement that the name "Psychology" could not serve as a title for the experience in his book.[4] World view is one of the most central concepts in German culture, and has a variety of philosophical and psychological meanings. The tension between "world knowledge" (*Welterkennen*) and "self knowledge" (*Selbsterkennen*) characterizes the different thinkers who clarified the issue of world view, including Jaspers. Great similarity can be seen between the perception of world views of Wilhelm Dilthey and Jaspers, to the point of doubting the originality of Jaspers's ideas. The viewpoint in which the book is anchored is clear already in the definition Jaspers gave the key concept "world view" (*Weltanschauung*).[5]

> What is a world view? Something whole and something universal. When this is knowledge (*Wissen*), this does not mean professional knowledge (*Fachwissen*), but knowledge as a wholeness, as a cosmos. However, a world view is not just knowledge, but it reveals itself in assessments, in life patterns, in fate, and in the experience of the hierarchy of values. In other words: when we speak about world views we have in our mind ideas, the ultimate totality of man—both subjectively as an experience, as power, and as knowledge, and also objectively as a world constructed tangibly.[6]

Unlike knowledge acquired within a defined professional setting that determines its boundaries and fixes objective criteria for its examination, the world view is presented as an expression of people's whole world: it portrays the variety of their concrete experiences and their ability to objectivize them and to construct from it a wide understanding of themselves in reality.[7] Just as Jaspers's discussion of mental illness was focused on the person as a real Being, so was his interest directed, in this context, at the subject who formed the world view instead of at world views as realities separate from their owners. Yet, while his early statements about subjectivity were characterized by generalization lacking real justification, in *Psychology* Jaspers distinguished between different facets of human beings revealed in his world view, and tried to express the new horizons that had opened up to him during the period since publishing his earlier writings.

Jaspers presented two basic components establishing the world view: subjective and objective. The subjective element refers to the concrete experience of individuals in the world, involving people's actions and the thoughts accompanying these actions.[8] These thoughts often reveal the distance between the early images they had about reality and their expectations from it and the concrete experience that does not always match them.[9] People are exposed to new phenomena that alter their knowledge regarding some aspects of human reality. However, the deeper the experience accompanying this process, and the more it relates to fundamental aspects of existence, the more it confronts individuals with themselves and can gradually lead to a more general change in their self-perception. The objective element in world views is reflected in people's tendency to objectivize their different experiences, and to use them to give meaning to the real reality in which they find themselves "existing there" (*Daseiende*). In *Psychology* the term "Existenz" usually denotes the individual's perception of reality. This term was destined to serve in the philosophical writings to denote the individual's subjective Being, while the term "Dasein" denotes there the concrete existence without the reflexive attitude the individual could adopt toward it (see the discussion in Chapter Three below).[10] But these objectivizations should not be seen as expressing the ideal of objectivity, on which the scientific viewpoint is based, since they are subject to concrete experience, and were intended to enable better self-understanding. In this respect, the objectivizations performed by individuals are subject to changes to the same extent that people's experiences change and vary throughout their life.

The change the terms of objectivity and subjectivity underwent in this context, compared with their perception in the early writings, is visible to the observer. During the psychiatric period, the physiological aspects reflected the objective aspect of the mental illness while the unique influence of these aspects on the person suffering from the illness expressed its subjective level. In contrast, in *Psychology* there exists no room for the early meaning of objectivity. This concept now refers mainly to the way subjects organize their range of experiences, while the term subjectivity expressed the experiential layer of the concrete experience even before being processed by individuals. Subjectivity is perceived in *Psychology* as a Being that constitutes itself through reflection on experiences in reality, but which after they are processed, become assimilated in its consciousness as different reflections derived from its selfhood as one whole. Jaspers not did distinguish between experiential and subjective experience and the action of its objectivization, nor did he draw epistemological conclusions from it.[11] Throughout objectivization, Jaspers wished to understand "which last positions (*letzten Positionen*) the soul takes and which forces motivate it."[12] He apparently saw these objectivizations mainly as an ontological representation of subjectivity in its particularity and the world view created by the subject as "a means of self-consciousness (*Selbstbesinnung*)"[13] or as a tool providing "clarifications and possibilities that can serve as a means for self-reflection."[14]

The discussion in this chapter of the explication of selfhood arising from Jaspers's discussion in *Psychology* will be based on this distinction regarding the centrality of the subjective element in world views. The perception of world views as a structured framework of experience negates the possibility of seeing world views as being merely a "product" of mental processes or an expression of the actualization of a "goal" people set themselves at some stage during their life. The argument in principle presented below is that the discussion of world views was essential to Jaspers for the understanding of people's subjective being, not only because at that time he perceived it as a framework where the people could express their experiences in reality, but also because, by the very constitution of a world view, individuals form their selfhood.

3. The Method in *Psychology*

A. The Framework: Object-Subject Relations

Jaspers's method in *Psychology* relied in principle on object-subject relations. As he says: "The thought of the multiplicity of connections between subject and object, and the multiplicity of meanings of the subject and of the object, as something that cannot be assumed solidly, is the basic thought of our search and systematic organization."[15] This statement expresses Jaspers's new awareness of the need to determine a general framework for the discussion of subjectivity, not typical of his approach in his early works, as we have seen. Jaspers revealed that he wished to find an anchor point for his search, an "Archimedes point," as he put it, outside the separation between objectivity and subjectivity. However, he claimed that this was not within the limits of human experience, although in his opinion the person's ability to move between different viewpoints could serve as a substitute.[16] In some respects, the person's mobility between viewpoints can soften the rigidity that can accompany the identification with a certain viewpoint that harms a person's ability to identify the horizons beyond the individual point of view. However, the ability of consciousness to widen its frame of reference clearly cannot rescue people from the basic limitations applying to them and existing beyond the boundaries of the personality experiencing the constitution of a world view.

The general framework of object-subject relations was mainly subject to the new meaning Jaspers gave in *Psychology* to the terms subjectivity and objectivity. This meant that most of his arguments aimed at clarifying the Being experiencing the constitution of a world view and did not deal with objects involved in this experience. This expresses not only his distancing from the fundamental perceptions of science, but also his basic affinity to Immanuel Kant's premises that granted the subject a decisive status in determining the nature and character of subjectivity. Jaspers noted that the status of the objects he deals with in *Psychology* was derived from the meaning the subject granted them.[17] In this framework Jaspers presented human experience as existing in a "latticework,"[18] in which each line represents a different aspect of it. The approach that the relations between objectivity and subjectivity are expressed in different ways served Jaspers as a basis for explaining the wide range of world views despite them being an expression of one fundamental phenomenon: people's aim to provide meaning to their experience of existence. This laid the first foundations for his perception of individuals as infinite Beings. However, while during the psychiatric period the infinity was reflected in the psychiatrist's personal view of the mental patient, in *Psychology* Jaspers portrayed it in the direct experience people have regarding themselves. The main significance Jaspers granted to the object-subject relationship being a fundamental feature of people's experiences did not depend on what it taught people about the external boundaries forced upon their human consciousness, but instead on what it taught them about themselves. The act of objectivization does not exclude individuals from the experience they are undergoing, but is part of their understanding of their personal experiences.[19] This act constantly expands people's frame of reference and establishes the link between their self-perception and their experiences in reality. Against this background, human experience is portrayed as a range of forms of expression of the totality spread between individuals as subjects and the world of objects around them, or as a mosaic of world views.

B. The World View as an Individual Case and as Part of a Multiplicity

Jaspers's discussion in *Psychology* was based on "two types of descriptions": the first dealing with the general and systematic description of the phenomenon of multiple world views, and the second focusing on the individual world view.[20] The first description, characterized by Jaspers as "the psychological point of view," is grounded in the general framework of object-subject relations and in the observation "the more we deal with the contents of world views, the more we notice analogous forms that are repeated again and again."[21] This discussion was interested in the objectivizations that people perform on their experiences in order to expose the structural patterns common to different world views, patterns that transcend the boundaries of the particular experiences of individuals in formulating their world views. The psychological viewpoint served as a means for making the particular objectivizations people perform as part of their consciousness into statements in principle of human existence as such, with the concrete contents expressing the individuals' experiences perceived as of secondary importance. The second description focused on the subjective being that formulated the world view. In this framework, the world view was perceived as an ontological expression of the individual's subjective being and as a medium in which the general exclusively becomes concrete.[22] Understanding the subject as a concrete Being aiming to understand itself pushed back the structural and general aspects typical of world views as such, as a general phenomenon, to the margins of Jaspers's discussion. The world view is perceived as a medium where objectivizations become consciousness itself, and this world view lacks meaning in the absence of its inherent link to the individual who constituted it from his concrete experiences.

The integration of these two descriptions of world views reflects the fundamental tension typical of Jaspers's thought at that time, which was to become more severe later on. He aimed at formulating a general perception of selfhood, but he also wanted it to express the particular and private Being of the individual as such. The difficulty in integrating these two viewpoints is clear, since they reflect different kinds of issues and require different types of discussion. However, we can also understand the difficulty Jaspers had in giving up one of these descriptions. The one focused on the private world view continues the trend indicated in his early writings, emphasizing the particular Being of the individual, and in a way now was his chance to give this aspect real expression. However, the description focused on the multiplicity of world views was also essential to Jaspers, since in *Psychology* he took his first steps as a philosopher and aimed to anchor his approach in a structured framework. In this double move,

Jaspers tried to respond to two contradictory requirements: to preserve the unique nature of the individual's experience as portrayed in his private world view, and at the same time to grant this world view general significance and validity, following which it would cease to be merely a private world view.

These different approaches reflect the two basic points of views through which Jaspers's thinking as a whole developed: the epistemological and the ontological. The epistemological viewpoint aimed at revealing the objective aspects of the subject under discussion. In this context it is expressed in the attempt to reach a relativistic understanding through illuminating the multiplicity of forms by which people can organize their experiences and grant them meaning. In the ontological viewpoint, the aim to find expression for the subjective and particular layers of the issue was more dominant. Here the main attention was directed at explicating subjective being as constituting a world view as part of a process of self-understanding. In his article "Comments on *Karl Jaspers's Psychology of Worldviews*" (1919–1921), Martin Heidegger argued that Jaspers's book contained two directions. In the first he created the science of psychology as a whole, and in the second he provided options for self-reflections using conceptual clarifications.[23] Along with the basic link between the expressions of these two viewpoints in this context and the way they were expressed in his earlier writings, we can also notice their modification in *Psychology*. The epistemological viewpoint, directed in this context at the phenomenon of the multiplicity of world views, examines the character of subjects by analyzing the objectivizations they perform on their experiences in reality. Although the origin of the objectivizations is subjective, the significance they receive is mainly general, and as such is also aimed at explaining other objectivizations of other subjects. The basic motive behind the ontological viewpoint is completely different. Unlike the epistemological viewpoint, this viewpoint aims a-priori to explicate individuals in their individuality, assuming that only by focusing on their private world view, revealing the necessarily particular way they experience reality, can full understanding of people as unique Beings be achieved. The epistemological viewpoint helps identify the general forms typical of private world views and present on their basis generalizations such as types of world views, while the ontological viewpoint serves as a basis for the explication of the contents of world views. This argument about the existence of these two world views can be established using Jaspers's words.

The epistemological viewpoint is reflected in Jaspers's statement "the meaning of the psychology of world views is less a straight single study (which is only in casuistry, which here is not desired) than a demarcation of the area which we at the moment perceive conceptually."[24] Jaspers clarified that his book did not deal with "the empiric case in itself" or in the "causal,"[25] involving a particular world view, but instead presented a "gallery of world views"[26] analyzed using each other and offered to the reader for selection. The multiplicity of world views, the "catalog" as he put it, was defined as a "relative scheme", awareness of which should guide the observation of each of the private world views included within the multiplicity.[27] The emphasis placed on the structural viewpoint and on the general aspects regarding the essence and role of world views in general expressed a distancing from the private world views to the extent of seeing each of them as representing a general "type" that serves as a blueprint for several private world views. The observation of world view types is focused on the question of the proper ratio between the concrete contents of the private world view and the type that represents a generalization of it. Inevitably, the uniqueness of the world view, grounded in the individual character of the personality that formed it, becomes irrelevant,[28] and this is the main disadvantage of this point of view.

However, the epistemological viewpoint has a clear advantage in enabling the formation of a rational understanding of the nature of world views as different expressions of a general phenomenon. This means that using this point of view we see that not only does the constitution of a world view not make the subject special as such—the particular world views individuals possess reflect only one of the possibilities they could have chosen in order to organize their experiences. Treating the world view as a possibility can help the observer discover moderation and openness toward some positions included in world views and form a wider perspective of world views as such. In this spirit, Jaspers stated that rational observation of the multiplicity of world views can serve as a "means of destroying a disguised and false form of existence"[29] typical of some world views. The understanding of a particular world view as one among several possible world views apparently determines the status of each world view toward the outside, as one of many, but it may simultaneously more correctly form people's attitude toward their personal world view as bearing a certainty that is not absolute.[30]

Just like Jaspers's position denouncing the methods that aspire to encompass everything contained in mental illnesses and as a result miss the contact with the patient as an individual,[31] so in this context he was aware that the very construction of types of world views could miss the essential truth of the private world view as such.[32] Jaspers did not refer to this problem directly, but we can find in his words a basis for confronting it. He stated in *Psychology*, "everything that is systematic remains in the flow" in which nothing is absolutely final, and that people should constantly aim to overcome the inflexibility typical of systems as such.[33] He also added the requirement "*to be constantly systematic and nevertheless keep attempting not to allow any system to gain control, thus* to enable as many systematic thoughts as possible—all of them if possible—to have influence."[34] These words express the two needs that create the fundamental contradiction that trapped his thinking in *Psychology*: people's need for an external anchor and affirmation of their experiences, and simultaneously the need to grant them a decisive status in granting significance to their experiences. The varied nature of human reality, the infinite character of the individual, and the world view aiming to connect these two elements apparently restrict the ability to be systematic in discussing the human experience in constituting world views. This restriction applies not only to the individual world view, since even the psychological viewpoint, the one aiming at the general, is subject to this restriction. As he wrote:

> It is futile to talk about unity. To prove it is impossible. To disprove it is equally impossible. It is an idea whose realization in a systematic order—while it attempts to be critical—must be a loose structure between a system and a catalog.[35]

Jaspers aimed his search for unity using the psychological viewpoint at enabling a wide perspective of world views that would grant them significance beyond that granted them within the boundaries of the experience of the subjects who created them. The difficulty in achieving such unity is given a positive significance. It testifies to world views containing an individual expression of a particular experience, and this by its very nature cannot be organized and generalized. This is not a restriction that can be overcome by changing the method, but the nature of the object on which the psychological method is operated: the subjective being of the individual. Defining the product of the psychological viewpoint as a "loose structure" portrays the difficulty and also the attempt to resolve it: it permits a broad perspective of world views as such, and serves as an instrument for their rational understanding. However, the psychological viewpoint tries to avoid where possible the diminution of the particular character of world views that results from their being an expression of the personal truth of the subjective being that created them.

The psychological viewpoint is revealed as a tool appropriate to the varied and contradictory nature of human reality that no system can overcome. The multiplicity of world views on which this viewpoint is based may serve to prevent the granting of an absolute status to some private world view, whether by individuals themselves or by others, helping both the individuals and the researcher of world views to be in a position of "relating to the essential in a fertile lack of clarity"[36]—a position Jaspers supported and described himself as holding. This stance of individuals facing the unity they seek but understand they cannot achieve expresses the difference between what Jaspers called "prophetic philosophy" and the psychology of world views. While "prophetic philosophy" provides people in advance with an organized set of values and meanings they can hold onto even without a real experience of a personal search process, the psychology of world views is merely a methodical viewpoint. As such, psychology gives the observer a purely relative understanding of the variety of possible perspectives of the world[37] embodied in the private world views.[38]

The difference between the psychological position observing the multiplicity of world views and the process of creating a private world view, involving constant intensive experience, does not allow us to consider the psychological position itself as a sort of world view. Consciously or unconsciously, Jaspers designed the observer's character as a phenomenologist observing the world views as phenomena. From this point of view, based mainly on avoiding judgment, the observer is perceived as aiming to identify the elements on which the world views rely, and to decipher their typical structure. However, although the relativistic viewpoint helped form a new, wider framework for discussion of subjectivity compared to that in his earlier writings, the second point of view shows that Jaspers's position in *Psychology* was not primarily phenomenological. The use of the term phenomenological viewpoint in this context assumes the Husserlian move of "phenomenological reduction" that fundamentally expresses avoidance of judgment regarding the ontological status of the object of the discussion. However, the phenomenological tradition that developed after Edmund Husserl (primarily that of Heidegger) criticized Husserl's position and aimed at formulating ontological positions.

Alongside the approaches expressing the epistemological viewpoint of world views, we can see in Jaspers's discussion arguments that express the ontological viewpoint, aimed at explicating the unique character of the private world view.

> Here we are not searching for the frequent or the average... We are searching for the specific patterns even if they are rather rare. Our area is not what we see when we examine for example one hundred people around us, but the material that comes into being when we see what we notice in the historical experience, in the living internal [experience] and in the [one] present in the peculiar (*Eigentümliche*), in itself unique, even if this only appears and is built as typical.[39]

The handling of the general and structural aspects typical of world views as such, which accompanied their observation as a multiplicity, is found in light of these words to be irrelevant to the explication of the self-experience at the basis of a particular world view. While Jaspers presented a rational test for the multiplicity of world views, he chose to establish the observation aimed at explicating private world views on instincts.[40] Relying on instincts as a source for explicating a world view not only stresses the commitment people show themselves from the subjective point of view, but also demonstrates more generally the centrality of the subjective experience in determining the significance of the experiences that led to the world view. What could have satisfied the psychological viewpoint—a "loose structure" instead of "unity"—cannot satisfy the observation aimed at explicating the private world view. As he wrote:

> In this act of ordering a person knows that it is not sufficient to create merely a superficial catalog, but that he must move himself around the thing. In this order—in which wherever he wishes to be, it would indeed become false—there is nevertheless something that must be congruent to the tangible thing.[41]

These words, clarifying the nature of the unity sought through observing the individual world view, restate the difference between it and the unity discussed in the context of the epistemological viewpoint, aimed at clarifying world views as a multiplicity. While the second arises from the methodical needs of the phenomenological viewpoint, aiming at providing significance to phenomena, the first depicts the basic image of selfhood as a Being that forms itself through its world view. The main philosophical effort aimed at clarifying the unity of the private world view was concentrated on the character of the selfhood that held it. The character of human beings arising from the philosophical discussion of the unity of the individual world view is obviously not perceived from the relativistic point of view, seeing the very constitution of a world view as realizing one among several options, but instead relies on a wider view of the range of forms of their life. What was called in the writings about mental illness "the desire for the mental," without which Jaspers thought people could not practice psychopathology,[42] is now expressed in this point where the private world view is perceived as an expression of the unique nature of the human personality. In a way, the desire for the mental and the observation of the private world view express the drive to achieve an ontological representation of what Jaspers perceived at this time as the original and complete human Being.[43]

The two viewpoints, the epistemological and the ontological, or more precisely the insights achieved through them, were essential for Jaspers's discussion of selfhood in *Psychology*. Each of them revealed different facets of the individual's subjective being that was the focus of Jaspers's discussion. However, the status of the ontological viewpoint is apparently more central. This interpretation is confirmed by Jaspers's statement that in individuals' attempt to organize their viewpoint of the world and in their frequent meeting with different world views, they discover that all world views have the potential of becoming part of their world view. The other world views are defined as "positions" (*Stellungen*) that people encounter and see as expressing the possible range of their biographical development,[44] and not as final possibilities they have to decide between. In this spirit, Jaspers added that all the individual approaches presented in his book were related to each other and should add up to "a continuum of positive substantial approaches of the soul,"[45] so that the revealing of the multiplicity of world view types presents the immanent parts of the private world view. This means that Jaspers's philosophical discussion in *Psychology* was not primarily intended to contribute to psychology as a field of knowledge, but instead to create a framework within which the subject's self-consciousness could become clarified. Further support for the interpretation that the ontological viewpoint is more central in Jaspers's discussion can be seen in words he wrote retrospectively about *Psychology*:

> This philosophizing is absolutely not purely observing just as the psychology of world views never was.... It wants in every description to make present (*vergegenwärtigen*), swear to, appeal to, namely turn itself to liberty.[46]

These clear words cannot be misunderstood. Jaspers's aim to closely represent the subjective being explicated in *Psychology* is obvious. Jaspers required the reader's personal involvement in the contents presented by the book:

> The book is meaningful only for people who have started to wonder, to reflect upon themselves, to see the doubtful things in existence. It has meaning also for those who are experiencing life as a personal, irrational and undeniable responsibility.[47]

Although Jaspers did not testify about himself in the first person that he was personally involved in the processes he described in *Psychology*, he did write explicitly "as much as we try to avoid any value judgment" and position ourselves purely as observers, "we cannot avoid value judgments always arising."[48] While in his discussion of the multiplicity of world views Jaspers saw fit to note the contribution of rationality to annihilating "a disguised and false form of existence," he added in the same context the inability of rationality to help design life[49]—a role preserved for the individual's private world view. Against this background it becomes apparent that Jaspers's interest in private world views stemmed from them being reflections of the selfhoods that had constituted them out of their different experiences. In this respect we can note that of the words "world view," Jaspers was more interested in the "viewer" than in the "world" seen through people's eyes, out of their different experiences.

Obviously, this interpretation, indicating the centrality of Jaspers's references to the meaning of the private world view, should not invalidate the importance of the relativistic position arising from the observation of the multiplicity of world views. The epistemological viewpoint contributes to a critical understanding of the phenomenon of world views, mainly in the subjective personality not being exhausted by the structural aspects typical of its world view, but becoming clarified by studying the concrete contents of the private world view. The limitations of the epistemological viewpoint in representing the subjective being in full will be indirectly clarified in the following discussion of the metaphysical elements of the world view.

4. The Metaphysical Elements in the World View

The main insights regarding the individual's subjective being, reached in the discussion of the two points of view toward world views and the relationship between them, make *Psychology* into an integral part of the explication of selfhood. However, Jaspers's discussion in this book contained much more. In the margins of his discussion and sometimes as background or as asides, some ideas appeared where Jaspers wished to anchor subjective being in a metaphysical perception whose meanings and implications transcended the discussion of world views or of the subject who constitutes them. We should clarify that we cannot extract a real metaphysical approach from Jaspers's discussion in *Psychology*, but instead we see evidence of some intuitions and ideas, which from the perspective of his entire work can be seen as the beginning of this approach that was developed only in his philosophical writings. The dependence of the "early" on the "late," discussed in the transition from the writings before *Psychology* in relation to the framework of the explication of selfhood, will also characterize the discussion below on the metaphysical elements of world views.

Our discussion of the metaphysical elements of world views will use as a starting point Jaspers's clarification that the concept of observation (*Anschauung*), usually denoting the activity of the senses, has a much wider place within the context of the discussion of world views. He says that observation exists where the contents of the object's consciousness has individual and even unmediated fullness that cannot be exhausted by concepts and definitions. The concepts, the symbols and everything the person experiences directly and indirectly can arouse this observation, although it will always remain the "unmediated that cannot be proven rationally."[50] Observation, as an unmediated entity (*Unmittelbares*), serves as a premise for every experience.[51] At this point, as in other places throughout the book, Jaspers is diverted from a description with a primarily rational context to describing an experience that is almost mystical. In this context, he writes that our essence has strong yearnings that observe and desire a spiritual body and aim to fill themselves with observable contents.[52] On the basis of this clarification of the concept of observation, Jaspers presented the aim of *Psychology*:

> We are trying to achieve a subjectively aimed feature. This is the task of describing the types of observation without relation to a particular world view and without judging a world view: thus we grant precedence to the undefined mass of observation spreading from simple sensory observation up to the intuitions that go beyond anything that can be perceived rationally or esthetically. This mass of observation of the intuitive approach is the material in turn perceived in specific forms by the esthetic or rational approach, but [perceived] in a way that the material forms will never become sovereign.[53]

The observation in which *Psychology* is grounded is located on the scale between, at one end, simple sensory observation, aimed mainly at objects, and at the other end, observation anchored in intuition, characterized by an experience of wholeness usually desired in the process of self-aware analytical consciousness. This location enables us to clarify the understanding of selfhood at the center of the discussion, which was not identified with the immanent contents of an individual world view, but was perceived as having depth that could not be objectified. Following his earlier position that intuition was essential for treating mental patients, his words in this context about intuition of the understanding of selfhood as a primary element, characterized by unity and wholeness, testify that consciousness cannot penetrate its first roots. However, the other end of the scale where *Psychology* was located, in Jaspers's words what "cannot be perceived rationally or esthetically," hints at the horizons beyond selfhood and finality itself. This insight is also reflected, in my opinion, in what he wrote retrospectively about *Psychology*, that: "my philosophical drive pushed, in the guise of psychology, toward the whole."[54] This statement draws a continuous line between the stage he was in during *Psychology* and the later stages of his thinking, where metaphysics became an overt, central theme. The turning point in Jaspers's thinking that led to the establishing of a new channel of philosophizing termed "the explication of Being" will be discussed in Chapter Eight. As becomes apparent later, this channel cannot contradict the basic tendencies of the framework of the explication of selfhood in Jaspers's thought. Not only will the metaphysical approach join the framework of the explication of selfhood from a more expansive point of view, but already at the early stage of the development of his thinking, that of *Psychology*, it enabled Jaspers to locate more accurately the starting point on which his perception of selfhood relied. As he put it:

> If a person is motivated by forces (*Kräfte*) of a world view, he can never remain in the concrete finite, since everything concrete has at the same time both a finite and an infinite nature. No matter what the essential [thing] for him, he always encounters ways to the infinite or the whole. He can find in the face of the infinite in the evasive mystical experience a limited satisfaction in time and in quiet. However, if he remains alert, if he remains in the split between object and subject, any infinity leads him to the abysses of the contradictions that are called antonymous.[55]

In these words, Jaspers expressed one of his most basic intuitions that was destined to become an explicit insight in the philosophy of Existenz that he developed after *Psychology*. According to this intuition, what appears in immanent reality is not exhausted by the understanding that separates objectivity from subjectivity, but also contains an aspect that transcends its character in the finite Being. While the immanent contents of world views reveal selfhood or in Jaspers's words "the finite and concrete," the term "whole" (*Das Ganze*) denoted the aspect beyond selfhood as perceived in *Psychology*. Jaspers did not attribute to the words "concrete" and "finite" the meaning they usually have in existentialist philosophy. His entire discussion was focused on human beings' consciousness of what he considered reality, and has no real reference to the existence of the world as immanent reality as a Being that has its existence. Such a reference appears, as we will see in the next chapter, only in the first volume of the trilogy *Philosophy (Philosophical Orientation in the World)*,[56] and it reflects a new period in Jaspers's thinking. This distinction contradicts Heidegger's interpretation that the object of Jaspers's search in *Psychology* was the phenomenon of existence,[57] and that he perceived the existence of the "self" as beyond experience that can be offered a "regional definition."[58] This interpretation misses the object of Jaspers's enquiry in *Psychology* and reflects Heidegger's personal philosophical point of view. Even when existence did appear as a reality external to the subject being in Jaspers's writings of the philosophical period, it was not accompanied by the premise at the basis of *Being and Time*,[59] according to which people could draw conclusions from the discussion of the self regarding existence. In any case, even later on, when he wished to deal with the question of the world's reality ("The Question of Being"),[60] unlike the typical idealist approaches, he did not see the "self" as constituting existence. Jaspers's dealing with this aspect does not contradict his basic commitment to anchor his discussion in the general context of object-subject relations,[61] but instead reflects the attempt to find an explanation that would give full meaning to the mental reality coming into existence in this division. Just as the perception of human beings as a wholeness, mentioned in *General Psychopathology*, reflected Jaspers's attempt to understand people beyond the physiological aspects typical of their mental illness, so in this context the idea of the "whole" expresses Jaspers's wish to go beyond the frame of reference controlled by the division between objectivity and subjectivity. This refers mainly to the vagueness and generality characteristic of his mentions of the "whole" in the first edition of *General Psychopathology* (1913),[62] and not to the extended interpretation of the "whole" in the fourth edition that was saturated in his mature philosophical ideas as formulated in his writings up to the appearance of the fourth expanded version in 1942.[63] In this respect, we can see the very appearance of the concept of the "whole" as a continuation of the general tendency of Jaspers's thought to expand the area of philosophizing.

Nowhere in his earlier writings or in *Psychology* did Jaspers clarify the meaning of the concept of the "whole" or its relation to the framework of discussion, but he integrated it into his words as if it were an agreed concept. From this, Heidegger probably deduced that the concept of the "whole" reflected an early "preconception" of Jaspers that explains the principle of the division between object and subject on which the whole book was based.[64] From

Heidegger's point of view, the idea of the "whole" as a preconception failed, both at the functional level regarding the aims he believed were at the foundation of the book, and also in terms of its role in achieving a harmonious vision of existence as a uniform Being.[65] He believed that this idea was unnecessary for the development of Jaspers's main themes in *Psychology*.[66]

However, in contrast with this interpretation, according to the interpretation offered here, Jaspers did not offer any definition of the "whole," which, paradoxically, indicates the basic nature of this idea that could not be turned into a separate object of thought, but that should be understood from the experience in which it was revealed, the framework of the explication of selfhood. The interpretation offered for the idea of the "whole" does not accord with that of Heidegger, who saw it also as an expression of an esthetical experience.[67] Jaspers himself, in his criticism of the esthetical point of view, chose to emphasize its isolation from the infinite "whole" and its tendency to perceive the separate and the isolated as "whole."[68] The understanding that any dealing with finality eventually leads to contact with the infinite, or more precisely "everything concrete has at the same time both a finite and an infinite nature,"[69] does not allow the discussion to remain outside the limits of the relations between objectivity and subjectivity. This framework leads to "the depths of the contradictions that are antonymous,"[70] and at this point the psychology of world views reaches the edge of its ability. In this respect we can see the appearance of the idea of the "whole," even in its raw form, as an expression of Jaspers's critical understanding of the very possibility of performing an explication that would be limited to clarifying the subjective being of the individual. Already at this stage of Jaspers's thinking the understanding that this possibility is groundless was becoming apparent. The idea of the "whole" expresses the understanding that selfhood is contained within an encompassing whole, without clarifying or at least being aware of which selfhood cannot be fully understood.

This interpretation, according to which the idea of the "whole" reveals the primary elements of selfhood and adds a metaphysical aspect to *Psychology*, can be illuminated from another angle using the division Jaspers presented by way of the three stages that lead to the constitution of a world view. Although this description appeared at the beginning of the book, it can only be understood after clarifying the main philosophical processes that formed the core of the explication of selfhood in *Psychology*. The observation of the multiplicity of the world views and the reflections of private world views. Jaspers described the first stage as the stage when individuals aim during their experiences to draw for themselves the "whole" that appears to them as a "clear horizon." This task, defined as a life task whose achievements are always fragmentary and unstable, contrasts with the existence of particular truths of private world views sometimes characterized by a closeness that denies everything existing beyond them.[71] Despite the vagueness of these statements on the part of Jaspers, they have a double importance in understanding the perception of selfhood Jaspers developed in *Psychology* and the interpretation of the philosophical writings that appeared later. First, they hint at the solipsistic image of selfhood that leaves no real room for the possibility of a wholeness other than that depicted in its private world view. The meaning of solipsism as one of the features of the perception of selfhood in Jaspers's writing will be discussed in the following chapter. These words also give some expression to the metaphysical aspect in which Jaspers's perception of selfhood was embedded already at its early stages. These distinctions will be clarified later as having meaning for the interpretation of his philosophical writings where Jaspers developed a real metaphysical perception.

The second stage of the constitution of a world view was presented by Jaspers as an attempt to find the psychological whole, through which "the person motivates himself to the most outward boundaries." At first this is done through the tools of general psychology, the principles, categories, and methods of general psychological consciousness. Afterwards, through the psychology of world views, defined by Jaspers as "moving man to the most outward horizons, to the ultimate forces, [and including] an indication of the boundaries in which our mental life took place for the view we have had up to here."[72] The terms "most outward horizons" and "ultimate forces" indicate that the object of the psychological method, the mental life, is not independent but relies on something else. Jaspers clarified that the psychology of world views, like general psychology, is subject to what is given to us for understanding.[73] But it is clear that the special interest the psychology of world views shows in the "whole" did not permit it to focus only on the methodical aspects involved in the process of clarifying the human soul. The desire for the positive contents of the soul itself, expressed in the discussion of the private world view, was also at the root of preferring the psychology of world views over general psychology due to its potential to reveal the aspect of wholeness in selfhood. Heidegger offered a different interpretation according to which the psychology of world views and general psychology are two equal options.[74]

At the third stage, according to Jaspers, a "crossing of the boundaries of our mental life" takes place.[75] This means that the psychology of world views has exhausted itself as a method of getting to know the mental life, and now a new perspective is required, one of the "whole," basically metaphysical, to complete what cannot be reached within the boundaries of immanent consciousness. Here the observer needs a dialogical observation of different world views to soften the differences between them and to focus on what Jaspers called in another context "the point of the pyramid at which are aimed" the different world views.[76] At the third stage the idea of the "whole" functions as a horizon beyond the immanent contents filling the different world views or the structural and general distinctions the psychological viewpoint achieves of the phenomenon of world views.

The idea of the "whole" might express the most mature stage of the explication of subjectivity from the point of view of world views, or that its very appearance in the discussion expresses a distancing or even an abandonment of this viewpoint. The first option leaves a basis in principle for a dialog between general psychology and the psychology of world views, while the second option sets a border separating them. From the point of view of the framework of the explication of selfhood, this is a significant difference with implications not only for the boundaries of the human search for self-knowledge, but also for the very possibility of conducting a complete philosophical explication of the individual's subjective being, without this explication leading to the establishing of a metaphysical approach.

As clarified in the Introduction, the aim to delineate the boundaries of the object of philosophizing and of the discussion is one of the basic features of this thinking. However, we should note that in Jaspers's discussion in *Psychology* we could not find any basis to decide between these two options, which in themselves express a hint from his words instead of an explicit element of them. However, the appearance of these two options is not only aimed at the basic tension between the immanent and the transcendent elements of the explication of selfhood, but later is also revealed as a foundation for the explication of Being in Jaspers's thinking. In a way, this tension has already been exposed through the distinction between the two viewpoints in *Psychology*: the epistemological and the ontological. The epistemological viewpoint revealed the immanent aspects of the individual's subjective being, while the ontological viewpoints implied its metaphysical aspects. This did not indicate that the epistemological viewpoint was marginal in *Psychology* or that people cannot explicate the individual's subjective being, but instead testified to the multi-faceted complexity of the framework of the explication of selfhood in Jaspers's thinking, and especially that it cannot be exhausted within its boundaries.

The tension between the immanent and the transcendental aspects of the perception of selfhood, like other aspects of this perception, matures and becomes explicit only at later stages of the development of Jaspers's thought, when it deals directly with the explication of Being and of Transcendence. See the discussion in Part Three of the book. This tension is not relieved, despite the modifications that take place in this thinking, which testifies to its continuity and to Jaspers's loyalty to the early intuitions that had accompanied him from his early days. However, for this stage of the explication, the most important understanding is that the perception of subjectivity cannot be exhausted in the explication of selfhood, neither from the perspective of the private world view nor through the one that sees world views as a general phenomenon. The minimalist interpretation, including the idea of the "whole" within the immanent perspective borders of world views also indicates the space to which the self-aware being is exposed. The idea of the "whole," even in its general and vague appearance, directed the explication of selfhood to clarify the experiences that transcend the limited context of object-subject relations that served as a starting point for the discussion.

The concepts of the "whole" and the "boundary," which on the formal level of language have contradictory implications, reveal the formative elements of human experience in the search for self-understanding. Human beings, so it transpires from the discussion of Jaspers's thought already at this stage of his development, not only search for a more complete self-understanding but also aim to form a relation toward a wholeness transcending the boundaries of their humanity. At this stage a clear understanding of the dialectical nature of the starting point of *Psychology* is achieved. It saw itself as obligated to identify with the viewpoint of subjects who perceive their world view as total, as able to provide meaning to every possible experience. However, since psychological observation was also aimed at clarifying the multiplicity of world views, it could not ignore the fragmentary nature revealed in private world views. The idea of the "whole" could serve as a framework for a more correct understanding of the ratio between the different world views and the private world view, or for clarifying what Jaspers called the "strings" and the "tangle."[77] After the discussion of the "whole" we can no longer be satisfied with the general understanding that the private world view is a particular expression of a general phenomenon or of the multiplicity of world views; now it transpires that wholeness cannot be achieved within the boundaries of a private world view, but requires a link to human wholeness that constitutes an element transcendent to world views as such, and the explication of selfhood is required to overcome the borders private world views place before it. This also changes the understanding of the relativity of world views, as not being the product of a comparison between different private world views, but of a clarification of their relation to the wholeness of the human soul as such—a wholeness that cannot be fully expressed in any particular subjective being. At this stage of the explication, the particular viewpoint at the basis of the private world view is shown in a different light, and in a way the difference between a viewpoint anchored in a private world view and one grounded in observing the multiplicity of world views becomes blurred. Jaspers demonstrated the dialectic that the psychological viewpoint was destined to reach when he described *Psychology* as "progress… from one experience of whole to the next."[78] What appears to the owner of a private world view as wholeness and totality turns out from the psychological viewpoint observing world views as a phenomenon to be a "relative whole."[79]

In light of this, we can reach a clearer understanding of the wholeness in which the explication of selfhood in *Psychology* was grounded. This wholeness denoted different levels transcendent to selfhood. On the first layer, the transcendent aspect portrayed the totality exceeding the boundaries of different world views. This totality was attributed to the private world view, and it reflected the attempt to adopt the particular viewpoint of the individual forming the world view in order to achieve its ontological representation. On the second layer, revealed through the discussion of the idea of the "whole," the transcendent aspect portrayed what exceeded the boundaries of world views as such and what is beyond what a person can experience, human wholeness as such. The distinction between these two facets of transcendent aspects presents the idea of the "whole" as a founding datum of self-perceptions in *Psychology*: it constitutes an implicit datum in the first stages of the explication of subjectivity and serves as a means for identifying the basic components of the discussion's starting point, "world view." Later the idea of the "whole" becomes a more overt aspect of the perception of subjectivity, not only helping sharpen the awareness of the limitations of the explication grounded in the subject's self-perception, but also placing human wholeness as a comprehensive and more general aim of the explication of selfhood.

The different stages within Jaspers's dialectic process in *Psychology*—from the psychological observation that studies the multiplicity of world views and formulates a relativistic position regarding it, through the adoption of the private world view as expressing the individual's subjective being, to overcoming the total nature of this viewpoint by revealing wholeness as a formative datum of the explication of selfhood—not only formed the individual's subjective being as the object of the explication, but also revealed the metaphysical aspects inherent to its being. The introduction of the idea of the "whole" into the framework of the explication of selfhood in *Psychology* created tension between the immanent and transcendent elements in the discussion. However, this tension was not decided and did not lead to a disputing of the premises of Jaspers's discussion, aimed mainly at explicating the individual's subjective being. The aiming of the subjects toward what Jaspers called the "point of the pyramid" did not harm the basic understanding of the world view as a framework that expresses their self-perception as particular beings. In this dialectical framework the value of the psychological viewpoint for formulating a rational understanding of the multiplicity of world views was also preserved. In any case, the aim of forming a trans-subjective unity, whose origin arose from the discussion of the idea of the "whole," was a temptation that would demand realization the more the metaphysical intuitions became established in Jaspers's thought.

Three

SELFHOOD AND THE WORLD

1. From Subjectivity to Existenz

Karl Jaspers's attempt to form a viewpoint of selfhood protected from the tendency to wide generalizations, which early in his career he had attributed to the positivistic trend in science, was expressed already in his early writings in the field of psychiatry. In *Psychology of World Views*[1] this effort found a wider realm for realization, with subjectivity examined through its self-perception, through its world view. The discussion of Jaspers's perception of selfhood, as presented so far, indicated that his interest in the being of the self was devoted mainly to revealing its particular aspects. However, as we will see, clarifying these aspects no longer satisfied his interest in the issue of selfhood. In the perception of selfhood he developed in his philosophical writings published after *Psychology*, he maintained the link with his early positions, but significantly expanded the boundaries of the discussion of selfhood, forming a more complex perception of it.

The discussion of selfhood in *Psychology* was an intermediate stage between Jaspers's abandoning his practical and scientific involvement in psychiatry and the beginning of forming his philosophical thinking. On the one hand, in *Psychology* Jaspers felt liberated from the restrictions imposed on the discussion by the scientific setting and placed at the focus of his discussion something that had previously deviated from it: the individual's subjective Being. In this context, he was able to fill the perception of subjectivity with contents, and it no longer remained an intuition referring to an enigmatic and elusive Being to which access was restricted. On the other hand, Jaspers's attempt to focus on the particular fullness of this Being was unable to rescue his approach from the basic problems he had encountered already in his early writings, the relation between the private and the general, between the individual and the multiplicity, and between the advantages and disadvantages of the system. The perception of subjectivity in *Psychology* made it difficult to examine selfhood in relation to other objects of thought, greatly restricted the possibility of predicating it, and eventually led to the isolation of selfhood from the world it apparently wished to observe.

The explication of these steps reveals the tendency to solipsism that was contained in Jaspers's early perception of selfhood. Selfhood was perceived as a Being that forms itself by reflecting on its experiences in reality, but after processing these experiences they become assimilated in its consciousness as different reflections derived from its selfhood as one wholeness. More precisely, Jaspers's solipsistic tendency at this stage did not develop into radical solipsism such as that of Berkeley, or into methodical solipsism like Descartes's, since Jaspers did not see in the contents of consciousness a single embodiment of reality or an exclusive source of certainty. This tendency was not primarily based on the metaphysical premises typical of the original solipsistic position, but was largely the result of Jaspers's wish to focus on the individual's subjective Being, and a result of the absence of tools to express additional aspects of human existence. This distinction, that to some extent moderated the solipsistic nature of the perception of selfhood presented so far, explains Jasper's ability to overcome it in the philosophy of Existenz that he developed later.

In *Philosophical World Orientation* (henceforth, *World Orientation*), the first volume of the trilogy *Philosophy* (1932)[2], Jaspers first contended with the possibilities for philosophical clarification of selfhood in relation to the reality of the "world" (*Welt*) and "formal knowledge" (*Bewußtsein überhaupt*). His early understanding of philosophy as dealing with questions about the reality of the world and the nature of consciousness made these the main axes around which the philosophical discussion of the individual's subjective Being was formulated. Jaspers's aim, as a person previously known as a psychiatrist and perhaps a psychologist, to enter the field of philosophy, was also expressed in the use of new terminology. The concepts of "mental," "self," and "subjectivity," typical of his early writings, were replaced at this stage by the philosophical concept of Existenz, which gained a central place in his writings. These changes reflected both the search for a new point of view in the philosophical discussion of selfhood, and also Jaspers's self-criticism of his earlier perception of subjectivity. In retrospect, Jaspers referred to *Psychology* as a "hasty book of my youth."[3]

One of the first questions arising from examining the work *Philosophy* regards the manner of its internal division into three volumes: *Philosophical World Orientation, Elucidation of Existenz*, and *Metaphysics*. In *World Orientation,* Jaspers dealt mainly with aspects related to the explication of Being, in *Elucidation of Existenz*, the focus of his discussion moved to selfhood, and in *Metaphysics*, he returned to discussing Being. The location of *World Orientation* after *Psychology* and the psychiatric writings and before *Elucidation of Existenz* apparently interrupted a thematic sequence of the discussion of selfhood. However, since the different parts of this book show his turn to philosophy as a new developmental stage in his writings, where he distanced himself from issues that had interested him in previous periods, the volume *Elucidation of Existenz* is inserted into a philosophical move related mainly to the explication of Being.

The discussion in the three volumes of *Philosophy* was constructed gradually by order of appearance, and this does not permit us to assume that Jaspers did not attribute any significance to their order, and the discovery of the internal logic of this sequence is essential for understanding both Jaspers's philosophical perception of selfhood and his perception of Being. The interpretation of Jaspers's philosophical perception of selfhood presented below is anchored in the understanding that at this stage Jaspers was unable to continue discussing Existenz without linking it to the question of the world's Being. The search for world orientation (*Weltorientierung*) reflects an attempt to orient in the world of Existenz as a "worldly Being." However, when explicating Being, the significance of the location of *Elucidation of Existenz* in the middle, between *World Orientation* and *Metaphysics*, was that Jaspers's turning to deal with Being did not involve abandoning the discussion of Existenz, but instead was part of his perception of selfhood. The maturation process of this approach, reflected in the philosophy of Existenz, was expressed in the understanding that the self-consciousness of Existenz cannot be exhausted by referring to itself, but must form a relation toward the Being existing beyond it. What seems like breaking the sequence of the discussion of selfhood will transpire during the discussion as part of what Jaspers wished to argue about the two frameworks of discussion around which his thinking was formed: the explication of selfhood and the explication of Being.

In addition to the question of the relation between the three volumes of *Philosophy*, we should also ask about the connection between this work and the earlier writings. Our discussion of the early works focused on the perception of selfhood that arose from them, but it also revealed some metaphysical aspects whose implications went beyond the boundaries of the explication of the individual's subjective Being. In *Philosophy*, two main issues of discussion are presented: selfhood and Being. The status of selfhood in the discussion changes, and with it the metaphysical aspects, which are no longer marginal, but are now formulated into an independent axis of explication. The overt presence of two issues of philosophizing will reveal, as we will discover, the tension between the two axes of explication that had only been implicit so far. In this respect, the philosophical explication, of Existenz and of Being, permits a more complete and encompassing understanding of the issues that interested Jaspers earlier on.

The discussion below focuses on Jaspers's philosophical perception of selfhood and illuminates the developments that took place in it and its relation to the perception that appeared in the early writings. However, the discussion will not be merely genealogical. The accumulation of insights on the individual's subjective Being allows us to form a thematic understanding of selfhood through comparisons with its early perception and an analysis of the links between it and other issues that appeared for the first time in Jaspers's writings. The interpretation of the philosophy of Existenz presented in this and the following chapter examines Jaspers's philosophical viewpoint regarding selfhood, being aware of the change that took place in the status of selfhood in his thinking with the establishment of a new axis of philosophizing, aimed at the explication of Being.

2. The Reality of the World as a Component in Elucidating Selfhood

The perception of selfhood that Jaspers developed in *World Orientation* originated in the meeting of the perception of subjectivity developed in his earlier writings and a reality whose factual existence was not derived from its character and needs, or exhausted by its representations in the individual's consciousness. This attempt not only expanded the boundaries of the discussion of selfhood beyond clarifying the particular aspects characterizing the individual's identity. The new viewpoint of selfhood was anchored in the understanding that "in any form of existence that has become known, I am in my foundations."[4] This means that the individual's self-consciousness cannot serve as a basis for explicating selfhood. These statements did not completely distance Jaspers from his early interest in the particular aspects of selfhood, but instead confronted his early perceptions of the individual's subjective Being with new aspects, whose entry into the discussion created tension with these perceptions. The philosophy of Existenz, presented below, was the outcome of handling the tension between Jaspers's early approaches and the early premises at the basis of the formation of his later philosophical perception of selfhood.

World orientation, which served as an opening point for the formation of the philosophical perception of selfhood, was based on two premises implicit in the discussion. The first premise was that Existenz exists in the world or is a world Being. This premise made the elucidation of the reality external to the subject essential for the explication of Existenz. The second premise was that the world's external reality is not exhausted by its representation in the individual's subjective consciousness, and so it must be examined beyond the boundaries required for the explication of Existenz as a world Being. Whereas the first premise stresses the commitment to explicating selfhood, and as a result of this has a clear connection to Jaspers's early views, the second premise marks the beginning of the axis of philosophizing aimed at explicating Being, which opened to this thinking new horizons aimed at the reality existing beyond the individual—immanent and transcendent.

Jaspers's handling of this complexity is reflected in the philosophical formation of the concept of "situation Being" (*Situationssein*), denoting both the liberty and the necessity that create the Being of Existenz.[5] While the liberty reflects the options of self-fulfillment available to Existenz, the necessity represents the factual data that restrict its ability to experience and act.[6] Jaspers grants the relevance of the concept of "situation Being" to the explication of Existenz on two levels. First, the situation as a concrete Being containing Existenz itself represents simultaneously both the liberty and the individuality typical of Existenz and the connection between it and the surrounding reality. The conscious presence of Existenz in reality grants it meaning. Were it not for the role of Existenz in designing the reality external to it as the "situation Being," Jaspers might have been able to define this reality using the general term "world," which is not primarily connected to self Being. Second, situation Being represents the external reality beyond Existenz—both as a separate entity and as a subject in relation to which its self-consciousness is formed. In this respect, we should see it as a necessity that the philosophical explication of Existenz must confront. While the liberty element of the "situation Being" shows continuity with Jaspers's early perceptions of the individual's subjective Being, the recognition of the necessity component shows the change in his approach.

This interpretation of the term "situation Being" limits the framework of world orientation to discussing the basic phenomenon of the individual's existence in situations. In this respect, the reality relevant to Existenz's self-perception is mainly related to the options for self-actualization that it identifies in the surrounding environment.[7] This reveals a fundamental insight regarding the nature of Existenz's experience in the world: it does not experience the world as an encompassing wholeness, but only some aspects of the concrete situations in which it participates—situations that are partly a result of the self-formation of its consciousness and partly reflect the reality in which it already finds itself contained.

The introduction of the term "world" into the philosophical discussion, so far mainly controlled by the particular parameters of subjectivity, required Jaspers to take into account factors that challenged the solipsistic status of selfhood. Especially against the background of the tendency to continue his early approaches, the evident confidence that usually characterized self-understanding through a world view was undermined. As a result, not only was there recognition that Existenz did not exist alone in the world, but the philosophization itself was required to re-examine the premises on which it had been based so far. However, the dismantling of the "world" into individual "situations" within the explication of selfhood facilitated the integration of a new term into the philosophizing framework so far almost totally controlled by Existenz, and even softened its perception as a solipsistic Being. The confrontation of Existenz with the "situation," which is by nature partial and dependent on the context in which it is contained and the meaning it forms, instead of with the "world" as a reality not dependent on the self-Being referring to it, is much less threatening to Jaspers's early perceptions where selfhood was presented as a being that perceives itself as whole and total.

The connection between the way Jaspers dealt with the concept of "world" and the philosophizing framework in which it was discussed becomes clear not only in this context, dealing with the explication of selfhood, but it is also apparent, as we will see later, in the perception of the "encompassing" relating to the axis of philosophizing directed at Being. The clarification of Jaspers's handling of the concept of "world" in the two main axes of philosophizing reveals two opposite tendencies. In the context of the explication of selfhood, Jaspers wished to dismantle the concept of "world" and presented Existenz as experiencing "situations" instead of the "world" as a whole. In contrast, in his discussion aimed at Being, the apparent tendency is to gather into the concept of "world" components that had previously been part of the explication of selfhood ("existence," "general consciousness," and "spirit") and to enable them to be viewed as different "methods" within the encompassing totality of Being. Within the explication of Being, where Jaspers strove to present a more encompassing wholeness than that of Existenz and the world combined, he did not need to "dismantle" the world—quite the opposite. In the more mature representation of Existenz, appearing in the concept of the "encompassing" developed in his later book, *Out of Truth*,[8] awareness of the limitations of self-awareness replaced the tendency to solipsism typical of his early thought. The process of Existenz becoming aware of its limitations is analyzed in Part Two of the book, *Transition Mechanisms*, Chapters Five, Six, and Seven. This awareness served as a basis for the formation of the philosophizing framework aimed at the multiplicity of objects—as Jaspers put it, "modes"—in which space was found for both the "world" and Existenz, whose main interest was in clarifying the relationship between them instead of reducing the tension or the threat that had not been created due to the shared presence of concepts with a general meaning within the same framework of philosophizing.

The concept of "situation Being," which filled crucial needs of Jaspers's perception of selfhood, was unable to satisfy Jaspers's interest in the "world," and he wished to obtain a wider understanding of it, which he defined as "world thought" (*Weltdenken*) or "world reality" (*Weltdasein*). An opposite trend appeared in his words, not aimed at limiting the concept of the world, but instead at expanding it. As he said:

> Situation becomes a starting point and a target, since it alone is real and present. But it itself becomes comprehensible to me only through thinking about the objective reality of the world. I must think again about this reality as self-standing, in order to keep returning and annihilating it. I cannot perceive my situation without progressing to the world thought, and nor can I perceive the world without always returning to my situation only in which the examination of what has been placed in thought occurs.
> .... However this motion is not absolute. There remains a connection in the limitation of existence and through the practice and habit of the person so far.[9]

Jaspers presents awareness of human experience in the world occurring within the limitations of defined and restricted situations as paradoxical. Although it enables us to understand the reality in which Existence finds itself, it is unable to silence the urge to think about reality as "self-standing," to form vis-à-vis the world an awareness that is not bound to the explanation of Existenz toward it. *World Orientation* served as a framework for the formation of a philosophical perception of selfhood, while at the same time the foundations were laid there for the philosophical axis aimed at explicating Being, and this largely explains the dialectic in which the "situation becomes a starting point and a target." It serves as a starting point for the explication of Being that was destined to establish a concept of "world" much wider than the "situation," but it served as a target for the explication of selfhood, which elucidates what constitutes reality for Existenz. The basic difference in the status of the concept of "situation" in these two frameworks of philosophizing reflects more generally the condition of the two frameworks within Jaspers's thought at this point. The one dealing with selfhood was at an advanced stage, enabling Jaspers to see the targets facing it, while the one dealing with Being was at its inception, and so he could only indicate its starting point at this stage. This distinction can explain why Jaspers was unable to formulate a uniform concept of "world," and he was required to present two concepts of world, or, more accurately, to split this concept into two, according to the needs arising from the two frameworks of explications. As he phrased it:

> When I say world (*Welt*) I must think of two meanings, which despite all the separations, remains connected through their movement toward each other: either *the world as a whole of the other* that can be investigated as one thing with general validity; or existence finds itself in its world as a self-Being (*Ichsein*), in other words, as a not-I (*Nichtich*) of itself and this, as a whole of the same time is a *world as my world.*[10]

These words well reflect the dialectic typical of Jaspers's attitude toward the world's reality at this stage of his thinking. We can see in them a two-stage development: the world that individuals recognize as "other" clarifies to them their private existence in their own worlds, but, at the same time, through these worlds, "other worlds" also become accessible, expanding the area of "otherness" surrounding the person's existence. The reality of the world is perceived by Existenz itself in two ways: as a reality concentrating all that is different from it, but referring to it, and around which its life is formed, or as a reality whose differentness and distance from Existenz make it into an object for it. Now the meaning of "world" is expanded, and it is not limited to "situations" in which the person participates.[11] However, the split into two concepts of "world" demonstrates Jaspers's real difficulty in assimilating into his perception of selfhood the independent existence of another Being at this stage of his thought. This difficulty leaves intact the basic link between the perception of objective reality and the way in which Existenz experiences its near reality, in situations. The two meanings of "world"—positive or negative—do not break through the boundaries of the philosophical explication of Existenz.

The dialectic was not resolved. However, we must stress that beyond the meanderings of Jaspers's thoughts it did recognize the reality of the world—whether this reality expresses the otherness that stands in contrast to the "self," where everything different to Existenz but related to it and forming its reality is concentrated, or whether portraying an otherness so deep it becomes an object of formal knowledge. This distinction does not expose an innovation in Jaspers's thought, since although in his early works he did not explicate reality, he did not doubt its existence. The interpretation inherent in Jaspers's philosophical moves in *World Orientation* aimed at giving meaning to the dialectical movement of Jaspers's thought itself, to the limitation of this relation to the boundaries of "situations," and to the expansion toward the "objective world reality." This was an aim whose full achievement his thought did not yet contain the tools to enable. Eventually the dialectic confirmed the observation that what was unresolved in *World Orientation* was not the very existence of the reality of the world, which was not under discussion at all, but the possibility of forming a philosophical relation toward this reality. At the same time, it became apparent that the nature of the relation toward the reality of the world reflects the boundaries of the explication of selfhood, and to a large degree also those of the explication of Being, which were in the early stages of formation.

Scholarly literature contains different interpretations trying to contend with the complexity characterizing this stage of Jaspers's thinking, when he aimed to form a philosophical perception of Existenz as a worldly Being, and at the same time to require the separate reality of the world. Most scholars, both those dealing with Jaspers's complete writings and those focusing on *Philosophy*, did not see the reality of the world as a key component in the development of Existenz. For example, Thomas Räber argued that Jaspers's thinking contains two basic meanings of the term existence (*Dasein*): the existence in the sense of "presence in general" where the objects are perceived as phenomena, and the subjective existence in which the world is perceived according to the meaning it has for the person.[12] Räber justifies the understanding of existence as a term denoting the presence in general using the medieval philosophical tradition that distinguished between *existentia* and *essentia*—a distinction on whose basis existence was understood as presence in space and time. However, in Räber's opinion, these two experiences eventually encounter "the same world"; these two concepts refer to the same reality.[13] In any case, he believes that the "supremacy of the I over the non-I" is maintained, since in his opinion the phenomena "have a concrete function in the praxis of the unmediated life of the self," and this function serves as a basis for the reality of the phenomenon itself.[14] The implications of Räber's statements about the meaning of world orientation are clear: the world as a real reality does not contain a reality separate from the Being of Existenz, and so there is no point trying to isolate the elucidation of the world from the philosophization aimed at explicating Existenz.[15] The two meanings Jasper presented for the concept of existence are united in Räber's interpretation, identifying the existence of external reality with the content of the consciousness based on it and active in it.

Alan M. Olson expresses an almost opposite interpretation of the framework of philosophizing in *World Orientation*. In contrast with Räber, Olson argues that the problem in this framework stems from the phenomenon of "separation," according to which the person is both part of the world and separate from it simultaneously.[16] Olson saw this phenomenon as a basic issue not only regarding philosophizing itself, but regarding thinking at all, and so in his opinion there cannot be a whole system of "transcending" and of ontology. Jaspers's opposition to ontology will be discussed in Chapter Nine below. In Olson's opinion, the perception of the "world" as "not-I" served as a starting point for a search for understanding that would deviate beyond the reality defined by object-subject relations, and, by implication, also beyond the existence where Existenz lives and acts. Even so, Olson stated that Jaspers's opinions in *World Orientation* show a materialistic understanding of the world relying on an empirical viewpoint, and this did not allow him to form a wider understanding of the concept of the world, in which the reality of the world and the reality of Existenz would not exclude each other. Eventually, Olson argued, the more this materialistic viewpoint was rejected, the more Jaspers was able to formulate what he termed a "unified world orientation." However, this took place after *World Orientation*.[17]

These two interpretations—the one that did not recognize the world's real reality as having independent existence, but only in its relation to the subject referring to it, and the other that could not see the world's reality as reflected in *World Orientation* as expressing what Existenz could see as its own world—are joined by Werner Schneiders's interpretation, which adds another aspect. Schneiders's main argument is that Jaspers was not interested in the concept of existence as a real Being, but instead in the explication of Existenz. According to Schneiders, even *World Orientation* did not discuss the connection between Existenz and existence, but mainly the relation of Existenz to transcendence.[18] In Schneiders's interpretation, too, we cannot find expression of the world's reality, although unlike the interpretations of Räber and Olson this reality was not rejected by Schneiders due to the centrality of Existenz, but instead thanks to transcendence—the Being beyond both the world and Existenz.

The sometimes vague and even paradoxical combination of the two different tasks of *World Orientation*, the meeting of the two explications within this discussion, created real difficulties in understanding Jaspers's positions. The different interpretations dealing with the issue of that status of immanent reality in the philosophy of Existenz testify that the basic tendency of most scholars was to decide in favor of the centrality of one of the components creating the difficulty. However, this type of interpretation is not satisfying, since it is not grounded in a wider, holistic understanding of Jaspers's thinking, and especially does not take into account the changes that occurred in his thinking upon the transition to *Philosophy*. The criticism of Räber's interpretation related mainly to it not expressing Jaspers's efforts to deal with the world as a real existence defined as "not-I," which may explain his not noticing the formation of a new axis of philosophizing, aimed at explicating Being and anchored in different premises than those of Jaspers's philosophy of Existenz. Räber's study, based mainly on Jaspers's arguments in *Philosophy* alone, misses the genealogical perspective, on which the awareness of the vast contribution of *World Orientation* to the understanding of the explication of Existenz largely relies.

We also find it difficult to accept Olson's interpretation, which stressed the materialistic character of Jaspers's treatment of empirical reality. This understanding does not accord with Jaspers's main motivation in emphasizing the element of "possibility" in the Being of Existenz that prevents its objectivization. Even the term "situation Being," representing concrete reality, was used by Jaspers to stress the element of liberty alongside the aspect of necessity. Jaspers himself stated in a different context that the idea of existence that is purely empirical and does not require the person's relation toward it does not agree with the reality of empirical reality itself. As he said: "Existence contains a pushing beyond itself" (In the original this appears as a title: "*Dasein birgt in sich ein Über-sich-hinaus-drängen*").[19] With these words Jaspers rejected the possibility of establishing a viewpoint toward reality without the involvement of reflection and a certain degree of criticism from the observer. The criticism of Olson's position provides an opportunity to clarify the fundamental difference between the meaning of existence (*Dasein*) in *Philosophy* and the meaning that appears in his later book *Out of Truth*. Olson identifies the concept of existence as it appears in *Philosophy*, where Existenz constitutes an essential component,[20] with the concept of existence as it appears in *Out of Truth*, where it is part of a completely different philosophical move, serving as one layer in the picture of Being Jaspers calls the "encompassing"—a move that according to the general approach at the basis of this study involved a limitation and restriction of the presence of Existenz within the setting of philosophizing. However, the criticism of these interpretations does not necessarily lead to accepting Schneiders's interpretation, which also did not view the world's real reality as a strong element.

In contrast with the interpretations presented above, the interpretation offered here stresses the innovation entailed in Jaspers's referring to the world's reality and the criticism implied in this toward his positions in his earlier works. We should see the discussion in *World Orientation* as a redrawing of the area of the explication of selfhood, and as an extending of its boundaries. As we have seen, in the psychiatric period Jaspers did not discuss the issue of the world's reality, and not only due to the more general context that did not suit such a discussion, but also since the distortion of reality was one of the expressions of mental pathology.[21] Even in *Psychology*, grounded in the object-subject relationship,[22] the objects, and even the world as a reality, lost their independent existence, and their meaning was confined to their representation in the subjective consciousness through the world view.[23] The concept of *Dasein* appears in *Psychology*, but there it is discussed in the context of creating values (*Wertschöpfung*), in which Jaspers believes the person has no trust in world events (*Weltlauf*). This concept was also discussed in relation to the human experience of antinomy.[24] For the first time in *World Orientation*, the subjective consciousness of Existenz confronted the real and separate reality of the world. In the attempt to examine the relation of Existenz to what was outside the marked boundaries of its selfhood as a closed space, Jaspers sought to give philosophical expression to his concept of selfhood. This attempt made the solipsistic understanding of Existenz, characteristic of his works before *Philosophy*, impossible. In the same context where Jaspers discussed the relation of Existenz to the world, he also dealt with the meaning of "science" and the "question of Being." The discussion of science appeared already in the psychiatric period, but since at the time Jaspers's formal occupation was scientific, at least according to his definition, his referring to it was not connected to the discussion of the world's reality as a philosophical problem. The question of the relationship between science and philosophy interested Jaspers throughout his writings, and has received extensive discussion in the scholarly literature.[25] The presence of these general issues in *World Orientation* may also contribute to the establishment of the interpretation that the interest Jaspers showed in the reality of the world at this stage was not limited to the significance it had for the understanding of selfhood, but was starting to be formulated independently.

3. The World as Real Reality and the Question of Consciousness

Jaspers's attempt to extend the boundaries of the discussion of selfhood and its perception was expressed in his question whether formal consciousness could help the explication of Existenz. The question presented in this context was whether, in addition to the subjective and particular aspects, Existenz had any sides accessible to the objective viewpoint of consciousness. Jaspers answered this question in the negative, but as we will see below, just contending with it helped him clarify, this time through elimination, the particular aspects of Existenz. His argument in this context was that since Existenz was not an object, but a "Being referring to its possibility, it does not exist as such for consciousness at all wherever it may be."[26] The perception of Existenz does not rely only on elucidating the possibilities it has already realized but also those it has not yet realized but identifies as belonging to it. This potential facet in the Being of Existenz is not accessible to formal consciousness, since it implements its abilities to organize and generalize on defined objects in the world.[27] Formal consciousness cannot identify the particular Being of Existenz, and in any case it cannot expose its objective and general aspects, if it has any. Instead of the objects it is used to, consciousness finds a "vacuum" when it examines Existenz.[28] To demonstrate to what extent consciousness is denied its ability to represent Existenz, Jaspers stated that Existenz places before consciousness a "border" that it cannot cross. In this context, as in others, the two basic meanings of the concept of "border" have relevance. Inwards, regarding what takes place within the borders of consciousness, the border indicates that the processes that take place there reach a barrier that constitutes the end of the range of activity of consciousness. However, since already in this experience a clear awareness is created of the existence of horizons beyond it, the experience of the border outwards indicates the existence of further possibilities of clarification where Existenz could achieve a fuller understanding.

The differences between the Being of Existenz and that of objects are reflected, in Jaspers's opinion, in their unique ways of being accessed. Objects are "knowable" (*Erkennbarkeit*), while Existenz is "elucidable" (*Erhellbarkeit*).[29] The use of the root "to elucidate" instead of "to organize" or "to illuminate" was aimed at demonstrating consciousness' stance vis-à-vis Existenz. While the action of consciousness expresses the person's activity, control, and planning, the consciousness directed at Existenz is mainly a disposition characterized by the ability to let it become elucidated by itself. In German this position could be defined as "*hell werden lassen*" (let [it] become clear). Gabriel Marcel noted that the use of the verb *erhellen* is not common in philosophical language.[30] This disposition is enabled after the viewpoints preventing access to Existenz are removed, although this does not guarantee the elucidation of Existenz. This is only achieved after Existenz is placed at the center of philosophical consciousness aiming at forming modes of expression that suit the particular nature of this Being. Jaspers perceived Existenz as a Being that revealed itself due to an internal impetus, and so demanded that the philosophical viewpoint should not force any criteria on it, but should show openness to the variety of modes of expression of Existenz. Even the philosophical viewpoint termed "elucidation" contains a degree of activity expressed in the attempt to find a way to overcome the gap between the general modes of expression of language and the particular expressions that it aims to represent. However, the main aspect of this activity does not involve external control of the object of philosophizing by examining it using general criteria. This activity is expressed in the effort to adapt the philosophical viewpoint to the particular Being at which it is directed.

This discussion of the differences between the different modes of access to object and to Existenz served Jaspers as a means of establishing the superiority of Existenz within the framework of philosophizing. As he put it:

> I as possible Existenz has decisive priority for the philosophizing that is in breaking through the circle of Being out of object-Being and I-Being. Possible Existenz is the movement to what in this circle is only by

> elimination being-in-itself (Ansichsein). It [Existenz] may open the way that in the world of objects is blocked to consciousness in general. This philosophizing, which for empirical existence is nothingness [and] for consciousness in general is an imagination that cannot be established, is for possible Existenz the way to itself and to real Being.[31]

Existenz is apparently not only different from the other things existing in the world, objects, and other people, but it also perceives itself through elimination. Its self-consciousness is precisely the awareness of the difference between itself and other people existing in the world. The viewpoint of elucidation, unlike that of formal consciousness, allows us to follow the two main expressions of Existenz: the formation of the relation toward itself and toward real Being. The formation of the relation of Existenz to Being will be discussed in Part Three of the book. The priority granted to the viewpoint of "elucidation" does not stem only from it not being subject to the borders of representation of formal consciousness, but also from its accessibility to what the objective viewpoint of consciousness is barred from representing. This statement does not make the discussion of "consciousness" within the context of the explication of Existenz meaningless, since the action of consciousness also expresses a stance regarding the existence that Existenz experiences. In this respect, Existenz is not created only through its unique stance toward existence, the search for possibilities for self-realization. The uniqueness of Existenz is revealed, by elimination, also through discussing the modes of existence where its uniqueness as an individual Being is not expressed. The positive aspect of this elimination will be discussed in the following chapter, in accordance with its place in the dialectical move of *Elucidation of Existenz.*

The rigidity Jaspers attributed to formal consciousness, as a framework referring only to objects, did not allow him to grant it a positive role in the explication of Existenz. The strategy Jaspers adopted in facing the tension formed by the introduction of new concepts into the discussion of selfhood—restricting their discussion according to their relevance to the explication of Existenz—was apparent also in his handling of the question of the possible contribution of formal consciousness to the explication of selfhood. Just as the discussion of the "world" helped the formation of Existenz as a worldly Being, so the discussion of formal consciousness clarified its perception as a unique Being in relation to all other objects in the world. Jaspers's discussion of consciousness as an extra-Existenz point of view was itself subject to the framework of the explication of Existenz. Consciousness' viewpoint transpired as essential for the explication of Existenz, despite the basic differences between it and the viewpoint of consciousness designed by the particular criteria of Existenz itself. In Jaspers's discussion of the gap between the Being of Existenz and the borders of expression of formal consciousness we can see the influence of one of Søren Kierkegaard's key ideas, namely, the idea that the Hegelian perception of the subject (in some respects equivalent in meaning to Jaspers's perception of the empirical sciences) constitutes a viewpoint that cannot help individuals understand themselves.[32] Several scholars of Jaspers's thought argued significant influence and even similarity exist between Kierkegaard's and Jaspers's perception of Existenz. Elisabeth Young-Bruehl, for instance, compared the philosophical ideas that Kierkegaard expressed through the persona of Johannes Climacus with Jaspers's perception of Existenz.[33]

The discussion of consciousness reveals the complexity of Jaspers's philosophical perception of Existenz, which feeds simultaneously from insights related to the early perception of selfhood, stressing the particular aspects of the individual's Being, and also from the perception of Being, which he started to formulate in his writings of this period. On the one hand, his negative attitude toward the possible contribution of consciousness to the philosophical understanding of selfhood is a continuation of his early criticism of the positivistic approach, which saw what was reflected through consciousness as all that existed. Jaspers hinted at this criticism in his argument that since consciousness was not the only medium through which the human being's experience in the world can be examined, it should not be used as the main means of evaluating the philosophical arguments of Existenz. In his words: "Existenz finds itself... in the world, without becoming knowable (*erkennbar*) as a world-Being (*Weltsein*)."[34] The inability of consciousness to express the specific Being of Existenz does not result from Existenz itself being outside the border of immanence and does not express a retreat from the perception of selfhood as a worldly Being, but instead from the basic limitations of consciousness that do not allow it to express the unique mode of experience of Existenz in immanent reality. On the other hand, dealing with the viewpoint of consciousness can be seen as a new beginning, announcing his reservations regarding the idealistic and mystical world views in philosophy—reservations that were destined to accompany his later philosophical writings, and especially influence his perception of Being. In contrast to the functional role granted to formal consciousness within the philosophy of Existenz, the formal viewpoint of consciousness was presented as an efficient means of elucidating some aspects of Being, which Jaspers called the "Encompassing." In any case, this change did not make consciousness into a medium where the reality of Being or its constituent components was determined.[35]

The discussion of the differences between the viewpoint of consciousness and that of elucidation, although conducted largely by elimination, helped Jaspers present a complex perception of selfhood, as a Being that presents different stances toward existence. Although the viewpoint of consciousness does not recognize the category of Existenz, it is relevant to the framework of the explication of Existenz. This is the case not only because Existenz as a worldly Being is anchored in the same world to which objective consciousness refers, but also since Existenz is a Being that experiences objective consciousness. A fuller self-understanding of Existenz requires it to be aware of different positions and to examine its ways of experiencing, including modes of existence in which it is not revealed in its particular Being. Accordingly, a complete explication of Existenz also requires observation of the modes of existence not expressing the additional residue where Existenz becomes what it is.[36]

Jaspers's attempt to form a philosophical perception of selfhood, expressed in the integration of the concepts of "world" and "consciousness" into the discussion of Existenz, did not permit him to continue focusing on the particular aspects of the individual's subjective Being. What creates Existenz is the consciousness of the uniqueness it has compared with other people, but beyond this is revealed its basis, shared with other people in the world: Existenz exists in a world whose external reality is not exhausted by the significance it has for it. It is also capable of understanding the formal language of consciousness just as other people understand it—Existenzes and non-Existenzes. In this respect, the perception of selfhood Jaspers formulated in *World Orientation* revealed general aspects that no longer permit identifying it with the formative uniqueness of selfhood as Existenz. Just revealing these aspects creates the philosophical perception of selfhood.

Jaspers's use of the method of transcending, made clearer and more tangible in *World Orientation*, is expressed in expanding his perception of selfhood beyond the borders typical of his early thinking, and including objective and general aspects that enabled Existenz to become an object of philosophizing. The use of the method of transcending enables the demarcation of the line dividing scientific world orientation and philosophical world orientation. The first, serving as the main instrument of science, is achieved by the application of pre-prepared methodical principles to empirical facts or objects. The second is grounded in a constant attempt to re-evaluate the general structures in which science operates, and to note the "*doubtedness* of a factual world orientation."[37] Philosophical world orientation is not motivated by the aim of softening the rigidity of objective facts or to ignore them in order to preserve the uniqueness and particular existence of the selfhood being explicated. Despite this, philosophical world orientation is expressed in the attempt to explicate the selfhood that recognizes the reality of an objective Being but refuses to see itself as one of the facts of this Being.[38]

The analysis of Jaspers's positions proposed here does not rely only on the positive contents that filled his main concepts, but also aims to reveal the motives that directed his discussion of these concepts. A study of *World Orientation* from this point of view showed that Jaspers's attempt to place alongside the existentialist viewpoint additional points of view was accompanied by a constant effort to preserve the separate status of Existenz among other objects in the world. This motive explains the partial and largely biased discussion of the concepts of the world and consciousness in *World Orientation*. This once more clarifies his commitment to the understandings he had achieved before integrating the concepts of the world and consciousness into the discussion of selfhood, and the difficulty in letting go of them became more acute. The depth of the method of transcending depended on helping Jaspers achieve a more complex understanding of selfhood without having to abandon completely the primary insights he had formulated early in his thinking. This interpretation may explain why although a new philosophizing axis started to appear in *World Orientation*, aimed at explicating Being, and largely pushing aside the status of Existenz from the center of the discussion, Jaspers again placed it at the focus of discussion in *Elucidation of Existenz*, the second volume of *Philosophy*, to be discussed in the next chapter.

Four

SELFHOOD IN ITS OWN EYES

1. Back to Existenz

Elucidation of Existenz was Karl Jaspers's last setting where selfhood constituted the main subject of discussion. Unlike the previous contexts, this time Jaspers examined it without the mediation of other issues (such as: mental illness, world views, and the world). In this respect, this framework of discussion can be seen as the climax of the philosophical move directed at the explication of selfhood in Jaspers's thought. The fundamental insights achieved regarding selfhood continued Jaspers's early perceptions of it, deepened them, and even gave them new validity. However, Jaspers only achieved this continuity through a dialectical move where the early perceptions were critically re-examined. The same insights that in *World Orientation* diverted selfhood from its central status did not prevent its restoration to the focus of philosophizing in *Elucidation of Existenz*. The return of Existenz to the focus of discussion, and the renewed interest in the implications of its perception as a worldly Being in *Elucidation of Existenz*, did not express a withdrawal from the basic insights achieved in *World Orientation*, but instead an attempt to complement them and to determine their importance in his philosophical perception of selfhood. After Jaspers had discussed, in *World Orientation*, the objective aspects that create the Being of Existenz—a discussion reflecting the epistemological viewpoint of selfhood—in *Elucidation of Existenz*, he tried to express the way Existenz views itself. In this context, the ontological viewpoint became more prominent, seeking to represent the particular aspects of this Being.

The following passage reflects the clear awareness of the restrictions imposed by external reality of the world that is independent of Existenz and of its options for self-actualization, but at the same time reveals Jaspers's difficulty in continuing the philosophical move that had diverted Existenz from the center of philosophizing:

> … What satisfies me in knowing the world is ambiguous: either the world is *desired* as my realized existence-wish; … [since] it is inevitable for me to desire the world in which my Being exists; but as an absolute drive this desire becomes destructive for me; against [this desire] I hear the demand

> from my possible Existenz: to detach myself from the world into which I am in danger of sinking. Or else I perform [an act of] transcendence within the world… in which I see, think, and act.[1]

Jaspers here reveals the two motives that Existenz could have for knowing the world reality external to it. It can aim to know it because it is the realm where it finds its existence. In this respect, the knowing of the world is motivated by a positive motive, and can be seen as part of Existenz's self-knowledge or as a complement to its self-knowledge. Existenz's attempt to know the world can also result from a negative motive, its wish to identify the differences between itself and the surrounding reality in order to establish self-awareness as a Being separate and distinct from the world. These motives lead to the two options facing Existenz. The first, appearing here implicitly, directs Existenz to see itself as part of the world and to act on this awareness. This option is derived from the basic view of Existenz as a worldly Being. The second, more explicit, option faces Existenz with the extreme possibility of detaching itself from the world, and should be understood in the context of its uniqueness as revealed through the discussion of formal knowledge. The discussion of the possibility of detaching Existenz from the world has consistently made its mark in the interpretations in the secondary literature about Jaspers's perception of Existenz, which tend to present his philosophy as extreme subjectivism.[2] These two options portray the two centers of gravity that were constantly and mutually tempting at this stage of the explication of selfhood. Considering his awareness of the limitations of objective knowledge as a tool for elucidating Existenz, Jaspers aimed at establishing a channel of discussion where Existenz perceived itself as separate from the world. However, since the perception of Existenz as a worldly Being became in his thought after *World Orientation* an undeniable datum, Jaspers tried to offer his version of the way Existenz is anchored in immanence.

2. Separating Existenz from the World

Against the background of clarifying Existenz's fundamental difficulty in expressing its particular uniqueness in the external world reality, Jaspers examined the possibility of detaching Existenz from the world. However, the perception of Existenz as a worldly Being, previously formulated in *World Orientation*, did not enable him to argue that separation from the world could constitute a real option for Existenz as a concrete Being. The question under discussion is apparently related to the nature of the existentialistic consciousness formulated in the face of reality. The question is whether Existenz can exist in reality, but at the same time perceive itself as detached from this reality. To what extent can the self-consciousness of Existenz ignore the necessity forced upon it by external reality?

The early writings contained no space to discuss this speculative possibility, and this is not coincidental, since the perception of selfhood formulated there was not grounded in seeing the external world as a factor in reference to which the self-consciousness of Existenz is formed. The perception of reality at the foundation of the different world view types in *Psychology* largely reflected fulfilling the self-understanding needs of the subjective Being.[3] Jaspers perceived the world *view* that served as a framework for the formation of the individual's self-awareness as more real than the *world* it apparently wished to view. However, the external world's reality and the restrictions that its formal knowledge imposes on its representations became founding elements in the philosophy of Existenz, and as such they could not be seen as barriers that could be removed or overcome by any particular viewpoint. This implies that the discussion of the possibility of Existenz perceiving itself as detached from the world, with which Jaspers opened *Elucidation of Existenz*, does not deal with its relation to the reality that was recognized as we learned in *World Orientation*, but with the reflexive process that accompanies the formation of Existenz as a self-aware Being. Jaspers's answer to the question presented above is therefore negative. Existenz cannot perceive itself as isolated from the world's reality.

Even at this stage, despite the deep modifications that had occurred in his views, Jaspers's thinking preserved the motivation to find expression for the individual's subjective Being. The clarification of the objective aspects relating to the Being of Existenz did not weaken this motivation, but merely focused the essential difficulty of realizing it within the boundaries of a philosophical approach. The method of transcending, which had already become an overt and conscious element in his philosophical writings, could not enable Jaspers to be satisfied with achieving transparency regarding the situation of Existenz in the world. This transparency itself served as a basis from which Jaspers wished to transcend. Jaspers's attempt to remain attached to Existenz's viewpoint is evident in his frequent usage of the first person to characterize Existenz, as if it were the one revealing the philosophical insights about itself. The reexamination of Existenz's relations to the world's reality, which at first appears to be an unnecessary repetition or a regression to the earlier stages of his thinking, was also aimed at illuminating the attitude of Existenz toward its situation, and in particular at preventing the possibility that the objective aspects of existential existence revealed in the discussion would be its bottom line. The return to the viewpoint of Existenz is demonstrated in the following passage:

> The dissatisfaction that I experience … is a negative source that allows me, while pulling Existenz from the world's reality, to feel the reality in this pull.… This dissatisfaction cannot be sufficiently established, it is the expression of the Being of possible Existenz, which when it expresses its lack of satisfaction does not understand the other, but itself.[4]

The experience of dissatisfaction described here relies mainly on the interpretation Jaspers offered to objectivity from the existentialistic viewpoint. His main argument was that formal knowledge that generalizes about objects existing in the world could not serve as an instrument for elucidating Existenz, which is a potential and unique Being. Here Jaspers expressed the Hegelian idea that self-awareness was formed by elimination and motivated by the experience of dissatisfaction.[5] However, unlike Georg Wilhelm Friedrich Hegel, Jaspers's rejection of the objective viewpoint was a positive facet that affirmed the particular Being of Existenz on the same level where the negation itself appeared: in the framework of the explication of selfhood.[6] The rejection of the possible contribution of formal knowledge to the explication of Existenz becomes in its eyes "its thorn of becoming,"[7] meaning that the dissatisfaction is a positive expression of Existenz's internal truth as a particular Being that perceives itself as separate from the world.

The dissatisfaction that Existenz experiences when it wishes to express itself becomes a starting point for understanding its stance vis-à-vis the world. This is not a surrender of the search for self-understanding of its place in the world, or an attempt to ignore the way the world and Existenz itself are perceived from the objective viewpoint of consciousness. Without these, Existenz would cease to be what it was. However, since the world's reality does not appear to Existenz as an arena where it can realize the possibilities it identifies as its own, it is obliged to form a consciousness that separates the world's reality and itself. It vacillates between two insights that both have strong significance for it. First, "the whole reality of the world is lost before the isolation of the possible."[8] The world's reality is not expressed in what Existenz considers the possibility that exists for it, and so this reality no longer finds a place in Existenz's consciousness, or is "lost." The second insight, which is merely the other facet of the first, is the ultimate demand Existenz makes of itself, "to be from the source of my selfhood."[9] This requirement projects Existenz on itself,[10] when it experiences isolation, disappointment, and detachment from the world in which it finds itself existing.

The presence of the formal viewpoint of consciousness within the framework of the discussion of Existenz did not merely fill a role in the perception of Existenz as a worldly Being experiencing types of existence that non-Existenzes also experience. It made more severe the aim to grant expression to the particular aspects of the self-Being. Those aspects that established the perception of Existenz as a worldly Being were capable of disputing its very reality. The philosophical starting point for the discussion of selfhood did not deny the position typical of Jaspers's early thought, but confronted it, and created contradictions and tensions that could not be resolved within the boundaries of the explication of selfhood. These were expressed in the different interpretations presenting Jaspers's perception of Existenz as a Being that was relativistic, irrational, idealistic, and unknowable by the scientific approach.

Otto Friedrich Bollnow interpreted Jaspers's philosophy of Existenz as an attempt to reveal the person's "last internal core."[11] In his opinion, Jaspers's opposition to the ontologization of the concept of Existenz through consciousness and the very possibility that it could be understood as a category capable of objective knowledge was intended to defend the aspect of freedom, which had served as the cornerstone of the perception of Existenz.[12] In Bollnow's opinion, these premises made Jaspers's perception of Existenz an "extreme radicalization of the original life philosophy," which in itself represents an extreme relativistic position.[13] Bollnow eventually argued that Jaspers's perception of Existenz shows the nature of human beings as contentless internality.[14] He argued that this perception cannot be understood at all, and is impossible as a philosophical position.[15] Like Bollnow, Joseph Lenz also understood Jaspers's perception of Existenz as an extreme form of the philosophy of life based on deep skepticism and leading to the perception of human Being as relativistic, subjectivisitic, and irrational. The understanding of existentialist philosophy as an irrational position appears consistently in William Barrett's interpretation of the philosophy of Martin Heidegger, Søren Kierkegaard, Friedrich Nietzsche, and Jean Paul Sartre (whose references to Jaspers were marginal). This interpretation is present in the secondary literature about Jaspers, to different degrees.[16] In Lenz's opinion, in human existence's "escape toward internality," Jaspers's perception of Existenz led to a narrowing of the area of philosophizing.[17] Similarly, F. Imle argued that the selfhood arising from Jaspers's view of Existenz is "closed contingency hinting at the absolute."[18] In his opinion, the positivistic statements made by Jaspers did not exceed the boundaries of the self.[19] However, the attempt to search for God within the boundaries of this subjectivistic thinking divided it between pantheism and vague theism, and made it and the other subjects derived from it incomprehensible.[20]

The interpretation that Jaspers's perception of Existenz was a sort of idealism continued the interpretations of Bollnow and Lenz, stressing the subjectivistic and unknowable aspect of Existenz.[21] However, this interpretation is established mainly by revealing the relations between Jaspers's thought and classical philosophical approaches, especially those of Immanuel Kant and Hegel. Leo Gabriel argues that Jaspers's perception of Existenz summarizes Kantian idealism and even extends it by the openness to transcendence.[22] On the one hand, this openness is not structured into a particular religious position such as Kierkegaard's, but on the other hand it does not arrive at a rationalistic position such as Hegel's.[23] Gabriel argues that already in *Psychology*, Jaspers discovered the boundaries of objectivistic thinking. Gabriel's interpretation shows that in using the different philosophical influences that fed his thinking, Jaspers sought to express the Being existing beyond the boundaries of the representation of the consciousness grounded in the dialectic of object-subject relations.[24] This attempt, which does not allow the classification of Jaspers's thought as merely transcendental philosophy, is reflected in the identification of the concept of Being with the concept of selfhood as a Being existing beyond consciousness, the concrete I, and reason.[25] Gabriel characterized this Being as "pure spontaneity of self-realization, absolute freedom exhausted... in the realization of the whole of the world through the I existing as Existenz."[26] According to Wolfgang Stegmüller, Jaspers presented an extreme version of Kant's theory of knowledge, centered on the claim that it was impossible to know the "thing-in-itself."[27] This attempt results not only in the concept of Existenz, but even in Jaspers's entire philosophy becoming incomprehensible and even dangerous.[28]

A study of Jaspers's philosophy from the viewpoint of philosophy of science leads to a conclusion similar to those of the interpretations anchored in the "life philosophy", and of the idealistic philosophies. Jürgen von Kempski defined Jaspers's philosophy as a "call" aimed at the individual Existence only.[29] In his opinion, this call, sounding beyond any binding scientific understanding, makes Jaspers's concept of Existenz unknowable. Werner Schneiders criticized von Kempski's interpretation, arguing that it was grounded in a progressive perception of science, aiming to apply it also to the field of philosophy.[30] However, what von Kempski presented as a criticism of Jaspers's thought, Jeanne Hersch considered as the advantage of this thought. She believed that the illusion accompanying philosophy from its inception regarding its ability to obtain objective knowledge ended in Jaspers's philosophy.[31] As an alternative to this illusion, she believed this philosophy offers a clear judgment in favor of the subject that is in a constant process of becoming self-aware. A similar approach guided the interpretations of Johannes Reis, Heinrich Knittermeyer, and Hans-Rudolf Müller-Schwefe, who argued that Jaspers's Being of Existenz expressed a judgment in favor of the subject.[32]

Jaspers's negative attitude toward the contribution of formal knowledge to the explication of Existenz, and his discussion of its drive to separate itself from the world, probably influenced the interpretations presented above. Perhaps the separation between *World Orientation* and *Elucidation of Existenz* was also seen as expressing a retreat from the perception of Existenz as a worldly Being. In any case, these interpretations did not usually identify the positive arguments Jaspers formulated from the discussion of the boundaries of formal knowledge in the representation of the uniqueness of Existenz. Nor did they express Jaspers's consistent effort to reveal the objective aspects of the Being of Existenz. All these indicate that Jaspers's discussion of Existenz's drive to separate itself from the world expressed for the holders of this interpretative approach a real option that existed for Existenz.

I believe that the difficulties these interpretations raise are the direct result of missing the dialectical element in Jaspers's concept of Existenz, and evidently of the formative tensions of the whole perception of selfhood. This statement is especially true of the sweeping conclusion that Jaspers's philosophy of Existenz was relativisitic. This conclusion originates in the lack of distinction between two types of relativism: as the philosopher's *starting point* and as the *conclusion* formulated from the philosophical discussion. The first type of relativistic position seeks to refer in a balanced manner to the different aspects of the issue it discusses, and overtly avoids determining a hierarchy among the different components composing the discussion. The certainty regarding the individual's unique subjective Being and the central status granted to its particular aspects already in Jaspers's early thought do not allow us to attribute to it the motivations typical of the first type of relativism. With hindsight, we can identify in Jaspers's concept of Existenz the second type of relativistic position—a position grounded in completely different considerations aimed at reaching positive statements about Existenz. One example of such a positive statement is the argument that human beings' formal knowledge cannot serve as a tool for representing the particular aspects of Existenz. Unlike the first position, the relativism in this position constitutes a conclusion of the explication. Schneiders phrased this well when he stated that Jaspers's presentation of Existenz was the highest authority for its self-evaluation and for examining what surrounds it in the widest sense of the word (objects, values, norms, etc.), and does not reflect the arbitrary nature of this philosophy, but constitutes an expression of what this philosopher saw as an inescapable necessity.[33] These words of Schneiders's appear as criticism of Reis's religious position regarding the role of conscience in Jaspers, but they appear relevant also to the typical critical position from the viewpoint of philosophy of science.

The interpretation presented below of the second possibility through which Existenz is examined, as acting in the world with a clear awareness that it is part of it, is grounded in the basic insights presented in the previous chapter regarding *World Orientation*. At the heart of these insights is the argument that with the transition to philosophical discourse, Jaspers could no longer hold the perception of selfhood as a Being closed within its own boundaries. Dealing with the objective viewpoint of consciousness and its perception of selfhood as a worldly Being is a formative element of Jaspers's philosophy of Existenz. This statement also confirms the interpretation that Jaspers's handling of the possibility that Existenz could perceive itself as isolated from the world was part of a dialectical move aimed at establishing its perception as a worldly Being. This argument can benefit not only from the detailed discussion of the first possibility that was rejected, but also from the attempt to trace the roots of the interpretation that views the second possibility as an exhaustive expression of Jaspers's philosophical perception of selfhood.

3. Returning Existenz to the World

The immanent starting point that anchored Existenz in the world of phenomena, or as Jaspers put it, in the "situation Being," served as the background for the philosophical move that "returned" Existenz to the world after examining the speculative possibility that it could perceive itself as detached from it. In this context Jaspers was unambiguous: "possible Existenz *differentiates* itself from the world in order to really enter it afterwards."[34] This means that the perception of Existenz as a worldly Being does not contradict its perception as a unique Being, but these two coexist. Even when he saw the chasm between Existenz and the world as perceived through formal knowledge, and even when he needed it to fortify the unique status of Existenz, the cracks that appeared in the early solipsistic approach to selfhood forced him to reestablish the status of the two objective aspects in his perception of Existenz.

We should not be surprised that when he sought to examine the possibility of returning Existenz to the world, Jaspers presented a positive attitude toward the possible contribution of objectivity and generality in clarifying Existenz. While *World Orientation* stressed the differences between the validity types of "knowledge in general" and "causal self-understanding,"[35] when he wished to reanchor Existenz in the world, Jaspers viewed positively the possible contribution of knowledge and generality in elucidating selfhood. Jaspers argued that since the explication of Existenz was aimed at concrete "situations," it required an objective examination of the possibilities existing in the world and standing before Existenz. Objectivity serves as a basis from which the thinking transcends in order to achieve explication of Existenz. In *Elucidation of Existenz*, Jaspers differentiated between two stages: in the *first stage*, called "first transference,"[36] objective thinking has a crucial role. It provides the philosophical thinking on which the elucidation of Existenz is based with the logical clarity essential for the implementation of the method of transcending, and it also "ignites the spark of selfhood."[37] Objective thinking is essential not only because it serves as a central tool for clarifying the immanent aspect of the Being of Existenz, but also because it eliminates the possibility of seeing Jaspers's attempt to separate Existenz from the world as a real option. It affirms the discussion of this speculative option as part of a dialectical move aimed at establishing the self-perception of Existenz as a worldly Being. In the *second stage*, called the "second transference," the choice of the concrete possibility happens as a space for realizing the selfhood of Existenz.[38] The same objects that earlier confirmed that Existenz was a worldly Being undergo at this stage a process of "being raised while being dismissed" (*Aufhebung*), they become a tool through which "Existenz rises."[39] At this stage, Existenz attributes to the objects a wider significance than that given to them by consciousness. It identifies them with the very possibility in which it will realize itself. The vagueness accompanying Jaspers's arguments in this context results from the explication of Existenz revealing the very existence of possibilities for Existenz, but not presenting them concretely or elucidating the way in which Existenz experiences them. Here we discover the basic difference between the philosophical viewpoint of the possibilities in existence and the one Jaspers attributed to objective consciousness. The first examines the nature of Existenz itself through the existence of different possibilities in existence, while the second makes a logical evaluation of the possibilities of realizing the options themselves. Even if Existenz becomes aware of the self-realization options available in the world through objective consciousness, it alone determines their meaning for it. As he says:

> If I want to know what I am, then my objective existence presents itself, in the thinking moves I experience, as a scheme of my Being. I perceive myself inside it, but I experience that I am not completely identical with it: *what thus becomes an object cannot attain absolute identity with me myself*, since in my expansion I must lose myself in this scheme.[40]

The dialectical discussion of the relations between Existenz and the world finds in these words one of Jaspers's most concise formulations. Existenz sees the reality outside it, or as he puts it "objective existence," as part of itself. The process of forming its self-consciousness does not occur in a vacuum, but with reference to the external reality forced on Existenz, in the presence of the "necessity" aspect that is an integral part of the "situation Being." However, Existenz does not identify itself with this reality, since no identity exists between the access ways for clarifying this reality, between the objective viewpoint of consciousness and the explication of Existenz. The objects can help Existenz in the process of self-clarification only after Existenz has applied to them its typical reflexive process, thanks to which it can identify them as related to its self-realization.

The perception of Existenz as a worldly Being now receives its precise meaning. Existenz exists in the world and is formed with conscious relations aimed at itself and at this world. However, the element of freedom—the other facet of the "situation Being"—enables Existenz to transcend the "necessity" involved in the situations where it already finds itself. The same "necessity," or objectivity, in which its perception as a worldly Being is grounded may also be pushed aside in favor of a speculative option that does not yet exist in reality, but which Existenz aims to realize in its existence. The potential entailed in the existential freedom to transcend situations thus prevents the identity between Existenz and the totality of the situations in which it finds itself. So we can describe existentialist existence as a conscious movement between the reality that actually exists and a possible reality, or as a movement between two languages—the particular existentialist language in which it refers to itself and the language of objective thought in which it refers to the reality external to it.[41] Jaspers presents this movement as a process spread across an entire lifetime, with the individuals experiencing it as long as they try to live as an Existenz:

> … The separation is always available to be performed again. For existence as such the purely empirical forces serve merely as a condition, [while] the existential [forces] reach consciousness and reality only through pressing and penetrating: the process of separation that in an eye-blink exists in full clarity to the world can never be fully completed.[42]

This *in-out dynamic* typical of Existenz's relation to the world, or what Jaspers termed "penetrating" and "pressing," demonstrates the struggle for supremacy, and perhaps even for exclusivity, arising in his discussion between the two representations of Existenz. This dynamic no less expresses the establishment of the philosophical insight that Existenz itself is anchored in the same world to which objective consciousness refers, and the relevance of objective consciousness to a more complete understanding of Existenz as a worldly Being. Although the discussion of the concepts of "consciousness" and "world" within the explication of Existenz undermined the earlier perception of selfhood that tended toward solipsism, the functional nature of the discussion of these terms affirmed this perception, or at least the difficulty in detaching from it. In any case, even if the detaching from the early perception of selfhood was incomplete, the tendency toward solipsism that typified it did not remain an innocent or unconscious position in Jaspers's philosophy.

Support for the proposed interpretation, according to which the reality of the external world and the objective viewpoint of consciousness became for Jaspers data he could not retreat from in his philosophical writings, is expressed not only in the perception of Existenz, as presented above, but also in Jaspers's perception of Being. The "encompassing" and the "cipher"—key concepts in Jaspers's perception of Being, to be discussed in detail in Chapter Nine and Chapter Ten—were grounded in the necessitating of the immanent world's reality and of the viewpoint of consciousness accessible to the objective aspects of this reality. But in the context of the explication of Being, where these concepts were clarified, Jaspers developed a metaphysical view of immanence, and in this respect immanence did not exhaust the meaning granted to the world's reality. In addition, the positive attitude toward the viewpoint of consciousness did not make it the main instrument on which the explication of Existenz relied. The immanent world's reality and the objective viewpoint of consciousness served for Jaspers as a basis on which he implemented the method of transcending, and his main object of philosophizing was beyond them. However, although Jaspers manifested toward these two components a functional attitude harnessing them to the purposes of the explication of his main object of philosophizing—first selfhood, then Being—they continued to accompany his philosophical writings and became stable elements therein.

4. Freedom as Will

The two alternatives facing Existenz, separating itself from the world and finding itself within the world, rely on the premise that it has the freedom to move between them. Apart from this concept expressing a central element in the Being of Existenz, discussing it constitutes another layer in the elucidation of Existenz's complex relations with the world. For Jaspers, will is the main expression of freedom.[43] Will is perceived as based on freedom, while freedom is embodied in will. However, the separation between will and its object, or between will and what is desired in it, did not make the objects of will into an independent subject of the discussion, but instead served as an additional means of making claims about Existenz itself and maintaining its dominance in the discussion. As he phrased it: "will is not the activity that pushes only forwards, but its freedom is [in] desiring *itself* simultaneously."[44]

Jaspers did not focus on the psychological phenomenon of will, on the expression of activity people show in a certain state of affairs as a means of achieving their aims in existence. His interest was directed at a different, more general, human experience, not necessarily restricted to a concrete situation; experiencing "will that desires itself," defined as one of the expressions of Existenz's self-consciousness. Jaspers believed that psychology could help investigate the unconscious and covert motives of will, taking account of the general urges and the individual conditionings, but stated that it could not help elucidate Existenz. This reflects Jaspers's criticism of his earlier position in *Psychology*, through which he aimed at expanding the boundaries of psychology using the method of "understanding psychology" (*verstehende Psychologie*).[45] Even the existentialist will manifests the activity that people conduct regarding themselves;[46] however, this activity is not directed at what is beyond Existenz, but at formulating its own selfhood. Jaspers referred to Kierkegaard, who argued that the more individuals want, the more they are themselves.[47] Jaspers clarified that experiencing the "will that desires itself" is possible only where "the deepest clarification of the mental background succeeds, where through self-reflection the will achieves clarity and strength from its original contents,"[48] where consciousness turns to elucidate the options Existenz identifies as belonging to it, but has yet to realize.[49] Only then does philosophy replace psychology, and a philosophical approach to the existential desire is enabled.[50]

From the viewpoint of the explication of selfhood, we can observe two facets of the existential desire through which people see themselves: the conscious facet and the metaphysical facet. The *conscious facet* of the existential will is revealed in the argument that will appears "only where there is clarity of the '*choosing*

I'."[51] The discovery of will depends on the existence of self-consciousness or conscious reflection of people about themselves. To the same degree that self-consciousness constitutes a condition for the arousal of the existential will, it also portrays self-consciousness, since self-consciousness guides it and determines its nature. The ontological Being represented in this concept of will is Existenz itself, revealed as a Being that is aimed toward itself. C. D. Rollins identified this directedness of people toward themselves (self-seeking) with egoism, which he considered one of the meanings of solipsism.[52] The anchor of the perception of Existenz in the immanent reality of the world does not enable us to see this will as a reflection of a fantasy in which people sometimes err. However, the statement "will as thinking consciousness makes the *distinction* between dream and reality significant"[53] serves as the basis for explaining the nature of the relation of Existenz toward this reality, a relation anchored in the immanent reality that serves as an arena for its realization.

However, the concept of reality has a wider significance not exhausted by its contrast to dream. The reality to which existential will refers is not only the one realized in practice, but it also includes possibilities not yet realized that Existenz identifies as belonging to it.

> [The will's energy] is a continuum in the meaning of continuity of sense; it does not perceive ad hoc aims, but perceives at once [aims] for life, the latter aims are desired in what is still outside everything that is known.[54]

The reality of the possibilities not yet realized by Existenz in existence is no less than that portrayed by the concrete reality. It seeks them for itself and sees them as "aims for life," although their existing outside immanence leaves them on the level of "what is still outside what is known." Existential will is grounded in the two facets of the situation Being that forms the concrete Being that Existenz experiences: the "necessity" that does not allow the existential will to err in false dreams, and the "possibility" embodying all that Existenz has yet to achieve but is entitled to desire. The perception of Existenz as a worldly Being is thus reconfirmed through the "will" constituting one of the more typical expressions of the Being of Existenz.

The *metaphysical aspect* of existential will is expressed in Jaspers's statement that will originates in "*wholenesses* related to each other and serving it as an inclusive thing in the one-time action of will."[55] Existential will does not rely on itself alone, but is itself an expression or a realization of an entity or Being more encompassing than it. While this facet of will also expresses activity, this is not the activity of Existenz, but as he says, it is "active certainty of Being that it desires something,"[56] of a Being or entity beyond the limits of its immanent existence. The conscious aspect of the existential will transpires as a partial revelation, like the tip of an iceberg, of an encompassing Being on which it depends. In the context of this discussion, aimed mainly at the explication of selfhood, this Being is only implied, and while the reality in the background is perceived as immanent, the infrastructure essential for its full elucidation is lacking. However, even this covert presence can be seen as a prefiguration of the metaphysical perception that was to develop later in his thinking, including a far-reaching understanding of the world of phenomena transcending to the layer of potentiality embedded therein. This perception, like that of Existenz, was to be grounded in the immanent reality. Just as this aspect of the perception of Existenz left a wide field for the realization of the existential will, so in the perception of Being the anchor in immanence will not serve as a barrier to the development of a metaphysical perception of Being that will also include transcendent aspects. The metaphysical perception of Being is presented in Part Three of the book.

The distinction between the two facets of existential will—the conscious and the metaphysical—reveals a fundamental contradiction regarding the degree of autonomy Existenz has in the reality it experiences. On the one hand, the conscious facet of existential will presents Existenz's ability not to be tied to the factuality of existence and to form itself in the more open spaces of the possible. In this framework, Existenz is perceived as a source of will and as an autonomic Being. On the other hand, the metaphysical facet is where the will is revealed as an expression of what is beyond it. As Jaspers says: "Only in the idea and from the idea can I desire."[57] From the point of view of the explication of selfhood, we cannot resolve this contradiction between the two facets of existential will. Only in the context of the explication of Being, where Existenz turns away from itself and directs itself at the more encompassing Being, can the contradiction be resolved, or, more precisely, it is revealed as only an apparent contradiction. It transpires that in the transition from the conscious layer of existential will to its metaphysical layer, the area of the realization of will is expanded, and with it also the autonomy of Existenz. As a result, existential will discovers not only the selfhood of Existenz but also the Being beyond it.

The epistemological viewpoint, which revealed the conscious aspects of the perception of selfhood, transpires against the background of the discussion of the concept of existential will as having a metaphysical depth that cannot leave the discussion solely in the realm of the explication of Existenz. Although this insight relies, for the time being, on the rather vague hints that accompanied Jaspers's discussion of will, the doubt that it awakened regarding the degree of autonomy that should be attributed to Existenz formed another crack in the solipsistic understanding of selfhood, even though Jaspers's philosophy had yet to mature enough to relinquish it. In any case, although the full implications of the discovery of the metaphysical aspect of will would only be clarified later on, its importance for the perception of Existenz stems from the tension it created not relating only to its attitude to the external world. It was revealed as the depth aspect of its most basic qualities. The separation between the two facets of existential will demonstrates a more fundamental tension typifying the Being of Existenz: between the immanent facet that anchors it in the world and its transcendent facet that is revealed in its attitude toward an entity that transcends the boundaries of its real existence as such. This interpretation, strengthening the dialectical understanding of the consciousness that forms Existenz as a worldly Being from another angle, indicates the nature of the consciousness that forms Existenz vis-à-vis existence as a reality independent of it. It perceives itself as part of it, but at the same time seeks to form a relation toward what is beyond it.[58] So the depth of philosophical clarification of the Being of Existenz stems from the really present immanent aspect both in *World Orientation* and in *Elucidation of Existenz*. This aspect not only explains the tension in Existenz's relations with the world and with consciousness, but also indicates the continued existence of the solipsistic perception of selfhood even at this advanced stage of Jaspers's thinking. The attempt to examine the character of Existenz through its own eyes following the insights that arose from *World Orientation* put the solipsistic approach to a difficult test compared with the challenges it faced when it was discussed with the mediation of other topics. There Jaspers had been involved in defending his perception of selfhood from viewpoints that appeared to him likely to lead to its misunderstanding. Conversely, when Existenz was confronted with itself in *Elucidation of Existenz*, its internal vortex was revealed and the meanings it had been granted might become worthless considering the acquaintance with the encompassing Being in which it was contained. Only a wider viewpoint than the one in which Jaspers's perception of selfhood was grounded could rescue Existenz from this concern. This point of view, typical of the writings published after *Philosophy*, not only reflected another significant distancing from the solipsistic perception of selfhood, but also enabled Jaspers to develop a new perception of Existenz.

The philosophizing that led to the perception of Existenz as a worldly Being, originating in Jaspers's discussion in *World Orientation*, and continuing in *Elucidation of Existenz*, would later transpire as an immanent infrastructure essential for Jaspers's perception of Being, also grounded in immanence. Just as the existential meaning granted to objects in the context of the explication of selfhood did not negate their immanent and objective aspect, but instead relied on it, so Jaspers was to claim in his perception of Being that immanence contained a metaphysical depth beyond what we are used to identifying with the boundaries of existence. The anchoring of metaphysics in immanence—as the consciousness of Existenz and as an expression of an entity existing beyond it—would later transpire as a depth aspect linking the two main axes of explication in Jaspers's thought.

5. The Tension between Objectivity and Subjectivity

The two viewpoints that examined the relations between Existenz and the world—the objective, presenting Existenz as part of the world, and the subjective, in which the world was perceived as the world of Existenz—were clarified as two sides of the same coin. This understanding was based on the wide genealogical vision of Jaspers's thought, hinting at the future directions where the contradictions that arose in the explication of selfhood would be resolved. However, this genealogical explanation cannot suffice for the framework of the explication of selfhood, since it lacks an integrative understanding that could connect the objective and subjective facets of Existenz. Without such an understanding, not only is the basis of the contradictions that refer mainly to Existenz itself undermined, but it is also impossible to defend the very existence of a real perception of selfhood in Jaspers's thinking, leaving only a few single insights that do not add up. This is exactly what happened in the interpretations of Jaspers's perception of Existenz presented above. In the absence of a thematic viewpoint aiming at consolidating the different aspects of the perception of Existenz, these interpretations were unable to progress beyond exposing the contradictions it contained. Also, in the absence of the genealogical viewpoint, they were unable to identify the points where the perception of Existenz prefigured his perception of Being, and the possibility of a comprehensive solution of the basic problems in the perception of Existenz as a whole. Either way, the sweeping conclusion was that Jaspers's perception of Existenz was incomprehensible and impossible as a philosophical position. In the following passage, Jaspers points to the difficulty in connecting the objective and subjective aspects of the Being of Existenz, but also indicated their connection:

> The result of the possible misunderstanding of the entire elucidation of Existenz (mistakenly replacing Existenz with the empirical individuality of the individual's existence, identifying the existential internality with mere subjectivity) is the result of seeing this philosophizing [as a perception that considers] objectivity as dismantled within subjectivity, as losing the world within the abundance of its existence…
> [However] *Existenz is always in objectivity and subjectivity*. It is revealed to itself only in the world divided between subject and object, in other words in the interrelation between them. This existential problem—which by meaning is dialectical and has no solution—is the source and the target, the philosophical beginning and the inability of the philosophizing to stop.[59]

This clarification that the explication of Existenz takes place within the boundaries of the split between objectivity and subjectivity leaves no doubt that the two alternatives through which Existenz was examined in *Elucidation of Existenz* do not represent two different directions to self-realization. These are two philosophical moves aimed at one target: elucidating the nature of Existenz as a worldly Being. So the location of Existenz at this stage of the range of possibilities between objectivity and subjectivity is not a return to the basic framework of *Psychology*, also committed to "the range of connections between subject and object."[60] The reality of the world as an external Being was not reflected in Jaspers's perception of selfhood in *Psychology*. The context of object-subject relations in which his perception of selfhood was at that time anchored—a framework that Jaspers defined as "our prison," from which we cannot escape, although "we would like to get outside ourselves and move beyond ourselves and find an Archimedes point outside any subject-object relations..."[61]—did not reflect the view of external reality as a significant datum for understanding selfhood.

For the first time in *World Orientation*, Jaspers acknowledged the world's reality, and in the context of his perception of Existenz he was able to show a positive attitude toward objectivity, and to view it as relevant to understanding the individual's subjective Being. In his words: "a philosophical clarification of Existenz must preserve... the meaning of objectivity within its truth,"[62] both as a source of stability for Existenz[63] and as a means of obtaining knowledge and a basis for its validity. Sebastian Samay provides an interesting interpretation of the German term *Gegenstand*. The word *Gegen* expresses the contrast in objectivity, while the word *Stand* represents the element of validity. Samay relied on Dufrenn and Ricouer's distinction between the two forms Jaspers uses to denote the term "object" throughout his works: *Gegenstand* and *Objekt*. I believe the first term denotes the meaning the object has for the subject, while the second denotes the meaning the object has for scientific knowledge.[64] This change of attitude toward objectivity did not change the element of contrast it contained just from being a method of "standing against" Existenz. Maximilian Beck argued that the contrast exhausts the meaning of objectivity for Jaspers. Ludwig Armbruster's perception of the meaning of object in Jaspers stressed mainly the pragmatic and empirical meaning that Jaspers attributed to objects. My position is closer to Samay's, presenting objectivity in Jaspers as multi-faceted and as having many meanings.[65] Samay expanded the meanings that Jaspers granted to objects in general. These were no longer perceived only as a "means of self-knowledge,"[66] but had additional aspects originating in the consciousness directed at the objects themselves.[67]

The new attitude toward objectivity did not make its discussion into an independent element within the explication of selfhood, where the boundaries of the discussion were still fixed on the issues accompanying selfhood according to their relevance to its elucidation. Jaspers made the relation toward objects in the world into part of the process of constituting Existenz's self-consciousness.[68]

Jaspers defined subjectivity as "consciousness in general" (*Bewußtsein überhaupt*), as "individual consciousness" (*individuelles Bewußtsein*), and as "consciousness of validity" (*Bewußtsein des Gültigen*).[69] The process of admitting the existence of a reality external to Existenz, which progressively expanded the viewpoint from which Jaspers examined Existenz itself, demonstrated the maturation of his perception of selfhood. Unlike his early perception of subjectivity, Existenz was no longer presented as a whole and uniform Being experiencing a divided world, but as a Being whose maturing self-consciousness enabled it to turn away from its exclusive occupation with itself, and to observe what was beyond it. This explicit understanding of the Being called Existenz allowed Jaspers to phrase the two possible forms of "betraying Existenz": The first reflects a bias toward subjectivity, expressed in the introspection of Existenz and the resulting rejection of objectivity from its world. As he says:

> The subject as an individual existence is not pleased with the multiplicity of objects of the world reality, the people who cross his path, and the aims in which he must participate. Where he wants to separate himself in the world, he has the urge to alienate himself. He attempts to close himself as subjectivity. However, a "Being for itself" that is not subject to any restriction is impossible. In his isolation [the subject] would become unsure, everything would be rejected from him. He would be unable to be decisive regarding things and would not be honest with himself. The self wish of sensory existence would have had to turn against itself and remain a vortex of the multiplicities of nothing without existence and without freedom.[70]

The second form of betraying Existenz reflects a bias toward objectivity expressed by "accepting the thing exclusively."[71] Jaspers described this betrayal as follows:

> The certain satisfaction that Existenz experiences in devotion to the multiplicities of objectivity has boundaries within Existenz itself. This is because *the origin* from which objectivity is perceived... remains Existenz. When the slide into violent objectivity subjects itself to blind obedience, Existenz is shocked where people surrender themselves to almost mechanical obedience. The fossilization of objectivity is the annihilation of Existenz.[72]

The integrative understanding of the subjective and objective aspects discussed in the explication of selfhood finds its direct expression in the two forms of betraying Existenz described in the passages cited above. At the peak of the explication of selfhood, Jaspers chose to adopt these two aspects, and at the same time to qualify them from each other. Now objectivity is no longer understood as the contrast of subjectivity, but instead as including within itself subjectivity that faces it and provides it with its meaning as objectivity. However, the recognition matured in Jaspers's thought that isolating subjectivity as a means of protecting it was no longer beneficial, since without the objective aspects accompanying it subjectivity has no existence as such.

This integrative insight could not remove the basic tension between subjectivity and objectivity that was no less typical of Jaspers's thought than handling the tension itself. The two forms of betraying Existenz contain a double anxiety. In the first form, the attempt to separate Existenz from its environment may prevent the discovery of its multifaceted nature that relies on its different relations with the things beyond it, and lead to a limited perception of Existenz. In the second form, the betrayal may lead to the identification of the world with the objects within it, preventing its perception as a whole anchored in the relation of Existenz toward it as a store of possibilities that exist for it. Jaspers's definition of the relation between objectivity and subjectivity as a polarity not only strengthens the observation of the continuing presence of the tension discussed in this context, but also demonstrates his commitment to his early intuitions that determined his solipsistic relation to Existenz and made it difficult for him to assimilate objectivity into his perception of selfhood.

The idea of polarity between objectivity and subjectivity did not first appear in *Elucidation of Existenz*, but already in *Psychology*.[73] Jaspers's handling of the solipsistic perception of selfhood, or more precisely the implications of this perception within the context of the philosophical explication of Existenz, determines the basic difference in the meaning attributed to the tension in these two contexts. In *Psychology*, the framework of object-subject relations was perceived as a datum existing beyond the boundaries of the philosophical discussion. Since the possibility of explicating the tension between objectivity and subjectivity was restricted a-priori, there was no choice but to seek an escape from this polarity, portrayed as other types of world views or in the "Spirit types."[74] In contrast, in *Elucidation of Existenz*, where awareness of the problematic implications of the solipsistic perception of selfhood already existed, Jaspers was able to conduct a real discussion of the meaning of objectivity and subjectivity for Existenz. This enabled the viewing of the tension between objectivity and subjectivity as an integral part of the complete Being of Existenz. *Elucidation of Existenz* expands the ability of Existenz to contain as part of its self-consciousness things different from it. Objectivity was presented as "pending" within the Being of Existenz,[75] while subjectivity was described as a space where objectivity itself finds expression and realization.[76] This avoided the possibility that the attempt to examine selfhood through adopting its own viewpoint of itself would lead to renewed entrenchment in the positions typical of his early thinking—a possibility that at the early stages of the discussion appeared real, and some of Jaspers's scholars have even understood it as such.

The attempt to examine Existenz by adopting its point of view transpired as problematic and dissatisfying for the Being of Existenz formed by the very clarification of the relation between subjectivity and objectivity as its two foci of attention. This insight paved the way for the elucidation of additional aspects related to human existence (such as "consciousness" and "world") within the explication aimed at Existenz. At this stage, Jaspers was able to overcome to some extent the influence of Kant's transcendental view of subjectivity that was apparent in *Psychology*, which eventually prevented any predication of "the thing-in-itself." At this stage of the development of Jaspers's philosophy, when alongside the viewpoint of Existenz new insights were added that were not directly derived from its selfhood, it was no longer possible to continue defining the split between objectivity and subjectivity as "polarity". Now Jaspers aimed to indicate the "unity from subjectivity and objectivity." As he put it:

> Such unity is in no place an *asset* that can be perceived *without misleading*. Only the push from the subjective to the objective and back is real: the stored internality becomes itself real when it achieves objectivization through the external.
> However, whatever exists as purely objective is known by the subject only through its assimilation through the translation into the subjective reality: the truth is for me only if I understand it, the world is only the one where I act or in which I am contemplative. The idea is only what motivates power in me.[77]

These clear words cannot be misinterpreted. They confirm Existenz's search for its self-exposure. In this process, subjectivity is not supposed to be denied, or in Hegel's terms "placed above" (*aufgehoben*), since objectivity is once more translated into the world of subjectivity and assimilated by it. Existenz itself is responsible for unifying objectivity and subjectivity, so that they have meaning for it. Recognizing the relevance that objectivity has for Existenz itself did not provide it with an independent status in the framework of the explication of Existenz. The union between these two foci of reference continued to be subject to the continuity of the philosophical praxis that every time would connect these two components, whose polarity appears not to have been completely blunted. The philosophical explication of selfhood as Existenz reflects Jaspers's continual vacillation between his commitment to his early intuitions regarding subjectivity and his aim to escape them due to their restrictive solipsistic implications. However, before the status of Existenz changed and before Being and transcendence became the foci of Jaspers's philosophical discussion, he was able to close already in the explication of selfhood the circle where the discussion in this chapter started: the same Existenz that was presented as apparently wishing to isolate itself from the world found its way back into it on the same path it planned to escape from it.

PART TWO

TRANSITION MECHANISMS

Introduction to Transition Mechanisms

FROM THE EXPLICATION OF SELFHOOD TO THE EXPLICATION OF BEING

The growing awareness of the problematic nature of an explication focused on a single object of philosophizing was at the root of Karl Jaspers's attempt to expand his framework of philosophizing and to open it to new issues beyond the boundaries of the explication of selfhood. The introduction of the concepts of "world" and "consciousness" into the explication of selfhood already challenged the fundamental trend in the early writings, where the individual's subjective Being was examined on the basis of its personal experiences. However, since these terms were examined mainly from the viewpoint of Existenz, while assessing their relevance to its self-understanding, they did not lead to a systematic undermining of the solipsistic premises. These reappeared at different stages of the dialectic, which continued to be part of the philosophizing aimed at the explication of selfhood. Even so, along with the constant expansion of the perception of selfhood and of the boundaries of its discussion, a search for an anchor for the person's Being beyond the realms of the world, consciousness, and even the self-consciousness of Existenz started to emerge. The seeking of Being and transcendence, which Jaspers attributed to Existenz, served as an infrastructure for the formation of framework of philosophizing that I will term the "explication of Being." When Jaspers dealt with clarifying Being and transcendence, a large degree of continuity existed with the perceptions he had developed regarding selfhood, but the new philosophizing framework that began to form in his writings was designed using new criteria.

This part of the book will examine the philosophical ideas that were part of the explication of selfhood, but that at the same time helped Jaspers formulate a new axis of philosophizing, from which he was able to find a direction to solve the problems that had arisen in his perception of selfhood, and to complete the aspects that it lacked. I will define these ideas as "transition mechanisms": the term "mechanism" denoted their nature as *tools* of philosophizing, while the term "transition" indicates the location of these mechanisms as mediating between the parts of Jaspers's whole philosophical move. In biographical terms, Jaspers discussed these ideas, concentrated in *Elucidation of Existenz*, the second volume of *Philosophy* (1932)[1] in the middle of his long period of creation (1910–1963). While these ideas have also been discussed in other contexts and not only in *Elucidation of Existenz*, their presentation as "transition mechanisms" in this study is not based on the meaning they were granted in those contexts, which will serve merely for comparison. Regarding the contents, the ideas discussed in this part of the book embody three types of otherness, through which Existenz transcends its involvement with itself and forms a relation toward the Being beyond it: in "communication" Existenz transcends to another Existenz; in "historicity" it transcends toward existence as the time and place that form its concrete reality; and in "boundary situations" it becomes acquainted with the boundaries of existence and reality that are fundamental for its perception as a worldly Being, and tries to transcend them. "Boundary situations" first appeared in *Psychology*.[2] "Communication" appeared as a central theme throughout *Reason and Existenz*,[3] and was later mentioned in many contexts in *Out of Truth*.[4] "Historicity" was discussed in *Metaphysics*, the third volume of *Philosophy*.[5] Although in these ideas Existenz forms its relation toward what is beyond it, they continue to be based on Existenz's viewpoint. The aspects relating to the explication of Being embodied in the ideas included in the transition mechanisms are not sufficiently clarified within the context of the transition mechanisms beyond the viewpoint of selfhood regarding them, so they constitute part of the explication of selfhood. However, once these ideas are placed at the focus of the philosophizing, they can no longer be viewed as part of the transition mechanisms, but instead as part of the explication of Being.

The discussion of the transition mechanisms will be aimed at clarifying the turning point in Jaspers's thought when he transferred his focus of interest from selfhood to Being. Additionally, the explication of these ideas will serve as an instrument for evaluating the interpretative process up to this point of the research, and its future relevance. The separation of the methodological discussion of these ideas from the book's Introduction and its location after the discussion of Jaspers's perception of selfhood has a double significance: the methodological clarification enables us to distance ourselves from the intensive involvement with the contents and to reexamine the interpretative process that has accompanied their discussion. At the same time, the renewed interest in the philosophical moves already discussed, essential in a study dealing with the development of thought, sharpens our awareness of the interpretative moves already made and helps formulate the future interpretative directions. The discussion of the transition mechanisms is based on one of the most important premises informing the interpretation of this philosophy, the premise that research methodology does not precede the research investigation, but develops during its process from the phenomenological study of the text.

With these things in mind, we can present the philosophical ideas defined as transition mechanisms as instruments that helped Jaspers exchange the object of the explication in his discussion and at the same time maintain a dialog with the previous object of explication. In this respect, the transition mechanisms also reflect the continuity typical of this philosophy that created from itself the tools that regulated the relations between its different topics in the different stages of its development. This understanding is formulated as a criterion determining the nature of the ideas to be included in this part of the discussion: they have to continue in some way the philosophical move of elucidation of Existenz, and in this respect they should be viewed as an integral part of the explication of selfhood. In addition, the ideas discussed here are required to have new aspects regarding selfhood that had not yet matured and that left unsolved problems in the explication of selfhood. This dual requirement is intended so that the ideas included in the transition mechanisms will help achieve a new integration of previous aspects, but at the same time serve as a framework for clarifying Jaspers's self-criticism of his earlier approaches, which in itself constitutes a basis for the further explication of his thought. The discussion of the philosophical ideas included in the transition mechanisms is aimed at clarifying the argument that the peak of the explication of selfhood and the first formation of the explication of Being are located at the same point of philosophizing.

The central argument at the basis of the interpretation offered here is that the transition mechanisms constitute a frame of reference in which Existenz is presented as being pushed to transcend its boundaries, from its maturing awareness that it is not exhausted within its own boundaries alone. This awareness denotes a high stage in the process where Existenz finds itself able to separate itself from its surroundings and so focus its attention on aspects outside its Being. The maturation and establishment of this awareness and also of Existenz's self-distinguishing and separating skills are expressed in expanding its horizons toward wider and more absolute aspects of reality: Being and transcendence. The viewpoint from which these ideas will be discussed is designed in accordance with their function in the suggested interpretation of Jaspers's thought as a whole. We can phrase this in two questions. First, how much did these ideas help rescue Jaspers's mature perception of Existenz from the solipsism that characterized it in its early stage? Second, to what extent did transcendence become a closer and more tangible horizon for Existenz with the help of these ideas? In this respect, the discussion of the ideas defined as transition mechanisms is not intended to offer a complete and extensive discussion of their philosophical aspects, but instead to reveal their overall role in the formation of the metaphysical consciousness formulated through them at the stage of exchanging the object of explication. This discussion will reflect the duality in the particular condition of Existenz at this stage of Jaspers's discussion—after it was discussed as the main object of the philosophizing, and before it was removed from its central position in favor of the explication of Being. These two facets typifying the condition of the Being of Existenz are contained in Jaspers's definition of it as an "origin." As he says:

> Existenz is not a target, but an *origin* of the philosophizing within which it perceives itself. The origin is not the beginning through which I [could]

> always search for additional beginnings… but *Being as a freedom* I transcend to *when I reach myself in the philosophizing from the unknown*. The helplessness of the philosophizing that is in doubt regarding the origin is the expression of the helplessness of my selfhood, the reality of the philosophizing at the beginning of the impetus of this selfhood. The *perception* of Existenz is thus a premise of the philosophizing that at first is only a desire for significance and for a support, which is turned away empty-handed to the doubt and despair regarding its very possibility and then appears as unperceived certainty that clarifies itself in the philosophizing.[6]

The idea of the origin contains two basic meanings. First, it indicates the self-stamina of Existenz as a real Being that can be understood from within itself without the mediation of external factors. Second, this idea expresses Existenz itself being a starting point for a discussion of something else, still connected to it, but indicating what is beyond it. In the first meaning, the connection to the intuitions typical of Jaspers's early thought is still preserved, but the second meaning is anchored in insights revealed only in the advanced stages of the explication—insights that pointed out the limitation of Existenz to continue creating its self-perception with reference solely to itself. The connection between Existenz's self-perception at this stage of Jaspers's thought and the understanding achieved regarding the nature of the relations between it and the external reality is expressed in the following passage:

> The world and Existenz are in *tension*. They cannot turn into one [thing], nor separate themselves from each other.
> This tension is presumed in the philosophizing from a possible Existenz. The world as what has become *knowable*, and an Existenz that becomes *clarifying*, are distinct from each other in a dialectical way and perceived again as one.[7]

Just as the perception of the maturation of Existenz does not enable the separation between the two facets of the idea of "origin," so also this understanding cannot detach Existenz's self-awareness from its awareness of the real and separate reality of the world. However, the two facets of the idea of origin and the two stances of Existenz toward the world—as separate from it and as part of it—are not identical in content. These stances internalize the presence of the objectivity[8] of whose formation the transcending of Existenz is an integral part. In contrast, the reality of the Being of Existenz is a datum on which the first facet of the Being of the origin relies, while the second facet already reflects its transcending beyond its own selfhood. It transpires that the perception of Existenz as an origin expresses Jaspers's more cohesive and mature awareness regarding the Being of Existenz compared with the description of the internal-external dynamic typical of its relations with the world; this approach, indicating the status of the self-awareness of Existenz as more crystallized, was enabled only when its recognition of the objective world reality matured and when it transcended it; only then does Existenz appear as a unity beyond the sum of its two facets expressed in its relations with the world. This unity is what enables it to form a relation toward what exists beyond it. In the following passage, Jaspers described the existential consciousness typical of stage of the explication of selfhood:

> Whatever can be objectivized from within me is valid due to my empirical individuality, and since it can be a phenomenon of my selfhood as an Existenz it certainly does not evade a final and defined psychological analysis; this boundary of the knowledge of myself indirectly indicates something else without this observation being able to force itself. Thus the clarification of Existenz is released but not filled with knowledge; it achieves space for me, but does not shape a substance through the expressions of a Being capable of objective perception.[9]

These words show that the placing of Existenz as a target and a goal in his thought helped Jaspers establish his detachment from the scientific-empirical viewpoint of human beings and of the world, and largely freed him from being tied to objective thought patterns in general. However, already at the stage when the achievement of this target appeared close, from the realm of Existenz another target beyond it became visible. His description of this goal using the vague words "substance" and "something else" testifies not only to the vagueness surrounding everything revealed to Existenz, but especially that this vagueness was perceived from Existenz's viewpoint, which at this stage had yet to achieve an explicit understanding of transcendence and Being.

The perception of Existenz as an origin, entailing the special condition of Existenz at the transitional stage from the explication of selfhood to the explication of Being, enable us to state more clearly the status of the explication of selfhood in the context of Jaspers's entire philosophy. It shows that selfhood is the first stage in the philosophizing that would not be completed until the transcendent Being viewed beyond it underwent explication itself. At the second stage of the philosophizing, revolving around the explication of Being, Jaspers dealt with new subjects, different in nature. However, since this axis of discussion arises from the dealing with the explication of selfhood, it can be seen as complementing and closing a circle for Existenz itself. Just as the viewpoint that enabled the formation of the explication of Being was on the one hand dependent upon the awareness of the basic limitation of the philosophizing aimed at the explication of selfhood, on the other hand it relied on the insights that were formed there. The explication of Being is not exhaustable within its own limits, but needs the explication of selfhood as "the other" as a foundation for it.

Five

COMMUNICATION

1. Existenz Facing Another Existenz

Karl Jaspers's aim to form an approach expressing the individual's subjective Being, but not based on general criteria, was at the basis of the explication of selfhood as presented up to this stage of the discussion. He wished to examine the human soul through the physical symptoms of mental disease, to track the founding subjectivity of world views, and to elucidate Existenz, while not being subject to the objective viewpoint of consciousness. The premise behind these attempts, each of which represented a stage in the development of Jaspers's thought, was that the complete exposure of selfhood as a particular Being necessitates placing it at the center of the discussion and turning it into a framework where the other concepts would also be clarified.

However, while in the writings discussed so far Jaspers was mainly interested in protecting selfhood from approaches that examine it from general viewpoints, when he discussed communication he started examining Existenz in light of another reality. The confirmation this gave to the existence of another reality apart from that of Existenz—in this context, the reality of another Existenz—forced upon it a new reality that detracted from the totality attributed to it, and fundamentally changed Jaspers's perception of selfhood. Some references to the existence of another reality had already appeared in Jaspers's thought even before he turned to communication. In *Psychology*[1] it was the subjectivity that formed another world view, and in *World Orientation*[2] it was the reality of the existence where Existenz finds itself as an existing Being.[3] The presence of the otherness in previous contexts, whose status in the discussion was marginal compared with that of selfhood, did not change the attitude toward selfhood as a singular Being, but mainly influenced the understanding of other concepts appearing alongside it. For example, the concepts of "consciousness" and the "world" became an immanent part of his discussion of selfhood, which determined the boundaries of the reference to them. Conversely, the perception of communication discussed in this chapter reflects a real and conscious transcending from the solipsism typical of his perception of selfhood when this was the center of the explication. Consciously or unconsciously, Jaspers himself listed the reasons for the change that occurred in his perception of selfhood, and in his entire thinking, a change that served as an essential infrastructure for dealing with the very possibility of communication:

> Against the tendency to self-sufficiency, against the satisfaction with the knowledge of general consciousness, against the individual's self-will, against the drive to self-closure in self-contained life, against wandering aimlessly in an existing tradition as a routine way of life, the philosophizing wishes to enlighten.... through communication the freedom that perceives Being in its origin.[4]

With these words in mind, we can more precisely define the two facets of the starting point from which Jaspers turned to clarify communication: it is aimed against the approach Jaspers himself had developed earlier, against the tendency to "self-sufficiency" or "self-containment" attributed to Existenz, and at the same time it is a continuation of the opposition to the viewpoint of consciousness regarding the human being. So this starting point reveals one of the basic qualities of Jaspers's thinking, that no less than aiming at what was beyond it and what it had yet to achieve, it was also aimed at and against itself. The achievement of goals that were transcendent to it involved a repeat elucidation of what was included in it immanently, and sometimes even a dispute with it.

2. Existential Communication

The perception of communication in Jaspers's thought is anchored in the basic distinction between "communication in existence" and "existential communication." Jaspers saw communication in existence, which can become an object for study to clarify its motives and the basic patterns in which it is expressed, as hiding the individual's unique selfhood and identifying it with the selfhood of others.[5] However, he defined existential communication, in which the explicit selfhood of the person is portrayed, as follows:

> ... The philosophizing wishes to clarify the freedom before which the threatening solipsism or the universality of existence always [stand] through communication that perceives Being. This philosophizing applies to me from myself to hold me open and then to take without condition the communication connection that was realized. It seeks to *preserve* the *possibility* mercilessly denied in the solipsism and the universality of general consciousness.[6]

The location of existential communication between two poles, solipsism on the one hand and universality on the other, reveals the two greatest threats to selfhood with which Jaspers wished to deal in his discussion of communication. Universality reflects an impersonal attitude toward human beings.[7] This approach relies on the premise that the scientific and objective viewpoint aimed at elucidating the Being of human beings and the world is capable of enabling an exhaustive understanding of them. Japsers' criticism of this approach argues that it detracts from the particular uniqueness of the individual's Being by treating it extremely formally and impersonally. In this respect, we can see it as a continuation of the fundamental insights formed in *World Orientation* and even in his earlier works, where he rejected any attempt to objectify people and developed an approach that saw individuals as unique and particular Beings.

In contrast, the solipsistic world view perceives human beings—either as an abstraction or as a reality—as relying on themselves alone. Jaspers's position regarding this perception of the individual was clear. He stated categorically that the very possibility of seeing individuals as isolated essences existing in their own right is a "boundary image."[8] This means that the perception of a person as distinct from the surrounding reality is beyond the boundaries of human thought, and also beyond the boundaries of philosophizing. This criticism of the solipsistic world view, formulated here for the first time, is a new position in Jaspers's writings. Even if we assume that he would not himself have defined the perception of selfhood created in his writings up to that point as solipsistic, the definition of communication as existing outside it shows a new awareness of one of the possible implications of his early view, and perhaps even an explicit criticism of it.

However, the *anti-solipsistic position* to which Jaspers committed in his discussion of existential communications will be shown below as a *dialectic* position that sometimes contained explicit contradictions. This anti-solipsistic position involved several aspects that did not accord with each other and sometimes even contradicted each other. At one point, this position placed existential communication at the service of Existenz, understanding that it could not stand alone. At another point, it directed Existenz to exceed its boundaries and to form a relation to what transcends its boundaries. The tendency toward these two directions simultaneously introduced into existential communication the tension expressed in this context, as it is throughout the entire framework of explication of selfhood, in an attempt to deal with two contradictory trends representing two aspects of one subject. In Jaspers's perception of psychiatry, the duality was reflected in the presence of two different facets in the discussion of subjectivity—the expanding and the restricting—(see Chapter One). In *Psychology*, the duality was expressed in the two different tendencies of the explication of world views as part of a phenomenon and as private (see Chapter Two). In *World Orientation*, it was portrayed in the tendency to detach selfhood from the world and in the drive to re-anchor it in the world (see Chapter Three and Chapter Four). Apart from this basic duality, the dialectic typical of the perception of existential communication reflects wider processes occurring in Jaspers's thought, gradually leading to the replacing of the central axis to which the philosophizing was aimed. Alongside the continuing tendency to explicate selfhood, the presence of the "other Existenz" in the discussion precipitated changes that resulted in the processes of explication crossing the boundaries of selfhood and being directed to horizons beyond it. There are two different trends in Jaspers's perception of existential communication: while the philosophical arguments included in the first trend are an integral part of the explication of selfhood, the second trend shows existential communication to be a *transition mechanism* from the explication of selfhood to the explication of Being. In accordance with the framework of this study delineated in the Introduction, the discussion will focus on the writings appearing in the second period (in this context, especially *Elucidation of Existenz* and *Reason and Existenz*[9],) in which it is presented as a metaphysical problem. We will not discuss the works dealing with communication published in the third period, which have received special attention in research.[10]

In the first trend, communication is perceived as another means of forming the selfhood of Existenz. In this framework, Jaspers continued dealing with the implications of the universal viewpoint of selfhood, but in his discussion the awareness of the influence of the solipsistic view of selfhood became increasingly prominent. In a way, the placing of the other Existenz alongside the Existenz undergoing explication reveals a concrete facet of the reality of its surrounding world, filling with real contents the perception of selfhood as a worldly Being. In this respect, we can see communication as a context for dealing with the basic duality typical of Existenz, between the tendency to isolate itself from the world and its need to establish its existence therein. The possibilities entailed in the idea of existential communication in this trend contributed to the development and deepening of the perception of selfhood typical of Jaspers's thought up to this stage. However, the solipsistic substrate, which continued to play a real role in it, diminished the possibility of breaking through the boundaries of the explication of selfhood.

Only in the second trend apparent in the perception of existential communication was its function as a transition mechanism expressed. Compared with the first trend that contained a noticeable influence of the epistemological viewpoint, aiming to obtain increasing knowledge regarding Existenz, this trend emphasized the ontological viewpoint, aiming at elucidating the Being of the Existenz that intends to form a relation toward transcendence. The innovation in this trend lies in its confronting the Existenz under explication with another type of otherness, meaning not only that of the other Existenz, but that of transcendence. What makes existential communication into a transition mechanism is the very awareness forming in Existenz's self-consciousness of the existence of transcendence—an awareness that would become a central feature of Existenz in the explication of Being. There is no doubt that dealing with the possibility of forming communication with another Existenz as a Being that has its own existence was a starting point for the search for a reality existing beyond the boundaries of Existenz—a reality that gradually became an independent object of philosophizing in Jaspers's thought.

3. Communication as a Means of Constituting the Selfhood of Existenz

The philosophizing aimed at the elucidation of selfhood, as presented up to this stage, referred to selfhood as an individual Being. The loneliness separating Existenzes was assumed implicitly in the processes of individualization aimed at constituting selfhood. The link between loneliness and the processes of individualization was characteristic of many thinkers in Jaspers's period. Erich Fromm criticizes this approach.[11] These positions were in the background of the development of the socio-political critique of the Frankfurt School.[12] Since communication appeared in Jaspers's writings after the formation of selfhood as an explicit Being, it was assumed that the perception of communication itself should not be based on the individualization processes, but should transcend them. The explicit condition of Existenz served as a basis for sharpening the distinction between the "Being of I" and the "Being-with-the-other."[13] In a more detailed passage:

> Communication is present whenever two that are connected but must remain separate reach each other from loneliness and still know only loneliness, since it remains in place in communication. I cannot become myself without entering into communication, and I cannot enter into communication without being lonely. In any suppression (*Aufhebung*) of loneliness through communication, a new loneliness grows that cannot disappear without me myself ceasing to exist as a condition for communication. I must want loneliness when I dare to be myself from its origin, and thus enter a deeper communication.[14]

Jaspers's perception of communication reveals an undecided dialectic: the contact with the other creates the sensation of loneliness, which leads to communication, and so on. It transpires that the experience of loneliness remains a permanent element in the experience of communication. The experience of loneliness influences two different directions: it deepens people's self-awareness as individuals, and at the same time it pushes them toward the other out of a deeper, more established individuality. This dialectic perception of the relations between loneliness and individuality also appears in Jaspers's early article "*Loneliness*,"[15] which was more psychological than philosophical. The psychological viewpoint is especially demonstrated by his use of the term *Ego* and his reference to the "understanding" (*Verstehen*) method[16] known from the writings preceding *Philosophy*. This article was probably written between 1915 and 1916, but was only published in 1983 by his student Hans Saner, who edited it, and probably chose to include in it ideas originating in Jaspers's writings from the different periods, especially regarding the concept of truth and the concept of communication, which appeared in his philosophical writings published from the nineteen-thirties onwards. To the best of my knowledge, the article has not appeared in its original, unedited form in any of Jaspers's books or the collections of articles published during his lifetime or following his death, and the discussion of this article will not be incorporated into the body of this chapter. Perhaps the difficulty in determining the degree of the article's authenticity explains why it has not been mentioned by any of the scholars discussing Jaspers's idea of communication, apart from Donatella Di Cesare, whose study dealt mainly with works of the third period.[17] The connection between the sense of loneliness and the processes of individualization, which encompass a person's entire lifetime, appears to be the final element in the Being of the self-aware person.[18] Ignoring the clear link between the necessity of individuality and the solipsistic infrastructure in which Jaspers's perception of selfhood was grounded is difficult. In this respect, we may state that Jaspers located communication between solipsism and universalism, and this did not indicate his escape from solipsism, but only a clearer awareness of its existence and influence on his thinking.

The central status of loneliness in Jaspers's perception of communication appears in Fritz Kaufmann's interpretation, stressing also the solipsistic aspects accompanying Jaspers's perception of existentialist communication.[19] Kaufmann went further and formulated on the basis of the idea of existential communication appearing in *Elucidation of Existenz* an understanding regarding Jaspers's perception of communication with nature[20] and with God.[21] He also linked Jaspers's perception of communication with the issues he dealt with during the third period of his writings. Against this background, Kaufmann presented communication as one of the expressions of Jaspers's social criticism. In his opinion, the anchoring of communication on the basis of individuals, which grants it an aristocratic flavor, showed an individualistic reaction to the age of the masses. Kaufmann links this aspect to Jaspers's attraction to Søren Kierkegaard and Friedrich Nietzsche.[22] Kaufmann's sweeping interpretation, which did not distinguish between the different senses of this idea in the contexts in which it appeared, turned the idea of communication into the central subject of Jaspers's thinking, and on this basis presented his version of the possible directions in which it could have developed, but not an inherent interpretation of the concept of communication as it appeared in Jaspers's philosophical writings. This criticism of Kaufmann's interpretation is similar to Werner Schneiders's criticism of it.[23]

The continued existence of the solipsistic aspects in Jaspers's perception of communication was not expressed only in the central role allocated to loneliness in this framework. The discussion of communication contained more direct arguments linking it to these aspects and more generally to the framework of the explication of selfhood. Jaspers defined communication as "an inner struggle for the possibility to exist solely in my own right."[24] The "struggle" Jaspers mentioned in this context should not be understood as directed against an external entity, but as expressing a struggle with the human tendency not to become an Existenz and to remain on the level of what Jaspers terms "mere existence." The word *bloß* in German has two meanings: mere and bare. In this context, I believe both are relevant. See Jaspers's use of the term *bloß Dasein*,[25] referring to the "fall" of Existenz from a state of realization. At this point there is similarity with Martin Heidegger's approach, seeing *Das Man* as a main mode of Existenz.[26] The argument that communication does not serve as a means of overcoming loneliness does not necessarily indicate the failure of communication. The reliance of Jaspers's concept of communication on a solipsistic basis does not leave room to expect that communication would guarantee the end of loneliness, or even make it a rarer experience. In the absence of real reference to the character of the other Existenz, communication appears as a speculative possibility whose meaning does not depend on realization. Communication constitutes one more of the possibilities through which Existenz can realize itself and deepen its individual identity, and beyond that we know nothing about it. In any case, the loneliness that Jean Marie Paul rightly defined as the "hermeneutics of selfhood" is revealed as a formative element of Existenz, and also of existential communication.[27]

On the Marxist critique of the dialectic between loneliness and communication in Jaspers's philosophy, see Günter Junghänel's criticism that "the pseudodialectic between loneliness and communication [reflects] an attempt to cover the objective social contradictions, and especially the class struggle." He says that the loneliness Jaspers described does not constitute a party in the dialectic existing in human communication, but is a by-product of the socio-material situation in the capitalist world, which only the social order offered by Marxism could solve.[28] This criticism ignores one of the most basic premises of existentialist philosophy in general, perhaps the most fundamental of all, that the different levels of existence do not characterize different social groups, but are different modes of existence of the same person who alternates between authentic and inauthentic modes of existence. Compare also Schneiders's criticism of Junghänel.[29] For further discussion, see Georg Lukàcs's interpretation, seeing Jaspers's philosophy as a reflection of the bourgeois elitist ideal lacking any social consciousness.[30] Jaspers responded to the Marxist criticism directed at his thought in his article "Reply to my critics."[31] Saner discussed the role of Marxism in the socio-cultural context during Jaspers's early period, and on the image Jaspers had of Lukàcs.[32] Manfred Gangl discussed Jaspers's character as a social critic.[33]

While clarifying the link between the perception of communication and the main motifs of the perception of selfhood, we may ask the question: why had communication not been included from the start in the framework of the explication of selfhood, appearing only as a transition mechanism? The answer to this stems from the basic ambivalence typifying the perception of selfhood that was behind the concept of communication in Jaspers's thought. As he put it:

> Regarding the question: why is there communication? Why do I not exist alone? To this an answer is possible that can be understood to the same small degree as [there is an answer] regarding the question about selfhood.

In his opinion, at this point we encounter "… the paradox of the becoming *origin* of selfhood, which was actually *from itself but still does not exist from itself and with itself alone*."[34]

These questions, which appear rhetorical when they occur in the context of a discussion of communication, demonstrate Jaspers's real difficulty in breaking through the wall of solipsism he had himself constructed around selfhood in the early stages of his work, but at the same time also his awareness of this aspect in his concept of selfhood. The hints of disappointment, or even despair, Jaspers expressed in this context stemmed from the conflict between the discovery that Existenz requires communication to constitute its selfhood and the original intuition, whose influence in Jaspers's thought was still present, that selfhood had the ability to "stand independently" in the world.[35] The awareness that communication is essential not only relieved the feeling of loneliness, but also made it more difficult to experience, especially since being aware of it became part of Existenz's self-perception. The paradox to which Jaspers was now exposed in his discussion of communication was not a solution, since individuality was one of the expressions of the maturation of Existenz's self-consciousness, but this maturity was expressed no less by the urge to communication. In this context, Di Cesare suggested that Jaspers did not achieve a balance between loneliness and communication.[36]

The new self-understanding being formed in Existenz's consciousness in view of the possibility of communication with another Existenz, that it could not exist only in itself and through itself, but required the human Being outside it, was expressed in the following words appearing under the title "the dissatisfaction in myself alone":

> If I perceive myself in the face of the refusal to communicate and experience consciousness where I rely on myself alone then the dissatisfaction… is worsened… I cannot find the real because what is real is not *only* what exists as real for me; I cannot love myself if I do not thereby love the other. I must become dreary if I am only I am.
> However, there is in me a real and original drive *to stand by myself alone*; I would still like to be able to live as retiring to myself…[37]

The refusal to communicate is no longer presented as an expression of the dominance or power of individuality, but as a lack or fault in selfhood that damages the freedom that is one of the typical features of Existenz, and eventually leads to its identification as a closed objective Being.[38] In the absence of communication, Existenz is removed to outside the boundaries of Being and finds itself as "homeless" in existence.[39] In this respect, communication is not perceived as a means of escaping from selfhood or as evidence of the flimsiness of selfhood. The maturation of Existenz's self-consciousness is now presented as "pressing within the external *willingness* toward communication."[40] Jaspers, who at no stage of his philosophy renounced his primordial insights, found it difficult in this context also to push aside his original urges to grant philosophical representation to selfhood as an independent and self-sufficient Being, or as he wrote, "I would still like to be able to live as retiring to myself."[41] However, this urge was overcome by the awareness that such an approach would diminish the ability to achieve a complete understanding of selfhood that was at the center of his philosophical commitment.

The connection between communication and Existenz's grasp of existence is not expressed only in the negative, but also in the positive. Just as in the absence of communication Existenz is removed from existence, so also the presence of communication strengthens its hold in existence. Jaspers's argument that communication helps Existenzes that form it to participate actively in ideas, tasks, and goals that arise from real existence in the world[42] strengthens the observation that the ability to form a relation toward another Existenz is one of the most crucial expressions of Existenz's hold on existence. Existenz's grasp of the immanent expressions of the world and its ability to form a relation toward other Existenzes embody the two main implications of Jaspers's distancing himself from solipsism. While the other Existenz is not necessarily part of the immediate reality of the Existenz examining the possibility of forming a relation of communication with it, its ability to recognize its existence and to confront the possibility of communication becomes an inseparable part of its self-consciousness as a worldly Being.

In a way we can argue that there is a basic similarity between the role allotted to the other Existenz in communication and the role objects occupy for formal knowledge. Just as a person's mind requires objects as a basis for forming its consciousness, so Existenz requires the existence of the other Existenz in order to form and develop its self-consciousness.[43] We would do well to compare the role of the "other Existenz" in communication for the Existenz forming its selfhood with the dialectic of the master and the slave in Georg Wilhelm Friedrich Hegel's philosophy. To the best of my knowledge, such a comparison has yet to be made, although the connection between Jaspers's thought and Hegel's philosophy in other contexts has been examined by Alan M. Olson.[44] The very discussion of communication takes place from the point of view of the Existenz being explicated in Jaspers's thought and not from the viewpoint of the other Existenz, which is not presented as a real entity with its own existence beyond the role it may play for the Existenz under discussion. Not only can communication take place only between Existenzes,[45] but the very meeting between the two is defined as responding to the same possibility of selfhood identified in the other.[46] Preserving the link to the viewpoint of the Existenz is achieved by reducing the difference between the two Existenzes, intended mainly to moderate the otherness of the other Existenz.

At this point, the instrumental nature of the relation Existenz forms toward the other Existenz is revealed. Existenz does not require the fullness of the Being of the other Existenz, or even its concrete existence, which was not even mentioned in the discussion, dealing mainly with the situation from which the Existenz that is forming its selfhood is pushed to communication. The presence of this aspect in Jaspers's thought probably served as a basis for a variety of interpretations that understood in some ways the philosophy of Existenz as a rephrasing of the traditional approach of *sui causa* regarding human beings. From this point of view, Jaspers's philosophy was understood as an expression of the extreme subjectivism of excessive and dangerous autonomy of the individual, and even of anti-social elitism.[47] The implications of these interpretations for the understanding of the perception of communication are clear; this interpretation negates the possibility of understanding Jaspers's concept of communication as an option that Existenz can realize in practice in its existence.

Like these interpretations, the interpretation offered here does not see Jaspers's perception of communication as expressing a real possibility. Here we also reject the possibility of seeing the concept of communication as part of a dialogical approach, as other interpreters of Jaspers's thought believed. The scholars who saw Jaspers's perception of communication as a dialog viewed it as evidence of a real experience of Existenz, instead of as an expression of Jaspers's dealing with a speculative option. Hans Urs Von Balthasar lists Jaspers along with Martin Buber as two dialogical thinkers of the period.[48] Heinz Horst Schrey included Jaspers's thought in what he termed "the philosophy of dialog."[49] Similarly, Elisabeth Young-Bruehl includes Jaspers in a list of philosophers, such as Buber, Gabriel Marcel, Franz Rosenzweig, and Albert Camus, who dealt with "the issue of communication or dialog"—two concepts she probably considered identical (she argues that Jaspers was unique in this context in linking communication with truth).[50] Michael Theunissen offers a more moderate interpretation of Jaspers's perception of communication, and shows similarities between Buber and Jaspers that indicate, in his opinion, Jaspers's proximity to dialogical thinking, but do not yet enable his philosophy to be included in it.[51] Harry Wardlaw claims that Jaspers's understanding of truth as communication draws heavily on Immanuel Kant.[52]

I still have difficulty accepting the interpretation that sees subjectivism as the be all and end all of Jaspers's philosophy, since it lacks a real explanation for the very presence of the idea of communication in his philosophy of Existenz. It conspicuously ignores the open discussion of the implications created by the possibility of communication in Jaspers's perception of Existenz, and misses even the viewpoint focused on Existenz in which these approaches were anchored. Jaspers described the implications of this possibility in the following words:

> In communication I become open to myself with the other.
> However, this opening is also for the first time the becoming real of the I as self. If I think that opening is the clarification of an innate character, then I abandon with this thought the possibility of Existenz, which is still creating itself in the process of opening where it becomes clarified.[53]

The "opening," or the ability to self-transcend that is typical of Existenz, which enabled it to become acquainted with the possible existence of another Existenz, revealed to it new horizons so far hidden from it. Even before it was exposed to what was beyond it—Being and transcendence—it reached better self-understanding. Now it transpires that the very possibility that Existenz could form a relation toward what was beyond it reveals the real nature of the infinity that, already early in his writings, Jaspers had attributed to the individual's subjective Being. The infinity does not depend on the absence of boundaries imposed upon it, but on the possibilities of its self-understanding in light of what is beyond it, and naturally restricts it. In this respect, we can argue that the very possibility of forming a relation to a transcendent entity testifies first and foremost to the nature of the Being called Existenz. The perception of communication as the "openness" and "opening"[54] of individuals toward the other in order to form their selfhood is rooted in German culture. It refers primarily to two central concepts in Hegel's philosophy: *Entävßerung*, which means rejecting or renouncing the other, and *Vergegenständlichung*, which means making the object to which the person refers more vivid and concrete. These two concepts denote individuals' ability to use what is around them, in the widest sense, to form themselves as spiritual and creative entities.[55]

We can summarize this stage of our discussion of Jaspers's concept of communication by arguing that we can find in it the traces of the solipsistic infrastructure that has generally accompanied the framework of the explication of selfhood. In this context, this infrastructure is expressed in the centrality attributed to loneliness in "communication." However, the introduction of the other Existenz into the realm of possibilities through which Existenz can realize itself deepened the cracks in the solipsistic perception of selfhood beyond the influence of the discussion of the world's reality and of objective knowledge. This change made Jaspers's perception of Existenz more flexible and opened to it new horizons including the possibility of forming a relation toward transcendence—an option that had not appeared in this thinking while the explication of selfhood had been the main axis guiding it. The possibility of forming a relation toward transcendence, which appeared thanks to the changes in the perception of Existenz, served as a basis for Jaspers's perception of communication being located outside the realm of the explication of selfhood, as part of the transition mechanisms.

The opening of Existenz toward what was beyond it, achieved in the context of what was called earlier the "first trend" in the perception of communication, was not realized in the form of relations with the other Existenz, but only in forming a relation toward transcendence, to be discussed in the framework of what we have termed the "second trend." The first trend formed the foundation for what would be realized only in the second trend, to be discussed below. Only when communication serves as a transition mechanism can we determine whether, or more precisely, to what extent, Jaspers's perception of selfhood was liberated from its early link to solipsism.

4. Communication as a Transition Mechanism

The entry of the other Existenz into the arena of philosophizing revealed the basic polarity of the Being of Existenz. On the one hand, it tends toward "excited devotion"[56] to itself, while on the other hand it continues to want to "hold itself from loyalty to loneliness," and to find ways to "help itself."[57] Steffen Graefe discussed the connection between the element of "excitement" in the existentialist view of communication, the "excited approach" appearing in *Psychology*,[58] and *eros* in Plato's philosophy.[59] As long as communication is perceived merely as a framework of relations between Existenzes, we cannot decide between these two poles, since to the extent that "*love, the substantial source of selfhood in the communication*, can grow from itself the selfhood as a motion of its opening, it cannot enable the arrival at a perfect conclusion."[60] The processes occurring in the self-consciousness of Existenz when it faces the possibility of communication cannot be exhausted within the explication of selfhood, precisely because they direct Existenz toward what is beyond it, to transcendence. Just as in the other transition mechanisms, in the discussion of communication Jaspers used transcendence before explicating it. However, its role in the context of communication is quite clear. As he puts it:

> You and I, who are separate in existence, are one in transcendence. There we do not meet and do not even miss each other, but here in the becoming of a struggling communication that is revealed and confirmed in danger. Where this unity exists, there is a leap from what is already incomprehensible to what cannot be thought absolutely.[61]

The transition, or more precisely the "leap," from existence to transcendence skipped the possibility of a meeting between the two Existenzes, which was not realized at all. More accurately, this possibility could not have been realized in principle, and we cannot even say it was missed. However, although the deep individuality that typifies them prevented a real meeting between the two Existenzes, Jaspers believed that they could share the aim to form a relation to transcendence as a Being existing beyond them. Jaspers did not clarify what the phrase "we are one in transcendence" meant, so his words lack an answer to the question whether referring to transcendence could serve as a basis for real communication between them, or whether it was merely a shared characteristic of Existenzes as such. One possible answer to this question is the argument that the unity of the Existenzes in transcendence is transcendental to both of them, and to the framework of their existence in the world, and it could even be existence out of communication. However, such a unity does not leave real traces.

Jaspers himself noted the complexity of his arguments, which directed the discussion in two directions at once, and even understood the potential for a contradiction forming from them. On the one hand, he wished to follow the changes occurring in the self-consciousness of Existenz in light of the possibility of communication with the other Existenz. On the other hand, he wished to establish out of these changes an approach toward what was beyond the Existenz and the other Existenz, toward transcendence. From the viewpoint of the Existenz being explicated we cannot separate these two channels, since the same opening to the other is itself the realization of itself as an Existenz. In his words, "This process of realization as opening does not take place in the isolated Existenz but only with the other. As an individual I do not exist for myself, not as a revelation and not as an actual."[62] However, from the objective viewpoint of consciousness we cannot attribute processes of opening and change to a particular Being even before it was an actual Being. As he says:

> For objective thought, certainly only what existed *before* can be revealed. However, the becoming open that brings the Being simultaneously with this becoming is like originating from the nothingness, thus it does not [remain] only in the sense of mere existence.[63]

Jaspers clarified that although the "opening [becoming open] and the reality are in a relationship that appears to be forming in the contrast between its existing from nothingness and its being self-bearing,"[64] the contradiction that is forming is only an apparent contradiction,[65] a contradiction resulting mainly from the continued presence of traces from the early perception of selfhood, according to which selfhood is a "self-bearing" Being. This is because transcendence is perceived as "resulting from the nothingness" only from the viewpoint of Existenz, or more precisely as long as the dominance of this viewpoint is preserved in the discussion and the possible existence of an otherness separate from Existenz itself is pushed aside. However, as the self-consciousness of Existenz matures and opens new horizons to what is beyond it, it transpires that the very acquaintance of Existenz with the existence of transcendence is based on the changes that occurred in Existenz's self-consciousness. Perhaps there is still room to define the transition from the explication of selfhood to the clarification of the relation Existenz forms toward transcendence as a "leap," even if only not to grant this transition a deterministic meaning where the "openness" of Existenz necessarily leads to the formation of a relation toward transcendence. In any case, the perspective of Jaspers's whole philosophy confirms this process, since eventually Jaspers moved away from dealing with Existenz and focused on explicating Being and transcendence.

The openness to the reality of another Existenz transpires as an essential preparation for the perception of communication as a transition mechanism. It deepened the cracks in the solipsistic perception of selfhood and opened new possibilities for Existenz that were an "unknown" for it at this stage of the explication. The vagueness and lack of clarity typical of Jaspers's arguments about transcendence in his discussion of communication demonstrate the condition of Existenz, at this point facing two new options for it: forming a relation toward another Existenz and forming a relation toward transcendence. In the process, it forms a self-consciousness that no longer allows it to maintain its self-perception as a "self-bearing Being," but Jaspers's thought still lacked the tools to bridge the gap between its early self-perception and the possibilities revealed by the discussion of communication.

As in other places, here, too, Jaspers apparently spoke in two voices and left his words undecided. Sometimes he appeared to strive to bring both Existenzes closer to transcendence, and at other times he appeared to see their existence side by side as helping each of them to eventually arrive at transcendence while preserving their individuality and sovereignty. Sometimes he appeared to wish to create a relation of continuity from the level of existence to transcendence, while at other times he appeared to distinguish between the different stages of presenting a Hegelian-natured process where each stage was an escalation compared to its predecessor, but at the same time also its negation. Either way, the shared presence of both "trends" revealed in the discussion of communication illuminates the general direction in which Jaspers's philosophy was moving. This thought was at this stage in a process where the status of Existenz as the sole object of philosophizing was being undermined, against the background and limitations uncovered in the explication of selfhood. True, in this framework, too, Existenz continued in its explicit condition to serve as an essential infrastructure for Jaspers's arguments. However, his main attention was no longer devoted solely to the explication of Existenz, but started to be directed to expanding the sphere of reference of Existenz that served as a basis for forming new axes of philosophy not dependent on the self-clarification needs of Existenz. To be more precise, the metaphysical consciousness, which was the fruit of deep modification processes occurring in Jaspers's thought, is not the consciousness of Existenz, but this consciousness itself was already based on something existing beyond it.

The interpretation of Jaspers's concept of communication offered here, according to which it is part of the formation process of metaphysical consciousness—or more precisely a stage where this consciousness became a conscious goal of Existenz—stands in contrast with most existing interpretations in the secondary literature. They understood Jaspers's idea of communication as an explication of a real experience of Existenz, or interpreted the possible reality of this experience as equivalent to the possibility of forming the Existenz itself, also often defined by Jaspers as "possible Existenz." The understanding that Jaspers's perception of communication reflected a real possibility for the Existenz has appeared, for instance, in interpretations that tried to derive humanistic norms and ethical values from it. Salamun, for example, summarizes four norms that arise from Jaspers's perception of communication: the daring for mediating-creating loneliness and self-standing self-consciousness; the requirement to open to the other; the cry for unqualified and non-egoistical willingness toward the other; and finally the willingness to recognize in principle the other as a possibility for self-actualization.[66] The fundamental difficulty in accepting the ethical interpretation of Jaspers's perception of communication stems from this interpretation almost completely ignoring the fact that the Existenz as another to which communication is directed does not appear at any stage as a real personality with its own world. The criticism is not that we cannot derive from Jaspers's approach any ethical meanings or discuss the implications of his thought in this direction, but instead concerns the understanding of ethics as the central and comprehensive motive in which his approach is grounded. A total interpretation like this not only does not present a reasonable explanation for the changes and developments that occurred in his philosophy, but it also ignores the metaphysical aspect that entered the ethical aspects themselves. Without referring to this metaphysical aspect, the ethical aspects are also only partially explicated. If Jaspers's approach contains an ethical meaning, I believe that it is anchored in the metaphysics that is progressively revealed as a basic infrastructure of his thought in its different periods. Even if we ignore the question of the reality of the other Existenz, we cannot ignore that in his discussion of the possibility of communication Jaspers presented an instrumental attitude toward the other Existenz. It was largely a secondary factor in the change processes experienced by the self-consciousness of the Existenz that continued to be dominant in the discussion. Schneiders, too, noted the problems in principle posed by the ethical interpretations of Jaspers's philosophy of Existenz. In his opinion, Jaspers's negative position in the argument about the very possibility of recognizing moral norms with the usual instruments of our reason could lead to the "crumbling of moral philosophy." Jaspers's position, in Schneiders's opinion, should not be viewed as the abolishing (*Aufhebung*) of moral philosophy, since this position limits in principle the possibilities of forming it in reality. Schneiders argues that it is no accident that Jaspers's claim regarding the impossibility of deriving "worthy actions" was a fruitful basis for studies in the field of legal philosophy dealing with the special meaning of objectivity and normativity of actions.[67] He mentions three works written in this vein.[68] These works are valuable not only in the field of law, but also in moral philosophy, which is currently considered as part of it.[69]

The role of the other Existenz was mainly symbolic. The other Existenz represented for the Existenz undergoing explication a different form of humanity, but the main meaning of this humanity depends on the possibility that it could help the Existenz become acquainted with hidden facets of its Being. In any case, the question remains unanswered how we can conclude from the perception of relations between people, which is *apriori* presented as a speculative possibility, any norms and values requiring realization in the framework of the concrete reality of human action. Even if the requirement for the realization of the norms that the ethical interpretation deduced from Jaspers's general arguments, we could still not view his perception of communication as anything other than a vague phrasing of *mental positions* that Existenz develops in the face of the speculative possibility of meeting another. We can be almost certain that Jaspers would not have supported this restricted outcome, if only because of the psychologistic image arising from it—an image that he consciously and actively wished to cast off even before publishing *Philosophy*. Jaspers stated in retrospect that *Psychology* was not a psychological book in essence, and that it became his unconscious path to philosophy.[70] The conditions for communication that Jaspers listed related only to the Existenz under explication and not to the other Existenz to which the communication relation was supposed to be directed.[71] To use Heidegger's terminology, communication is an aspect enabling Existenz to reach a more advanced development of its selfhood, which deepens in view of the idea of transcendence, functions as an *Existenzial*, and should not be seen as representing the layer of the *Existenzielle* that portrayed for Heidegger the layer of realization.[72] Finally, the other Existenz remains in Jaspers's perception of communication a speculative element whose realization is at least not a consideration in the philosophizing, and perhaps does not exist at all.

As in the ethical interpretation, the interpretative direction characterized by an anthropological-philosophical orientation also contains an understanding of the perception of communication as an expression of a real option for Existenz. William Earle, who in general understood the existential elucidation as a rational framework, saw the perception of communication as an essential means for achieving a rational estimate regarding the reality in which we live. While rationality does not cancel the essential and unbridgeable polarity accompanying the Being of Existenz in its experience of communication, as a result of which it is condemned to live in a paradox, in his opinion reason and objective consciousness are able to help resolve it.[73] Urs Richli did not go as far as Earle in arguing that Existenz could be understood using the instruments of rational thought. However, from the same anthropological orientation, Richli, too, tried to deduce from the perception of communication, and in general from Jaspers's perception of Existenz, principles regarding the "correct humanity" that he believed was embedded in Jaspers's thought.[74] In a way, we could state that the anthropological position, satisfied with drawing general principles regarding people from the perception of Existenz, including Jaspers's perception of communication, without aiming to phrase from these principles any ethical requirements, does not harm the principle of freedom that was a founding element of the Being of Existenz. However, like the ethical interpretation, this interpretation, too, was characterized by understanding communication as a descriptive condition applying to the ontological reality in which Existenz is contained. The criticism presented to the ethical interpretation can equally be applied to the anthropological interpretation. Taking into account the understanding of the ethical and anthropological interpretations of the idea of communication as an expression of a real experience of Existenz, it is no wonder that they did not grant real importance to the role of transcendence in Jaspers's perception of communication, and were unable to explain the metaphysical depth of Jaspers's perception of communication and his philosophy as a whole.

The interpretative approach based on understanding communication as a concrete and realizable idea did not solve real problems arising from Jaspers's alternating between the other Existenz and transcendence, each of which represents a different Being of the "other." This interpretation was also unable to offer an explanation for the nature of the connection between Existenz and transcendence arising from the perception of communication. In contrast, exposing the two directions of philosophizing within the idea of communication, defined above as the "first trend" and the "second trend," has enabled us to follow Jaspers's attempts to escape from the perception of Existenz as a solipsistic Being and to reveal the transitional function entailed in his perception of communication.

The continuation of the tendency to achieve the explication of selfhood within the discussion of communication and the absence of a real explication of transcendence testify to the greater proximity of communication to the explication of selfhood than to the explication of Being. However, as transcendence and Being become central issues of philosophizing, there will hardly remain any trace of the idea of communication as a possibility of meeting between two Existenzes. This will clarify not only the functional status of the other Existenz, also harnessed to the self-explication of Existenz, but also the functional nature of the entire perception of communication that serves mainly as a means for the replacing of the axis of philosophizing—from the one aimed at selfhood to the one that was to be directed at Being.

Six

HISTORICITY

1. From World Orientation and Communication to Historicity

The perception of Existenz as a worldly Being, which started to form in *World Orientation*,[1] reflected Karl Jaspers's aim to provide his discussion of selfhood with a philosophical nature. The introduction of the concepts of "world" and "consciousness" into his discussion undoubtedly created a real change in his perception of selfhood. It no longer appeared as a Being detached from any context and link with the reality external to it, but became a worldly Being. While selfhood was still the main object of the philosophical explication, the discussion of the implications of this change was restricted to the relevance of the world's reality to the self-perception of Existenz. In a way, only in the perception of communication can we find a more direct handling of the implications of the perception of selfhood as a worldly Being. When Jaspers was discussing communication, he was not conducting an independent discussion about the world as a real context in which the meeting between Existenzes takes place. In the discussion of the concept of historicity (*Geschichtlichkeit*), on which this chapter focuses, Jaspers was able for the first time to consider the concept of the world as a Being that had independent existence that could be examined beyond the implications it had for the self-consciousness of Existenz. In this context, too, he added insights to the framework of the explication of selfhood, and therefore presented it here as one of the transition mechanisms. However, since historicity expresses a deeper otherness than that of the other Existenz discussed in communication, the clarification of this concept created a further distancing from the solipsistic perception of selfhood and made real progress toward the explication of Being. Unlike the concepts of communication and of boundary situations (to be discussed in Chapter Seven below), the concept of historicity has rarely been studied by scholars.

2. Between Historicity and History

The idea of historicity is based on the classic Hegelian distinction between the two meanings of the German word for history (*Geschichte*): history and story.[2] The first denotes the objective meaning relating to historical events, on whose basis the science of history was created. The second denotes the subjective meaning of this area, stressing the decisive role of the human factor in forming the past consciousness of people as a basis for their self-understanding in the present.

Against the background of this distinction, of which Jaspers was aware, he attempted to differentiate between historical consciousness and consciousness of historicity. People's role regarding *historical consciousness* is limited to their ability to observe past events and learn about different historical periods from them. These events do not necessarily have any relation to their personal lives. In any case, in the mental activity involved in historical consciousness, the person's presence is not the individual's presence, with all the subjective factors characterizing that selfhood, but the presence of someone gifted with an abstract reasoning ability, or what Jaspers called "consciousness in general." Not only is the individual's private personality not perceived as a factor influencing the process of understanding through "consciousness in general," but there is a deliberate effort to distance it based on the assumption that it could bias and even damage the understanding. In contrast, in *consciousness of historicity*, which is part of the consciousness of Existenz, it perceives itself as an entity forming in time. This means that Existenz perceives its existence in the present as a continuation of previous forms of existence, and as part of a reality that will continue even after it ceases to exist. At the center of the consciousness of historicity is an awareness of the temporal aspect of existence in its many expressions, an awareness that turns the existence of Existenz into one point on the time axis, and that requires a wider understanding of existence of which Existenz is only one part.[3] The consciousness of historicity naturally acts to reduce the importance attributed to the existence belonging to Existenz and to undermine the solipsistic self-understanding.

Jaspers's concept of historicity contains two main components: first it denotes the physical aspect of time as a continuity on which the objective examination of time in science relies. The general meaning of this is that every present point of time was preceded by another point, and will be succeeded by another point. This facet is relevant to the discussion of Existenz as a real Being in concrete time. The term "historicity" also represents the experience of reality through consciousness, in the process of constructing the individual's personal identity, which lasts throughout a person's life. This aspect relates to Existenz as a Being aiming at achieving awareness of the facts of its existence and its patterns of dealing with them. The consciousness of historicity, attributed first and foremost to Existenz, but present in all human beings conscious of their experiences, reflects the constant involvement of Existenz with its origins; its life story; the question of the relation between the life story and its current situation; and the way it perceives it. The combination of these two meanings of "historicity" enables us to understand the idea of historicity as expressing a process whereby people understand themselves as part of a surrounding human Being characterized by the continuity of concrete existence in time. This understanding is based on reflection aimed at clarifying the data and circumstances of the past on the objective level, but at the same time granting them subjective meaning relating to the concrete personality. The consciousness of historicity serves as a framework for a broad, independent clarification of existence, but also for Exisentz's dealing with the meaning this clarification has for its self-perception. The connection between the objective and the subjective aspects, or between the datum discovered and the reflection performed upon it to derive meaning from it is expressed in the following words from Jaspers:

> Here [in the consciousness of historicity] are originally connected in an inseparable way Being and knowledge... Without knowledge, meaning a clear perception and being inside it, there is no historistic Being, and without a reality of historicity there is no knowledge.[4]

The two components of the consciousness of historicity, "knowledge," and "Being," or the objective and subjective aspects of time, illuminate from a new angle the epistemological and the ontological viewpoints, which have been revealed as establishing elements in Jaspers's philosophy. The epistemological viewpoint, focusing on the question what can be known about selfhood, directs Existenz in this context to examine its past and to ground its self-perception in a wider view of the data of existence, understanding that only some of them can have some expression during its lifetime. In contrast, the ontological viewpoint, aiming at expressing the entity of selfhood as a Being present in the world, is reflected in the discussion of historicity in Existenz's effort to understand itself as part of the wider entity of existence. To be more precise, the anchoring of the ontological viewpoint in a wider awareness of the temporal aspect of existence is not exhausted by the perception of Existenz as a worldly Being that transpired from the discussion in *World Orientation*. There Existenz was still discussed as a Being that forms its existence and examines it according to the possibilities it entails, while the concept of historicity portrays a more mature self-perception of Existenz, seeing itself as part of a wider Being whose boundaries extend far beyond its individual existence.

In a way, only in the discussion of historicity, at least to a greater extent than in the discussion of communication, does the inability of the two viewpoints, the epistemological and the ontological, to fully describe the perception of selfhood start to become apparent. The epistemological viewpoint is required to expand its horizon and examine the whole of existence, the relevance of historical knowledge to the discussion of historicity. In contrast, the anchoring of Existenz in an existence whose boundaries extend beyond the concrete existence of Existenz requires the ontological viewpoint not only to examine the entity of Existenz, but also to present a broader entity. Up to this stage of the interpretation of Jaspers's thought it was possible to discuss the contribution of each of these viewpoints to the analysis of the subject, but we now require a new understanding that identifies the point where they meet. The knowledge achieved through the ontological viewpoint will no longer be perceived as external to the reality of the ontological Being of Existenz, but as inseparable from its reality, which cannot be exhausted merely by observing the concrete existence to which it is directly linked. The continuing undermining of the solipsistic intuition did not allow Jaspers to continue to see Existenz as a Being whose existence and self-consciousness could rely only on themselves. As we will see below, widening the frame of reference of the two viewpoints to the existence whose boundaries extend beyond those of Existenz softens the distinction between historical consciousness and consciousness of historicity and helps expose the connection between knowledge about Being and Being itself.

3. Consciousness of Historicity as a Means of Elucidating Existenz

A. Existenz and Historical Knowledge

Jaspers's handling of the possible contribution of historical knowledge to the clarification of Existenz raises anew questions that have already been discussed in previous contexts. In his early writings, Jaspers sought to determine the relation between the physiological aspects of mental illnesses studied by the science of psychopathology and the character of the individual mental patient; in *Psychology*[5] he discussed the question of the possible contribution of general psychology to understanding the mental life of a person as a subject; while in *World Orientation* he discussed the relationship between science and philosophy. Jaspers's argument all along was that even if psychopathology, general psychology, and science could contribute to understanding a person, the uniqueness of selfhood is not revealed except through the viewpoints that also contain awareness of the particular dimensions existing in the individual's Being. This awareness is apparent in the meanings he gave to the founding terms of the explication of selfhood: "mental," "world view," and "elucidation of Existenz." Jaspers not only tried to form a point of view through which the individual's subjective Being could be elucidated; he also devoted considerable effort to distinguishing between it and other viewpoints, which appeared to him to miss the point. Presumably, this principle would also apply to the distinction between historical consciousness and consciousness of historicity. Only consciousness of historicity would be relevant to the elucidation of Existenz. This premise was the basis for Elisabeth Young-Breuhl's interpretation, defining historicity as a concept of the Existenz that as such is outside the object-subject dichotomy, and reflects an inexpressible certainty of Existenz and of the reason that clarifies it. Along with historicity, she also listed the concept of freedom and the concept of communication as concepts of the Existenz. She also argues that there exists a link between Jaspers's idea of historicity and Immanuel Kant's perception of time.[6] However, the innovation entailed in the concept of historicity, and more generally in the ideas defined as transition mechanisms, is the change in the pattern that had accompanied Jaspers's thought up to this point. Unlike his previous discussions, in this context Jaspers aimed to make the gap between Existenz and what is beyond it more flexible. In his attempt to harness as many viewpoints as possible to the philosophical discussion, he was able to note the partial, limited nature of a viewpoint as such, and at the same time to move away from the idea that one exclusive point of view could reveal the fullness of the object of philosophizing to which his thought was directed. In the concept of historicity, this change became apparent in the effort to harness the mental skills involved in forming a historical consciousness, which were mainly aimed at establishing the scientific nature of history as a realm of knowledge serving the consciousness of historicity, and in turning it into an integral part of the self-perception of Existenz. As he puts it:

> From this historistic (*gechichtlichen*) source the *historical* also becomes for the first time really historistic. Without it, it would only mean a particular event attributed to the existence of the present evaluated positively or negatively. However, my theoretical knowledge from history becomes through the whole science of history a function of the possible Existenz, if its contents and images aim themselves at me, face me, demand from me, or push me away from them, not only as distant patterns existing as closed within themselves, or in other words: if it is *assimilated* to the function of the eternal present of the things that exist within the philosophical-historistic consciousness.[7]

It transpires that the idea of historicity entails the understanding that the historical knowledge itself does not reflect a mere generality, but also contains an existential element, and meeting with it may help the explication of Existenz. Existenz's observation of historical knowledge is not characterized by an unmediated, unbiased view, usually considered as a precondition for knowing things, but instead it perceives it a-priori as facing it, and it sees it as a fertile source for elucidating its selfhood. The viewpoint of Existenz regarding historical knowledge creates a transformation in it that expropriates its general, impersonal aspect, restructures it, and turns it into a tool through which it organizes its story of becoming.

On the face of it, these claims of Jaspers's contain no real innovation. As in previous contexts, here, too, he tried to harness the issues that arose in his discussion, in this case, historical knowledge, to the purposes of the self-elucidation of Existenz. As in his criticism of the science of psychopathology or of general psychology as formal frameworks of knowledge that could not enable access to the fullness and uniqueness of human Being, here, too, was implicit the assumption that general and formal historical knowledge could not serve as a source for the self-understanding of Existenz. We could even say that historicity granted historical knowledge the same role that the other Existenz had in communication—another means for establishing the selfhood of the Existenz being explicated. Just like in communication, so in historicity the specific features of the "other" were denied and assimilated into the press of the self-elucidation of Existenz, which apparently did not lose its dominance in the philosophizing.

Jaspers discussed the consciousness of historicity after presenting his perception of communication, and this could be crucial in revealing the motivation for this consciousness. Jaspers described in this context the mutual fertilization between Existenz and historical knowledge. On the one hand, the viewpoint of Existenz regarding historical knowledge shows new, unfamiliar facets of it, enriches it, and reveals its dynamic aspects; rescues the historical knowledge from the generality that typifies it as a framework of formal thought and encourages the creative forces it contains, which without Existenz would have remained silent and dormant. In this respect, we should not understand the argument that Existenz removes from historical knowledge its general element as an expression of its distorting influences, but of its ability to produce from it what is sometimes missing in the historian's view. Jaspers noted that through Existenz, "[historical knowledge] proves its power in the ability of its results, to be replaced by real historistic consciousness of the self existing in the present."[8] On the other hand, historical knowledge serves Existenz as a source for meaning and a broader self-understanding in existence; thanks to it Existenz does not perceive itself as an autonomic Being existing outside any context, but as a Being existing in a place and time and as part of a Being that existed before it and will continue to exist after it.

Clarifying the mutual relationship between historical knowledge and the existence of which Existenz is part served as a basis for Jaspers's claim that people's handling ofthe element of historicity in their Being requires them to become acquainted with other forms of objectivization through knowledge.[9] The meeting with these forms opens for Existenz a window on complete entities of realities beyond itself, through which it learns that its concrete existence takes place alongside other forms of existence, not necessarily existential ones, and is subject to the same conditions as the rest of them. This understanding does not make the general, objective viewpoint the main instrument for elucidating Existenz's experience of historicity. However, since historical knowledge becomes for it a criterion by which it examines everything around it, it is encouraged to identify the existence of general aspects applying to it as a Being existing in time, aspects that can also find expression in other Existenzes, but also in other entities that are not Existenzes at all. Contrary to the tendency to emphasize the otherness of Existenz compared with other objects in the world, in the process of becoming acquainted with its historicity, it learns that general, objective knowledge also relates to crucial aspects of its existence, which undermines the thought that Existenz is opposed to any form of generality and objectivity.

It is hard to ignore Jaspers's vacillation between the effort to grant expression to the particular element in the story of self-formation and the urge to make a general claim regarding the temporal nature of human existence as such. True, the historicity of a person does not express any more than the story of the birth and establishment of this person's selfhood as an Existenz—a Being that is not considered by Jaspers as identical to the sum of phenomena accompanying its existence in time. However, the dialog Existenz conducts with the possibility that this story could itself become knowledge, with all the implications of this, serves as a basis for the understanding of historicity as a "framework story"—the "story" being the sum of all the private experiences, and the "framework" also containing general aspects whose relevance exceeds the boundaries of the individual story of the concrete Existenz.

Against the background of this interpretation, I argue that the mutual relationship formed between historical knowledge and Existenz in the framework of historicity constitutes an innovation and development in the shape of Jaspers's philosophizing. In the explication of selfhood, the boundaries of the discussion of the different subjects were fixed according to their degree of relevance to the character of Existenz, and even in the perception of communication the element of mutuality in the relations between Existenzes was hardly discussed. In contrast, in the clarification of the influence of Existenz on historical knowledge, we find a clearer recognition of the reality of an otherness separate from the Existenz. Since the otherness of existence in time, which transcends the concrete existence of Existenz itself, is deeper than that of the other Existenz, which has the same structure as the Existenz being explicated, I argue that in the discussion of historicity, Jaspers's thought moved another step further away from the solipsistic perception of selfhood, beyond that enabled by the perception of communication.

B. Existenz and Existence

The pair of terms in the title above may appear tautological, but this title refers to the examination of the attitude of Existenz (*Existenz*) toward existence (*Dasein*). The argument discussed in consciousness of historicity, according to which Existenz is in concrete existence in time, appears to have no innovation compared with the insights Jaspers has reached so far. Already in *World Orientation*, Jaspers dealt with the meaning of determining the reality of the world for Existenz, and in *Elucidation of Existenz* this discussion was deepened. However, when it became apparent to Jaspers that separating Existenz and the world was impossible, the recognition of the reality of the world still posed a threat to the self-perception of Existenz. This demonstrated Jaspers's difficulty in abandoning the solipsistic image of selfhood that was fundamental to his early thought, leading to his inability to conduct an independent discussion of the world that was not subjugated to the purposes of the self-elucidation of Existenz. In the discussion of historicity, for the first time Existenz was presented as having relations of unity with existence:

> Being as *detached* [absolute] Being, whether transcendence or selfhood, is inaccessible to me. When I want to realize it by *distinguishing* it from existence, I lose it...
> I become certain of my own selfhood, and thus of transcendence, only *in existence*. The given, the situation and the tasks receive their meaning in *their fixity and particularity* to become for *me myself*... The contents of my essence are real only in a phenomenon and not outside it, in imaginary selfhood separated by abstract transcendence. *This unity* of myself with my existence as a phenomenon is my *historicity*, and awareness of it is *historistic consciousness*.[10]

The definition of Existenz as being in *unity* with existence should not be understood as evidence of Jaspers's moving away from understanding Existenz as a particular Being that he worked throughout his writings to establish. The consciousness of historicity as existential consciousness reflects the freedom of Existenz to form a conscious relation toward existence. In any case, its being subject to this existence does not contradict its typical uniqueness and particularity within it. Similarly, the recognition of Existenz being "subject to existence," which is an integral part of the consciousness of historicity,[11] does not express the perception of existence as a necessity forced upon it as expressed in the other contexts already discussed in previous chapters. See especially the discussion in Chapter Four, in the section "Detaching Existenz from the World."

The explicitness typical of Existenz's consciousness at this stage is revealed as having two facets. On the one hand, it is reflected in the self-understanding of Existenz as subject to the factuality of existence that places borders and boundaries around it, while on the other hand it knows that it is not exhausted merely by the boundaries of existence, and "... in this understanding Existenz realizes its essence through its fate."[12] In this respect, being part of existence, and even the access to historical knowledge and the uniqueness of the Being of Existenz, do not appear at this stage of Jaspers's philosophy as excluding each other.

Existenz's recognition of its reality in existence and the connection between this perception of existence and its self-perception establishes and deepens the activity and sovereignty Existenz shows toward itself in the ongoing process of self-explication. Compare with Alan M. Olson's interpretation, according to which transcending to transcendence occurring in historicity is based on the individual's life-practice (*Lebenspraxis*), determining the dialectical nature of freedom and will.[13] These expressions reflect the understanding that the existence to which Existenz is referring is not laid out before it as an absolute and complete element that it could accept or reject as a whole. Quite the opposite, the freedom typifying it as an Existenz encourages it to see those incomplete aspects of existence as an opening that enables it to perceive existence itself as a space where it might realize itself. As in the other contexts discussed in the explication of selfhood, the discussion of historicity also shows that Existenz is able to design existence to suit its character and needs. However, the innovation in the consciousness of historicity compared with the consciousness of Existenz formed up to the transition mechanisms is that at this stage Existenz recognizes that the elucidation of the basic data of existence is a necessary condition for determining the boundaries in principle in which its selfhood can be formed—a recognition that arises as a positivistic consciousness of Existenz regarding its dependence on factors beyond its control. Historicity as a framework where the attitude of Existenz to existence and the boundaries of the freedom it has within it is revealed as inseparable from the basic processes that were typical of the discussions in *World Orientation* and *Elucidation of Existenz.*

The maturation of Existenz's attitude toward existence that arises from the discussion of historicity reflects not only that it is not required to leave its selfhood in order to create the consciousness of historicity. From the point of view of this study, the importance of the idea of historicity is first and foremost in that it expresses Jaspers's deepening awareness of the problems in the solipsistic understanding of selfhood; in this way the perception of Existenz as a worldly Being is filled with real contents. However, the main importance of this idea is that it represents the stage of Existenz's reconciliation with, and acceptance of, itself and the world. Historicity, which assumes Existenz's awareness of its characteristic particularity against the background of the existence in which it finds itself, and also its ability to establish a consciousness of distinctness from it, does not negate the previous stages. The inclusion of the idea of historicity in the transition mechanisms creates integration between different insights discussed separately in previous contexts; on the one hand it enables maintaining Existenz's central position in the philosophizing, and on the other hand it opens the wide horizons of transcendence.

4. Transcendence in Consciousness of Historicity

The consciousness that started forming already in the explication of selfhood, according to which Existenz is not free of limitations and preconditions created outside it, has been fundamental to Jaspers's discussion of the perception of communication and the idea of historicity. In communication this consciousness was reflected in the confrontation with the possible reality of the other, while in historicity it was expressed in the attempt to become acquainted with existence from a viewpoint transcending the boundaries of existential existence. Existenz's awareness of its dependence on factors external to it, and as a result to the problems typical of the solipsistic approach, became more penetrating in the context of consciousness of historicity. While the isolated existence of Existenz was revealed in communication only through the other Existenz, whose perception was largely derived from the way Existenz perceived itself, in consciousness of historicity the dependence of Existenz on what is beyond it is clarified as having wide dimensions transcending the boundaries of its personal existence. As the awareness of the Existenz's dependence deepens, and as it achieves a clearer self-understanding, new horizons are opened to it, which Jaspers's early perception of selfhood had blocked due to its total nature. Recognizing the other Existenz that is close by and the boundaries of existence that extend even beyond it becomes a corner stone in the process of the formation of existential consciousness regarding transcendence.

As in the other transition mechanisms, in the discussion of historicity Jaspers's usage of the term transcendence did not rely on a real explication, which demonstrates that the ideas discussed in this framework were an intermediate stage prefiguring aspects that only later would become the focus of his philosophizing. While the consciousness of the dependence of Existenz on external factors reflects Jaspers's continued effort to leave the solipsistic viewpoint, the absence of any real elucidation of the concept of transcendence indicates that the consciousness of transcendence had yet to mature into a central object to which the philosophizing was aimed. Unlike the perception of communication, the discussion of historicity already shows some progress in clarifying the concept of transcendence. For instance, the description of transcendence as the world's Being of nothingness[14] indicated its location outside the world of phenomena and stated as fact the essential gap between it and existential existence, and existence in general. In any case, transcendence was presented as relevant to Existenz. As he said: "Any betrayal of transcendence exists for me in the pattern of betrayal of the *phenomenon of existence*, whose price is the loss of the Existenz."[15] Although as part of the world of phenomena Existenz is distant from transcendence, its uniqueness as a particular Being is expressed in its typical effort not to be limited to the boundaries of this world and to form a relation toward the transcendence beyond it. The argument that "historicity as existence in time is for me the only way in which the absolute Being is accessible to me"[16] grants the concept of consciousness of historicity its accurate meaning: being a consciousness forming in and directed at existence, it aims to understand people as a phenomenon of existence in general, including the existence that preceded it; consciousness of historicity establishes the perception of Existenz as part of existence. Since the consciousness of existence and of itself exposes Existenz to the horizons beyond it, consciousness of historicity becomes a viewpoint that bridges, first, between Existenz and transcendence as an absolute experience and, second, beyond existential existence and existence in general. Jaspers expressed these two aspects of consciousness of historicity in the following passage:

> Thus in historicity the duality of my consciousness of Being becomes clear to me, which first in the agreed unity is true: I exist only as existence in time, and I myself am not temporal. I know myself only as existence in time, but in a way that this existence becomes for me a phenomenon of my non-temporal selfhood.
> ... I and my phenomenon separate themselves and identify themselves the more I reflect about the ways or immediately exist with myself.[17]

Although the references to transcendence in the discussion of historicity did not exceed the granting of preliminary meaning to this concept, they were sufficient to clarify that historicity constituted an integral part of Existenz's self-consciousness. Jaspers went further, arguing that without the existence of a relation of Existenz toward transcendence, it would be risking the loss of its selfhood.[18] The dialog between existence and transcendence and the formation of both through each other in the discussion of historicity became crystallized in the concept of eternality, which Jaspers defined as an endless duration of time. The fixing of Existenz's grasp in eternality that remains connected to the world of phenomena of the present[19] compressed the consciousness of historicity into an eye blink.[20] Compare this with Jaspers's historical discussion of the eye blink (*Augenblick*).[21] Individuals as Existenz became aware that they were no more than a passing phenomenon in existence. Through this phenomenon itself, which has depth in the past and horizons in the future, the eternal was revealed to them. The eternality of human Being is not the sort of religious claim referring to the person's survival in life after death. Nor does eternality appear in this context as an expression of the realization of values. In my opinion, the main point of eternality is that it indicates people's ability not only to direct their future but also to design the past of existence, which has apparently already been decided, in such a way as to allow them to claim from it the story of Existenz's formation. Jaspers described the two temporal directions on which consciousness of historicity acts simultaneously as a paradox:

> The paradoxes of Existenz's consciousness of historicity, that the disappearing time contains the Being of eternality, does not mean that eternality is supposed to be somewhere outside the place where it appears temporally. In contrast [it means that] in existence, Being does not simply exist, but it appears as that which is already decided, and indeed what has been decided is eternal.[22]

In many ways, the meaning granted to existence in the consciousness of historicity may be compared to the meaning of "situation Being" in *World Orientation.*[23] See the discussion of the term "situation" in Chapter Three. In Chapter Seven below this term will be discussed from an additional angle. In these two contexts, existence was presented as a blend of necessity, meaning of data whose origin is external to Existenz, and of freedom or possibility that reflect Existenz's ability to act and to form itself. While for Existenz the wide consciousness of the world entails becoming aware of its dependence on factors beyond its control, its ability to achieve orientation within this world is revealed as a lever for self-realization. The perception of Existenz that appears for the first time in the discussion of historicity as being in unity with existence now receives its full meaning. The consciousness of existence and of formation in time does not lead it to view itself as confined to the boundaries of existence forced upon it as a worldly Being. Jaspers's interpretation of the concept of eternality enabled expanding the meaning of the idea of possibility beyond its appearance in *World Orientation.* While before it had been perceived mainly as having a meaning regarding the future of Existenz, in the discussion of historicity it refers also to its past, and not only the future but also the past appears here as an incomplete element for it. This means that the consciousness of historicity provides Existenz with a new meaning for events in its past, and it is not only subject to them but they appear as data that can be formed and acquired.[24]

In the absence of a real explication of the concept of transcendence, Jaspers found it difficult to separate this concept and its implications for the perception of Existenz. This difficulty is apparent in the argument that the unification of existence and Existenz in the consciousness of historicity is a *personal perception* Existenz reaches.[25] The perception of Existenz still finds it difficult to contain simultaneously both the particular elements and the new awareness of extra-existential, independent dimensions revealed in the discussion of historicity. Also, the insights achieved regarding transcendence in the discussion of historicity had not been independently conceptually formulated, and transcendence could be significant only for the Existenz that had experienced it.[26] Even if historicity as existential consciousness contained a degree of awareness of transcendence and exposed Existenz's ability to refer to what was beyond the boundaries of its concrete existence, the deviations did not breach the boundaries of existentialist consciousness, based first and foremost on its selfhood.

> The unity of Existenz and existence, as a phenomenon in its historicity, is as such only by the standing of selfhood in existence before its transcendence, whose absoluteness I cannot know outside the ciphers of its historicity.[27]

The difficulty in starting the clarification centered on transcendence, typical of Jaspers's perception of communication, remains largely in his discussion of historicity. It transpires that the gradual distancing from the solipsistic perception of selfhood—as expressed in becoming aware of the existence in which Existenz is anchored, its relation to the possible existence of another Existenz, and even in awareness of wider aspects of existence—was still insufficient to direct the path of philosophizing toward transcendence. As the clearer consciousness of the boundaries within which Existenz moves becomes formed, so does a more vivid awareness of their rigidity and the difficulty in breaching them without undermining the importance of Existenz in the philosophical discussion. The tendency to expand the philosophizing typical of Jaspers's thought as explicated up to this stage becomes a real threat to Existenz, which was already on the verge of being deposed from the center of the discussion.

The consciousness of historicity is formed in light of this situation of Existenz and designed by Jaspers as a controlled instrument aimed at providing a solution for this stage of the philosophizing. On the one hand, it demonstrates for Existenz the isolation and detachment imposed upon it by the attempt to form its selfhood only on the basis of introspection, and reveals to it the barren closedness of the solipsistic selfhood. The appearance of new horizons of philosophizing, emerging from this consciousness, opens for Existenz room to refer to the Being beyond the boundaries of the world of phenomena. On the other hand, because it has yet to achieve explication of these horizons, it is required to remain constantly alert for the possibilities at its disposal as an Existenz, so that expanding the boundaries of the existence in which its life is conducted would not lead to its uprooting from existence.

Seven

BOUNDARY SITUATIONS

1. Expanding the Boundaries of Existence from "Situation Being" to "Boundary Situations"

The attempt to expand the framework of the discussion of selfhood, whether by new points of view or by clarifying the connection between it and additional topics accompanying it, was typical of Karl Jaspers's approach to the issues of communication and historicity. The concept "boundary situations" is undoubtedly one of Jaspers's most original and fruitful, and we will see that not for nothing did different scholars and philosophers argue that even this term alone could have established Jaspers's status as a philosopher.[1] On the face of it, we should not expect the discussion of boundary situations to indicate the continuation of the tendency to expand Existenz's boundaries of existence, since in them people are exposed uncompromisingly to their finality and to their inadequacy in the face of the factuality to which they are subject in existence. These are not situations that a person can initiate, plan, or avoid, only "encounter."[2] Experiencing boundary situations, which shakes the foundations of a person's existence, is not part of daily life or of what Jaspers termed the "situation Being" shared by all people; even Existenz does not experience boundary situations continuously. However, the interpretation I will present below shows that the attempt to expand the framework of philosophizing is expressed also in the discussion of boundary situations, although in a different way to those we have seen so far. In communication and in historicity, and more generally in the explication of selfhood, the expansion was "horizontal," meaning that it exposed Existenz to new horizons that enabled it to refer to aspects of existence that had previously been hidden from it. In contrast, in boundary situations, the expansion of the limits of philosophizing is "vertical," meaning that it deepens people's ability to experience their familiar existence, which they have already identified as belonging to them, and enables them to become acquainted with some aspects that, Jaspers believed, contained the meaning of human existence.

As in the discussion of the concepts of communication and historicity, the interpretation presented here will also aim to express the *role* of the boundary situations in assisting the transition from the explication of selfhood to the explication of Being, and therefore the discussion will not detail the concrete contents of each of the individual boundary situations. In *Psychology*, Jaspers listed four boundary situations: struggle, death, chance, and guilt. In *Elucidation of Existenz*, he proposed a different division and added a boundary situation of suffering. "Struggle" and "guilt" were presented in greater detail, and for the first time two more general boundary situations that exist in the background of all human experience appeared: "chance" and "particularity" (*Bestimmtheit*). For a detailed discussion of the specific boundary conditions, see Edwin Latzel.[3] However, while communication and historicity were discussed mainly in *Elucidation of Existenz*, the boundary situations also appeared earlier, in *Psychology*. This not only provides us with a special opportunity to examine the development of Jaspers's philosophical insights in the period between the two appearances of this concept in two different periods of his writing—the medical-psychological and the philosophical—but also enables a wider examination of the general conception of transition mechanisms that located them in *Elucidation of Existenz*.

2. Boundary Situations in *Psychology*

The starting point for the explication of selfhood, on which Jaspers's discussion in *Psychology* was based, was anchored in observing world views as a phenomenon and especially as a framework for processing the subjective experiences of the individual. The world view the individual constituted served as a framework for the processing of these experiences, but at the same time also as a major tool through which the subjective Being is revealed in its uniqueness and fullness.[4] In this context, Jaspers presented boundary situations as follows:

> These situations, where we feel, experience, and think at the boundaries of our existences in general, we thus term "boundary situations." What they have in common is that in the tangible world, always divided into subject-object, there is nothing stable and absolute that cannot be doubted, and there is no grasp point that could withstand every thought and every experience... These boundary situations, as such, are unbearable for life, and thus they almost never appear in complete clarity in our experiences of life, but indeed we almost always have a grasp point when facing boundary situations. Without it life would cease.[5]

As the experience of boundary situations sharpens people's awareness of being, as a finite entity, bound to the split between objectivity and subjectivity, so the boundaries of the world view as a framework for elucidating their experiences and constituting themselves become more tangible to them. Indicating the permanent presence of the infinite aspect of human experience exposes the person to contradictions, or more precisely antonyms, which world views cannot solve. This discovery was capable of undermining the evidence of the wholeness of world views in general, and could even have created a crisis in the perception of subjectivity relying on it. As he put it:

> As long as man is motivated by the forces of world views, he can never remain [only] in the concrete, since every concrete thing has simultaneously both a finite nature and an infinite nature. To deal with what is essential for him, he always encounters paths to the infinite or the whole. He can find, in his escape from the infinite to the mystical experience, a temporal limited satisfaction and peace. However, if he stays alert, if he remains in the split of object and subject, then all the infinity leads him to abysses of the contradictions called antonyms.[6]

The antonymous and contradictory nature of the experience of boundary conditions on the one hand, and people's difficulty in containing them and dealing with them using the tools at their disposal from normal existence situations on the other hand, make it difficult to see it as a source for explicating the individual's subjective Being as a whole. The meaning of "boundary" in these situations is expressed in the argument that the contradictions in world views are real and constitute "something absolute."[7] This means that there can never be any solution to the contradiction between the experience of these situations and the other experiences in a person's life. The antonymous nature typical of the experience of boundary situations and the accompanying dead-end experience are presented as evidence of the basic limitations of human beings in providing a more encompassing meaning and significance to their experiences in reality. The antonyms arising from the boundary situations indicate not only the edge of the boundary of the world view, but also of human experience at all.

Latzel argued that the explanation for the antonyms created by the boundary situations originated in Jaspers's decision to adopt the method of "descriptive psychology," for which the antonymous structure of existence serves as a convenient starting point for discussion.[8] It is difficult to accept this explanation not only because the descriptive method is marginal in *Psychology*, serving at that time as only one of the viewpoints through which Jaspers examined the individual's subjective experiences. In light of the experiences occurring in boundary situations this interpretation is difficult to accept, since these demonstrate not only the limitations of this method, but also the limitations of any possible explanation of a person's experiences at all. The boundary situations reveal the undecipherable element of human experiences as such. In his words:

> This doubt appears with the awareness that there may still be other life forms. The conscious experience of boundary situations, which were previously covered by solid patterns of taken-for-granted objective life forms, in world pictures and images of faith… led *to the disintegration of*

> *these patterns*. These patterns were previously unconscious, and now it transpires more or less what is a pattern and this has been experienced as a binding, as a restriction and as a doubtful thing that does not have the power to give a grasp point.[9]

These words show that in addition to the experiencing of boundary situations facing people with the real possibility of their annihilation, it also exposes them to the helplessness of world views to give them meaning within the range of their other experiences. Experiencing boundary situations apparently throws individuals outside the protected boundaries of the private world view, which they achieved through hard work, and demonstrates for them the partial and unconscious nature of a world view forming within the imaginary reality they created for themselves. Experiencing boundary situations may remove the cover that the private world view spread over the actual reality that is full of opposites and contradictions, and over people's expected demise. In the absence of the security that their world view was supposed to provide them, those who experience a boundary situation stand exposed and freezing at the edge of the abyss, filled with the keen awareness that no world view exists that could fill the abyss that has opened between their self-perception in existence and the possibilities implied by these situations. The increasing doubt regarding the reality of the self Being that the world view aimed to represent threatens to turn the world view itself into an empty vessel.

The connection between boundary situations and the processes of self-constitution and rational criticism that Jaspers presents in *Psychology* is central to Kurt Salamun's interpretation of boundary situations in their early appearance. In his opinion, these situations lead to the loss of the sovereignty and confidence people have in their life routine, and to the denial of the value of all the rational solutions and knowledge they possess about the reality in which they live. As a result of experiencing them, these situations throw the person into what Kurt Salamun terms "the unobjectivizable core of his internality." However, in his opinion, the boundary situations are also granted a positive meaning in *Psychology*, since they are perceived as directing people to become acquainted with the depth aspect of their Being—an aspect where their decisions are not determined by an objective perception of a systematic world view claiming general validity. Against this background, he notes that boundary situations reflect the freedom and independence of selfhood in its decisions, and also the individual's very possibility of finding the strength for life's actions without turning them into an objective and compulsory thing.[10]

The centrality of antonyms in the presentation of boundary situations in *Psychology* receives an interesting illumination in the interpretation of J. Rudolf Gerber, who argued that the contradiction between reason and intelligence, appearing in Immanuel Kant, contains a sort of depth aspect on which Jaspers's terms in general, and also the boundary situations, rely. He claims that these situations bring the antonymous elements in life to a climax, and in order to produce the desired insights from them, people must "renounce the effort to escape the tension between the limiting *Verstand* and the aspiring *Vernunft*."[11] I find that these words of Gerber's explicate mainly the early version of the boundary situations, apart from his argument that through these situations the individual becomes aware not only of the boundaries of existence itself, but also through elimination, of transcendence that is perceived as "an existing 'Unknowable'."[12] Since consciousness of transcendence forms from *Philosophy* onwards and is not mentioned at all in *Psychology*, I believe that Gerber's interpretation does not enable us to understand the later version of boundary situations. My interpretation of this version appears later in the discussion. Erich P. Grünert presented another comparison between Kant's basic principles and those of Jaspers.[13]

In my interpretation, I will argue that the connection between the concept of boundary situations and Kant's concept of antonyms is prominent in their early form, while in their later appearance in *Philosophy* there is a noticeable influence of Kant's term of border (*Grenze*). As we recall, Kant's concept of antonyms indicated a logical contradiction between two premises, each of which was capable of being proved by disproving its opposite, and the law of contradiction could not decide regarding the validity or invalidity of either of them.[14] Kant understood this contradiction as expressing a stage where although a person's reason has achieved sophistication and maturity, it is not capable of formulating a consciousness regarding its selfhood. Similarly, in the idea of boundary situations Jaspers also expressed people's difficulty in containing the gap between the infinite aspect of existence to which these situations hint and the finite reality as a source for constituting their world view. Under Kant's influence, Jaspers described antonyms as contradictions that cannot pass the boundary of consciousness,[15] and the antonyms are also revealed as a boundary situation portraying the problematic nature of the objective aspects of the world views that do not accord with the reality to which they refer. We can also indicate a general similarity between the role of reason for Kant and the role of the world view in Jaspers's thought. Both are intended to help people obtain a more complete self-understanding aimed at overcoming the division between objectivity and subjectivity: for Kant it is reason that achieves a critical awareness of itself, while for Jaspers it is the world view that has to express what people perceive as the boundaries of their experience of the world.

The link between Kant's concepts of antonym and reason, and the contradiction in world views, revealed in the discussion of boundary situations, testifies that their main meaning in *Psychology* did not depend on criticism of rationality as Salamun believed.[16] This criticism accompanied Jaspers's thinking from its inception, and is not especially stressed in the discussion of boundary situations. The epistemological viewpoint, expressed mainly in Jaspers's discussion of the phenomenon of multiplicity of world views and its general aspects, guided Jaspers in formulating the concept of boundary situations in *Psychology*. This viewpoint emphasized the conscious aspect of boundary situations, and in a way its very presence in the discussion can be seen as an attempt to use rational tools to deal with situations in which the absence of rationality is central.

Assuming that the experience of boundary situations reveals sides of the human experience that nobody can avoid, Jaspers used them to classify people on the basis of the different behavior patterns they show when encountering them.[17] He presented three types: people who when becoming acquainted with antonyms experience an extreme destabilizing and lack of confidence that could end in paralysis of the ability to act and of their consciousness;[18] others try in any way to avoid such experiences using different forms of compromise and denial of the contradictions appearing in existence;[19] while in contrast to these two types there are those who harness the antonyms to their search for the infinite in life and apply the different contradictions as means of affirming life.[20] The parallel between the three patterns of reaction and the move whereby Jaspers's thought developed from his study of psychiatry up to becoming a philosopher in his own right is quite clear: Jaspers presents first the pathological reaction pattern, which cannot integrate the different experiences. Then he turns to the reaction pattern of denial and avoidance, a pattern we may assume to be most common. Even if this pattern is undesirable, it appears not to disrupt the normal life routine of people who choose it. The psychological viewpoint that sees world views as a framework anchoring the contrasts and contradictions in "something whole"[21] may be effective for understanding the people who have chosen this reaction pattern. Finally, the third pattern reflects the viewpoint of spirit types, to be clarified below, where the contrasts arising from the boundary situations serve as a positive element of experience itself, which regains the support for its existence. This classification also shows that boundary situations, just like world views, provide an opportunity for meeting the basis of the human Being.

We cannot conclude from the statement that the very constitution of the concept of boundary situations reflects an attempt to deal with these situations using rational tools, that different people show a uniform coping pattern with these situations or that the particular component in their handling of it is marginal. The presence of the ontological viewpoint in *Psychology*, aimed at elucidating the processes of the individual's self-constitution within the context of the private world view, also stresses Jaspers's attempts to express the particular aspects typical of the process of forming a world view. Even if some components implied by Salamun's criticism are expressed in the concept of boundary situations as appearing in *Psychology*, they do not reveal their main meaning, which is people's difficulty in constituting a coherent world view that can help them deal with the range of their experiences in existence and especially with those that contain an irreconcilable antonym. So, in the boundary situations in *Psychology* we encounter the boundaries of the world view as a tool for constituting selfhood. Perhaps we can see the early appearance of this concept as the first inklings of the limitations of the perception of selfhood or even of the self-perception that relies only on elucidating the individual's subjective experiences. In this respect, the boundary situations in their early appearance in *Psychology* prefigure the development that was about to occur in Jaspers's thinking, when its center of gravity was shifted from selfhood to the explication of the metaphysical infrastructure on which this selfhood relies.

I believe that when he wrote *Psychology*, Jaspers, who was endeavoring to write a book that would describe the human soul from the viewpoint of normality, was unable, or perhaps could not allow himself, to face the destructive potential of experiencing boundary situations in relation to the philosophical process that took place in *Psychology*.[22] The attempt to find mental patterns and frameworks that could contain his perception of selfhood, apparent already in the adoption of the world view as a framework for explicating the individual's subjective Being, continued to guide him, as we will see below, even when he wished to resolve the crisis that boundary situations created in his thinking at that time.[23]

> We ask what the condition is for them [boundary situations]... not being expressed at all. Thus we encounter the center of the spirit types. What grasp point (*Halt*) does man have, how does he have it, how does he search for it and find it, and how does he maintain it—this is the typical expression of the forces living inside him. When we ask about the spirit types we are [actually] asking where a person has his grasp point.[24]

The assimilation of the boundary situations as a positive element in the "spirit types" (*Geistestypen*) transpires as a substitute for the support granted by the world view, which was destabilized following the experience of the boundary situations. The definition of spirit types as "forces" in which the infinite perfections granted to human beings intuitively are represented[25] accords with the need to anchor the individual's experiences in a wider infrastructure—one where each single component will find its place in a more encompassing perfection than that granted by the individual's particular world view.[26] Jaspers presented several spirit types: nihilism, skepticism, rationalism, liberalism, authoritarianism, and others. The intuitive element in the spirit types makes it difficult to elucidate them using language, which in this context was described as "freezing" and "fixating,"[27] but at this point the world view can complement them as a more structured and conscious setting. The anchor world views have in the spirit types enables them to continue to serve as a framework that provides meaning to most of people's experiences. The advantage of the spirit types in comparison with the world views is that they contain the boundary situations within them, as a horizon viewed from the range of human experiences as such, although these situations reflect the coming annihilation of the person. The complexity and flexibility typical of the spirit types enables dealing with a wider range of experiences and prevents a single experience or an experience of a boundary situation from turning into a total experience on which a person's self-perception will exclusively rely. Unlike the world view where the antonyms in boundary situations became an absolute experience, entailing the possibility of denying the existence of the selfhood that had experienced them, in the spirit types the antonym is surrounded by what Jaspers called "life forces" that moderate it and harness it to the purpose of constituting a more conscious and stable self-perception.

In a way, the influence of the spirit types over the boundary situations expresses the success of the world view to expand the capability of human experience, so that people manage to observe beyond the boundaries of their world views the boundaries of existence itself. The maturity of the processes of self-constitution, reflected in the experiencing of boundary situations, does not enable the person to be satisfied with the world view without clarifying the general and perhaps hidden elements on which it is based, which Jaspers called "spirit types." The understanding of the boundary situations from the perspective of the explication of selfhood contrasts with other interpretations of this concept in secondary literature. William D. Blattner's interpretation, according to which the boundary situations in *Psychology*, reflects an ontological interest.[28] The boundary situations are portrayed against this background as a sign of the metaphysical aspect present in the processes of self-constitution, which is hidden from whoever is still undergoing this process. Experiencing boundary situations spurs people on to investigate the intuitive and metaphysical aspects on which their world view is based, a process whereby they become aware of the boundaries of the world view itself or of the type of experience with which it can help them deal. The spirit types aim at the same original purpose that was the basis for the constitution of the world view, elucidating the subjective Being of the individual. However, the advantage of the spirit types in relation to this purpose is that through them the person is able to deal with the boundary situations without completely abandoning the world view or undermining the basic insights achieved in *Psychology*. In this respect, the perspective of spirit types allows a more efficient coping with the crisis instigated by the boundary situations in people's confidence in their world view. Just before the entire conception on which the perception of selfhood formed in *Psychology* collapsed into the abyss created by the boundary situations, the spirit types helped reaffirm this conception. However, from the perspective of Jaspers's entire philosophy we can state that the spirit types only postponed the crisis the boundary situations created in the perception of selfhood to a later stage in his work; until it could contain the tools to face the disruptive element in them and from this formulate a wider understanding of the individual and of the reality that could contain them as a positive element.

3. Boundary Situations in *Philosophy*

The new discussion of boundary situations in the philosophical period of Jaspers's writings raises the need to examine the differences between the meanings bestowed upon them in the two contexts and to present an explanation for his reexamination of this issue. The central argument in which my interpretation of the boundary situations in *Psychology* was anchored also applies in the interpretation presented for their appearance in *Elucidation of Existenz*, namely, that there is a clear link between the meaning of boundary situations and the more general context in which they appear. In this respect, the two versions of boundary situations serve as a mirror to the wider perception of selfhood in the context in which each of them appeared: while the appearance of boundary situations in *Psychology* showed the main motifs of the perception of selfhood that was anchored in observing the world views, the concept of boundary situations as appearing in *Elucidation of Existenz* portrayed the dialectic typical of the relationship of Existenz toward consciousness and the reality of the world. As Jaspers said:

> These situations, like those I always exist within, that I cannot live without struggle and sorrow, that I accept upon myself inevitable guilt, that I must die, I call boundary situations. *They do not change*, but only their appearance; in their reference to our existence they are totally valid. *We cannot see* beyond them; in our existence, we do not see [anything] behind them. They are like a wall that we push and walk into. They cannot be changed through us, but we can only bring them into clarity without being able to deduce them or explain them from something else. They exist with existence itself.[29]

The understanding that sees boundary situations as referring to existence and as given along with it affirms the argument in principle at the basis of my interpretation of the boundary situations in *Elucidation of Existenz*. According to this interpretation, the concept is anchored in the general insights Jaspers held during that period, centering on the perception of Existenz as a worldly Being. Like the discussion of boundary situations that appeared in *Psychology*, Jaspers's handling of this issue in *Elucidation of Existenz* also brought about a crisis in the perception of selfhood. However, in this context it led to significant changes in the basic concepts on which the philosophy of Existenz relied. The most significant change is apparent in the status of Existenz within the experience, or more precisely, the weight it was granted in the formulation of its existence. This change was an outcome of the basic difference between the ordinary situations Existenz deals with and the boundary situations. The first, as presented in *World Orientation*, have two characteristics that define Existenz's framework of experience in the world: the necessity enforced upon it by circumstances beyond its control, and the freedom it still has in this context, thanks to which it can choose from among the possibilities it identifies in existence the one that appears as a source for fuller self-realization. See the discussion of "situation Being" in Chapter Three. The freedom component, so central in Existenz's "situation Being," is completely absent from the boundary situations, which appear to it as absolutely valid, with it having no influence on them whatsoever. Jaspers stressed the absence of existential freedom in the boundary situations when he described the feeling of Existenz in them as a "game ball."[30] This term demonstrates the arbitrariness accompanying the experience of these situations, and to some extent also the replacing of the activity typical of Existenz in existence with impotence.

Neither Existenz nor human consciousness as such has access to these situations or influence over them. In Jaspers's words: "A boundary situation is not another situation for general consciousness, since consciousness as knowing and as purposeful deals with them only objectively, or else avoids them, ignores them, and forgets them."[31] This description is aimed, in my opinion, not only at emphasizing the limitations of formal knowledge or of human reason in general, which was not Jaspers's concern in this context; it expressed the way that Existenz experiences its existence in the boundary situations. In the following passage, Jaspers clarified the main implication the experience of boundary situations has on Existenz's perception of existence in general:

> Boundary situations bring in their wake… a perspective in existence where it is doubted as a whole thing and is considered a possible, impossible, or differently possible [thing]. Existence in general is perceived as a boundary, and this Being experiences within the boundary situation that reveal that the world Being and my own Being within it are doubtful.[32]

In Existenz's experience of boundary situations, it is drawn into the particular form of experience portrayed, for example, in suffering, guilt, chance, and recognition of the necessity of death. Unlike people's general experience of different situations, usually occurring alongside other experiences, the boundary situation is unique in the extreme intensity typifying it, turning it into a total representation of existence for Existenz. The particularity of each boundary situation and the way it is experienced by Existenz destabilize the possibility of seeing the everyday existence experienced by Existenz through ordinary situations as a complete thing. Paradoxically, the routine situations that serve as a basis for a person's orientation in the world are perceived as partial, as hiding the total and infinite aspects of existence, and everything they show about the worldly Being becomes doubtful. In contrast, it is the boundary situations, in their extreme particularity, and in the absence of the person's ability to maneuver in them,[33] that are perceived as expressions of infinity. The inability to understand the boundary situations and the resulting helplessness Existenz experiences in the face of the abyss before it become fundamental data of its self-perception. The totality typical of the experience of these situations is responsible for the irrelevance of existential freedom when facing boundary situations not being attributed only to the experience of the boundary situations, but also percolating into Existenz's self-perception and perception of existence in general.

The vague definition given to the concept of boundary situations earlier on, whereby these situations "have [something] else but at the same time: this... does not [exist] for the consciousness in existence,"[34] now receives its precise meaning. The boundary situations illuminate the limitations of human beings in existence and at the same time they hint, from the boundary point where Existenz stands when experiencing them, to another Being beyond them. The experience of boundary situations projects in two opposite directions: on people's existence in general situations, now perceived as limited, and on the Being beyond them, regarding which they mark the boundary from which it spreads out. See the distinction between Kant's two concepts of boundary in the Introduction. Jaspers expressed the two facets of this experience by stating that "the boundaries appear in their real function, to be immanent and already to indicate transcendence."[35]

The argument that boundary situations influence another understanding of people's existence in situations in general does not, according to the interpretation offered here, make boundary situations into the sole test of Existenz, since just like existence, so boundary situations, too, have many facets. Interpretations viewing boundary situations as Existenz's constituting situations, such as that of Gabriel Marcel, were probably based on a misunderstanding of Jaspers's statement that "experiencing boundary situations and existing are the same thing,"[36] as if only in them can the leap from Existenz to existence take place.[37] This is because the ability to re-examine itself and its place in existence is one of Existenz's qualities par excellence. Most people may experience during their lifetime some aspect of some boundary situation, but they will usually return to the forgetfulness-inducing routine of existence, without this experience leaving any real traces in their self-consciousness. So, Existenz is unique not because it experiences these situations with greater force, but because this experience creates a fundamental transformation in the way it perceives itself and its surrounding. This means that the consciousness of self-constitution, its uniqueness, and particularity is pushed aside in favor of a new consciousness where it appears to itself as one of the phenomena of existence and everything that applies to them applies to it; this consciousness, percolating into the self-consciousness of Existenz in the different boundary situations, does not lead it to doubt its existence, or even its existence as an Existenz, although this does not appear to it to protect it from the abyss these situations has opened before it. Against this background, common to all boundary situations, we can characterize the consciousness Existenz has as a result, and present it as follows: Existenz becomes aware of the unavoidable factuality of the struggle and suffering in human existence; it knows that every day it approaches its inevitable death, which may be the result of an arbitrary accident, although this is insufficient to excuse it from the inevitable sense of guilt in these situations.

It is difficult to overestimate the power Jaspers attributed to the experiencing of boundary situations as appearing in *Elucidation of Existenz*. This is not the discovery of experiences that reveal to Existenz particular aspects that could have been assimilated into his philosophy of Existenz without undermining its basic insights. While in *Psychology* he was able to overcome the difficulties that the boundary situations raised regarding his perception of subjectivity and to leave it standing, in *Elucidation of Existenz* they undermined the most fundamental infrastructure on which the philosophy of Existenz relied. The question was not whether the contradictions between the way Existenz perceives itself and what it becomes acquainted with when facing the suffering, death, guilt, and chance in human experience could be reconciled, but whether Existenz could exist at all in these situations. The doubt naturally arises regarding the value of the self-constitution processes, in face of the cessation and end heralded by the boundary situations. As with the other ideas included in the transition mechanisms, so also in the discussion of boundary situations the emphasis was on the implications of Existenz's self-consciousness instead of on explicating the metaphysical horizons reflected by these experiences or those of transcendence, which were discussed only in the explication of Being. However, the uniqueness of the boundary situations as a transition mechanism was in their discussion bringing closer the end of the dialectic between the solipsism typical of Jaspers's early thought and the perception of selfhood as a worldly Being. This dialectic appeared as useless casuistry that changed nothing regarding the absolute and uncompromising finality emerging from the boundary situations. This is perhaps the greatest antonym people can experience as conscious Beings: they want to continue living forever, but when they become aware of this, they realize that they are approaching death with every passing moment.

Compared with *Psychology*, the awareness that the boundary situations constitute an inseparable part of the experiences occurring to a person as a conscious Being penetrated Jaspers's perception of selfhood more deeply in *Elucidation of Existenz*. However, it is probably the awareness of the deep undermining of the basic insights on which this consciousness relied that motivated Jaspers to try to moderate as much as possible the threat and negation of the very relevance of the philosophy of Existenz entailed in them. Such an attempt is also apparent in Jaspers's handling of the boundary situations in *Psychology*, where he wished to assimilate them into a more complex, flexible framework that enabled him to maintain the perception of selfhood anchored in world views. The difference is that in *Elucidation of Existenz* this attempt was imbued with the awareness that the changes brought about by the exposure of the boundary situations as a given element of the Being of Existenz were irreversible. Jaspers's effort at this stage was not aimed at overcoming the challenge to the basic insights of the philosophy of Existenz arising from them, but at searching for ways to help him handle them. His aim was to show that although the experience of boundary situations instigates essential changes in Existenz, it does not turn its characteristics into an empty vessel. He indicated the particular nature of the existentialist experience of boundary situations. He also stressed that the freedom of Existenz was responsible for the experience of the necessity in boundary situations not being perceived as absolute, but as opening a window to the horizons beyond the boundaries of existence in which it was contained.[38] The boundary situations deepen for Existenz the awareness of the limitations typical of its existence in the context of different situations, and so it is pushed to search for a more encompassing metaphysical Being, beyond the boundaries of existence. Existenz harnesses the very drives that motivated it in the process of its self-constitution to the search for a metaphysical Being, which the experience of boundary situations has made tangible, and whose elucidation had become essential for Existenz's self-understanding.

In my opinion, this approach of Jaspers's shows that the changes regarding the status of Existenz within the boundary situations do not lead to relocating it outside the boundaries of the philosophical discussion—not at this stage, and as we will see later, not in the framework of the explication of Being. What Existenz is denied is the very possibility of changing or avoiding meeting the boundary situations, but what remains open to it is the possibility of expanding the boundaries of its awareness in such a way as to allow it *in its existence* to give meaning to what is revealed to it following the boundary situations, or more precisely the Being perceived as spreading onwards from the boundary situations.

The question "*Why is there existence at all?*,"[39] demonstrating the agitation the acquaintance with boundary situations in *Elucidation of Existenz* caused, was not fully answered at this stage of Jaspers's philosophy. However, in his statement, "The Being exists only when there is existence, but existence as such is not the Being itself,"[40] he gave a partial reply, or perhaps just a direction for the answer to this question that would be the focus of his philosophical interest later on. Already now Jaspers could testify that the existence in which Existenz found itself was not the be all and end all, although it was clear to him that it was pointless to search for meaning in isolation from the individual's experiences in existence.

The discussion of boundary situations in *Elucidation of Existenz* created deep changes in Jaspers's perception of Existenz. However, this discussion continued to rely largely upon it, and perhaps was even meaningless without it. Not only the ability to withstand these situations, but the very acquaintance with them, depends on the existence of an explicit self-consciousness from Existenz's point of view.

Perhaps this observation was in the background of different interpretations that saw the "boundary situations" in *Elucidation of Existenz* as a framework where Existenz could realize itself. Salamun, for instance, argues that the descriptions of the types of human existence in the face of boundary situations, ranging from "nihilistic despair" to "internal appropriation" to "composure with the knowledge of death," are aimed at creating an autonomous picture of human beings whereby individuals can develop life patterns that will accompany their existence and turn them into the people they are.[41]

Another interpretation with an ethical orientation is that of Latzel, who argues that the boundary situations are a sign indicating an inconceivable depth, but containing the possibility of the self-realization of Existenz in transcendence. In this respect, Existenz, as a Being aiming at realizing itself, should be interested, in his opinion, in experiencing boundary situations.[42] Latzel argues that the boundary situations bring Existenz into an unresolved paradox. It has to want the impossible—self-realization in transcendence—and only by this can it achieve the possible—self-realization in existence—which it cannot want and cannot find satisfactory. In his opinion, only if Existenz does not try to escape the boundary situations and does all it can to avoid failure to realize itself, which is in any case an inseparable part of its existence as such, can this failure serve as an authentic Being for its self-realization.[43] Jaspers's concept of "foundering" will be discussed in Chapter Eight.

Beyond the difficulties that are raised more generally by the ethical interpretation of Jaspers's perception of Existenz, there is a particular difficulty in accepting it regarding boundary situations, as presented in both *Psychology* and *Elucidation of Existenz*. First, the question of self-realization is relevant mainly to the perception of the boundary situations in *Psychology*, when Jaspers's thought was focused on the processes of constituting selfhood; but the ethical interpretation is based mainly on the discussion in *Elucidation of Existenz*. As we have seen, in *Elucidation of Existenz* Jaspers's effort to constitute a philosophical approach is apparent especially regarding what was beyond the boundaries of Existenz's self-realization—an attempt that involved dealing with new aspects of his thinking that significantly threatened the basic insights on which his philosophy of Existenz was based. Against this background, it is clear why it is difficult to accept the central argument in the ethical interpretation, whereby it is in the boundary situations that Existenz can realize itself. The long journey the perception of selfhood had undergone in the period between the publication of *Psychology* and that of *Elucidation of Existenz*, expressed in the profound changes that occurred in Jaspers's perception of selfhood, could not apparently be expressed in the majority of the existing interpretations of boundary situations. These did not attribute any real significance to the very discussion of boundary situations in two different contexts, or to the contribution of the context to the meaning given them each time. Latzel argues that the meaning granted to boundary situations in *Philosophy* is a continuation without any real addition of the young Jaspers's original philosophical intuition from the period of *Psychology*.[44] However, the interpretation offered here regarding the boundary situations is anchored in the understanding that the Existenz, having been formed as a Being that constitutes a more complex relation to what exists beyond itself (existence, the other Existenz, historical time, and so on), is significantly different from the character of the subjective Being as portrayed in *Psychology*. This development, apparent also in the gradual release from the need to anchor the discussion of selfhood in the defined mental patterns that had served as its anchor (such as world views), enabled the introduction of new concepts and aspects to the arena of philosophizing, including the integration of new aspects, such as existence and transcendence, which had a decisive influence on the formulation of the concept of boundary situations in *Elucidation of Existenz*.

Against the background of the fundamental differences between the meaning granted to the boundary situations in *Psychology* and the meaning they received in *Elucidation of Existenz*, I wish to argue that Jaspers's writings contain two different versions of this concept, and that each one reflected the more general insights characteristic of Jaspers's thinking at that period. The first version shows the solipsistic version of selfhood, while the second version expresses the effort to escape from this approach due to the limitations it imposes upon the wider understanding of selfhood and the attempt to constitute a metaphysical relation to what was beyond the boundaries of Existenz's self-consciousness. In this respect, this interpretation reflects the division of Jaspers's work into periods presented in the Introduction. The metaphysical aspect revealed in the discussion of selfhood does not appear exclusively in the later version of the boundary situations. As we have seen, it was apparent already in his early writings dealing with psychiatry. However, in *Philosophy*, when transcendence already appeared as a significant component in Jaspers's discussion, the metaphysical aspect was not limited to the relevance to the process of constituting Existenz. Jaspers's repeated reference to the issue of boundary situations in the same context where he makes his first steps in forming a philosophical relation toward transcendence serves as the very basis for understanding the later version of the boundary situations as part of the transition mechanisms.

Just as the early perception of the boundary situations was an outcome of the perception of subjectivity typical of Jaspers's thinking at that time, so also their later version in *Philosophy* reflected the perception of Existenz, which at that time was imbued with awareness of the boundaries of its existence and focused on the effort to grant them a more comprehensive metaphysical meaning. The gap that is so noticeable between the perception of Existenz as an autonomous Being that constitutes itself and determines its relation toward existence and its helplessness in the face of the boundary situations led to a reshuffle in Jaspers's perception of selfhood. One of the clearest expressions of this development in his philosophy is demonstrated in the later version of the boundary situations where Jaspers tried to reverse the perception of existential freedom, arguing that these situations that reveal the boundaries of Existenz's experience and existence are the very ones that open a window for it to continue experiencing, and also a future space for self-realization in freedom. While it is possible in principle that the relation toward transcendence could later be translated into accepting an ethical or even religious value system, this would reflect a positive position existing beyond the boundaries of Existenz's consciousness in the boundary situations. The boundary situations in their later version place Existenz on the zero line: between becoming aware of the individual's expected demise and becoming aware of the existence of transcendence. The first erodes the difference between Existenzes and non-Existenzes, while the second distances Existenz from the center of the philosophizing arena.

4. Boundary Situations as a Transition Mechanism in Comparison with Communication and Historicity

The location of boundary situations as the final link in the transition mechanisms raises the need to compare them with the other two ideas in Jaspers's thought that helped transfer the center of gravity of the philosophizing to the explication of Being: communications and historicity.

A. Boundary Situations and Communication

On the face of it, we could assume that in light of the difficult experience of boundary situations—the struggle, suffering, sorrow, guilt, and death—communication might be a sort of relief to the person experiencing them. Jaspers's discussion of boundary situations includes no mention of communication at all. But this is not surprising considering the proposed interpretation. As we have seen, this interpretation did not view communication as a real possibility for Existenz, and stressed the influence of the solipsistic viewpoint on the relation Existenz forms toward the other Existenz, which was just one of the means Jaspers's thought placed at its disposal in order to deepen its consciousness as an individual Being. So, the disadvantage of communication in the boundary situations where a person especially needs it supports the offered interpretation of Jaspers's perception of communication, which was not dependent on the constitution of real relations with the other, but largely on its contribution to the broader self-understanding of Existenz and its preparation for forming its relation toward transcendence. Existenz stands alone in face of the boundary situations, and this is not only an expression of the essence of these situations where a person has no support or escape, but it indirectly implies that the perception of communication in Jaspers's thought did not deal mainly with relationships between people, but was a metaphysical category.

Understanding communication as an idea that could be realized by Existenzes also projected upon the interpretation of boundary situations. Salamun believed that communication and boundary situations represented different forms of self-realization that are interlinked in some complex way. Against this background he suggested a few alternatives for understanding the relations between them: first, that boundary situations and communication portray two basic situations in which people can realize themselves; second, that loneliness in the boundary situation implies the possibility of being in communication with people; and third, that it is the very lack of satisfaction Existenz experiences in communication that shows the possibility of self-realization from the loneliness in the boundary situation.[45] However, considering that Jaspers himself did not refer to the issue of communication during the discussion of boundary situations, it is difficult to accept Salamun's interpretation, which appears as structured into his ethical viewpoint. The experience of dissatisfaction by the Existenz—the experience that served as the starting point for the discussion of the ideas included in the transition mechanisms—leaves no doubt regarding the centrality of *loneliness* in the experience of communication, in the constitution of consciousness of historicity, and in boundary situations. Each of these experiences helped significantly expand the philosophizing framework beyond the one typical of the explication of selfhood, where Existenz was presented as a Being closed within its boundaries. However, the person standing as an individual in face of the different experiences remained unchanged. Even so, the advantage of the boundary situations compared with communications and historicity is that it sharpens Existenz's awareness that the loneliness it experiences is way beyond the absence of another human being to complement it. This is the harshest loneliness a person can experience: loneliness from transcendence. At this stage it is not possible to establish this statement, since transcendence has not yet been elucidated within the transition mechanisms, but has been experienced mainly as a Being other than that of Existenz, which proved false as an enduring source of meaning and significance for existence in the world. The transition mechanisms are presented in the interpretation offered here as an integral part of the elucidation of transcendence included only in the explication of Being, based on the functionality typical of them as a means of rescuing the philosophizing from the explication of selfhood. Finally, we can state that the boundary situations are unique in comparison with the other transition mechanisms in that they indicate more clearly that the self-realization horizons of Existenz are anchored in a metaphysical Being whose boundaries cross immanence.

The question of the relation between communication and boundary situations has also been discussed in the interpretation of Latzel, who stressed, unlike Salamun, the role of transcendence as a factor in the experience of boundary situations. In his opinion, the boundary situations constitute a sign indicating an inconceivable depth that contains the possibility for Existenz's self-realization in transcendence, and this raises the problem of the "announcing" or communication and turns the boundary situations into a medium in which it is clarified.[46] Latzel does not clarify whether in this context this is the problem of communication between transcendence and Existenz, or whether it means the inability of Existenz to report to another Existenz the nature of that "inconceivable depth" revealed to it by the boundary situations. The first problem relates to the nature of transcendence as such, while the second to the relations between Existenzes. However, the clarification of these two problems implicit in Latzel's interpretation does not contribute to the understanding of the boundary situations in their later version. First, Existenz's handling of the transcendence in boundary situations is not primarily related to its difficulty in establishing an explicit consciousness of it, and the awareness of its control cannot accompany the experience of these situations, which involve an extreme experience of helplessness. Second, the burning difficulty Existenz experiences in the boundary situations relates mainly to the inability *to contain in itself* what it becomes acquainted with, meaning the reality of its expected annihilation, an end that it as an Existenz cannot ignore. The power of the experience of the annihilation transpiring as a real horizon from the boundary situations relies largely on the Existenz knowing that the death is its personal death, while any discussion of death with another person could turn it into an event that is objective and external to the Existenz—removing it from being a boundary situation at all.[47] The necessarily subjective nature of the experience of boundary situations makes clear that communication is not a means of handling them. It is highly likely that the development of an interpersonal discourse about these experiences would distance Existenz from their real meaning that is accessible to the individual in loneliness. Even if dealing with communication in the context of boundary situations contributes to their explication, this contribution is not achieved thanks to the function of knowledge transfer constituting part of the experience of communication. But beyond the contribution of the criticism of Salamun's and Latzel's interpretations to further sharpening the interpretation of communication and boundary situations presented above, it also helped understand that these two original ideas of Jaspers's are part of one philosophical process: the perception of communication does not rescue Existenz from its loneliness, but reflects the seeing of the other Existenz as a means of transcending existence. The boundary situations, experienced by that Existenz that already knows that the possibility of communication would not rescue it from its loneliness, help it transcend existence once more and distance it another step from the rigidity of the solipsistic perception of selfhood.

B. Boundary Situations and Historicity

A connection exists between historicity, meaning the process whereby Existenz becomes acquainted with the roots and the wider boundaries of the existence to which it is subject, and the awareness forming in boundary situations whereby beyond its existence, which is expected to end, another, different Being exists. As Jaspers put it:

> *Existence is historistic* because it cannot be complemented in time; it causes itself restlessly since there is no agreement in any situation. The antonymous view is the one that in time-reality (*Zeitdasein*) [raises the requirement] to become (*Anderswerden*) another.[48]

Against this background we can state that although the explication of Existenz deepened in the boundary situations and was exposed to more significant threats than those it encountered during the discussion of historicity, Jaspers perceived these two ideas as part of one philosophical move. However, this statement does not accord with other expressions of Jaspers's, such as the argument that a person is destined to live with an irreconcilable split between the existence in different situations and existence in boundary situations,[49] and that "the power of this contradiction, if it does not weaken any side, is the truth of Existenz."[50] These sentences may indicate that boundary situations bring Existenz closer to constituting a metaphysical consciousness transcending existence more significantly than that enabled by consciousness of historicity, which is anchored in a deeper connection to concrete existence. In this respect, the contradiction reflects the great distance separating historicity from the philosophizing typical of the explication of Being to be presented later, compared with the boundary situations that are closer to this framework. But in another respect we can understand Jaspers's dealing with the link between the idea of historicity and the boundary situations as evidence that the connection of these ideas to the explication of selfhood was still significant, also showing the boundaries of the experience that still did not enable Existenz to constitute a relation toward Being. The limitations that required Jaspers to withdraw to the familiar thought patterns of the explication of selfhood were present also in his discussion of boundary situations in *Philosophy*. Either way, we cannot see the proposed options for understanding as an expression of Jaspers's contradiction or inconsistency, but as a demonstration of the special condition of the philosophizing during the transition mechanisms stage—a framework where on the one hand there is an expression of the distancing from and maturation of the early perceptions, while on the other hand there is an attempt to set the path where the new insights will be clarified. Jaspers's definition of boundary situations as amounting to their "immanent function"[51] clarifies the complex condition of his thought at this stage:

communication and historicity, and especially boundary situations, implied the inability to continue discussing Existenz within the boundaries dictated by the explication of selfhood. The discussion of these issues brought the philosophizing closer to the explication of Being. However, the distancing from the explication of selfhood, characteristic of the ideas in the transition mechanisms, transpired as insufficient to constitute a real link to Being and to transcendence.

TRANSITION MECHANISMS: A CONCLUDING OVERVIEW

1. Three Forms of Otherness

The maturation of the awareness of the limitations of the self-perception constituted only out of the elucidation of its personal experiences led Existenz to recognize its need for the "other," not only as a means of constituting a broader self-perception, but also as a Being without which its continued existence as an Existenz was threatened.[1] This is reminiscent of Georg Wilhelm Friedrich Hegel's statements of principle regarding the spirit's self-awareness.[2] Hegel connects the spirit's ability to achieve self-consciousness with its becoming aware of another self-consciousness and placing itself opposite it. The discussion of the three transition mechanisms shows that the aim to expand the boundaries of Existenz's Being through the other was accompanied by the fear of its annihilation and the fear of the collapse of the explication of selfhood. The discussion of the ideas included in the transition mechanisms was based on the fundamental insights achieved during the explication of selfhood, and it largely revealed the same points that had accompanied the study from its inception. However, the uniqueness of the discussion of these ideas lies in the integration between the different aspects that had appeared in earlier contexts and the criticism of these earlier ideas that it contained. The difficulty in detaching the expressions of the epistemological viewpoint from those of the ontological viewpoint was reflected at different levels in the discussion of these ideas. The distinction between the new facets revealed in Existenz and its reality as an existing Being now became almost impossible. The more we learned about Existenz and especially about its limitations, the more real a Being it became.

A comparative look at communication, historicity, and boundary situations from the perspective of transition mechanisms—in light of the question of the extent to which they helped transfer the focus of the philosophizing from selfhood to Being—shows that they represent three stages of distancing from the solipsistic selfhood typical of Karl Jaspers's early thought. This process was apparent in the dependence of Existenz on factors external to it and perhaps more powerful than it, and in its exposure as a Being in a process of constant formation anchored in its drive to transcend itself. The deeper the degree of otherness of the other with which Existenz had to deal, the more Jaspers was able to expand the framework of philosophizing and base it on concepts whose meaning was not limited to their relevance to the explication of selfhood. The interpretation behind the viewing of the three philosophical ideas as linked to the same developmental stage in Jaspers's thought did not rely only on exposing the functional facet they shared as a means of helping Existenz transcend itself, but was also anchored in clarifying the links of contents between them. My proposed interpretation of the philosophical ideas I included in the transition mechanisms did not grant them an independent status, and they were examined from the perspective of the two opposite horizons seen from either side: the explication of selfhood on the one hand, and the explication of Being on the other.

In *communication*, Existenz's perception of otherness was largely sculpted in accordance with the boundaries of Existenz's self-understanding, which was already in advanced stages of philosophical explication. In a way, the other Existenz can be seen as a sort of mirror Existenz placed before itself, to enable it to examine its character from another angle. But it was predictable that the explication of the idea of communication would reveal that what the Existenz saw was merely its reflection as elucidated in the clarification of Existenz. The idea of communication presents a minimal model of the other, a character largely reflecting the role Existenz had intended it for. In the end, the transcending to the other Existenz remained purely formal, and as such it preserved the obligation to the original Existenz at which the framework of the explication of selfhood was aimed.

In *historicity*, the otherness with which the Existenz was required to deal was deepened. This was no longer the formation of a relation toward a similar Being, but an attempt of Existenz to form a relation toward existence in the widest sense, and not just to adapt it to the needs of its self-understanding as we saw in *World Orientation*. In existence, as a whole reality spreading over the past and the future, there are constraints and forces that have their own dynamics that do not influence Existenzes differently from not-Existenzes. The consciousness of historicity expanded Existenz's viewpoint only regarding the boundaries of the time and space where it existed anyway, while Existenz itself remained the focus to which the wide boundaries of existence as historicity referred. The confrontation with existences as other was an encounter with a real and different thing, but in the negotiation that developed around the awareness of this existence, Existenz's familiar effort to understand itself was still expressed in many ways.

In *boundary situations*, as in the discussion of communication and historicity, Existenz confronted the reality of the other, but the contents of the otherness arising from these situations related tangibly to the possibility of Existenz's own annihilation. No doubt exists that through the boundary situations Jaspers marked the upper limits of Existenz's ability to experience, limits that also denoted the borders of its explications. Jaspers did not cease searching for the existential meaning of these situations, and sought to translate the experiences Existenz had in its encounter with the boundary situations in a way that would moderate or at least distance the annihilating possibility arising from them. The philosophical effort aimed at harnessing the boundary situations to the life forces for Existenz greatly softened their absoluteness and made their boundary into one with which Existenz could live. In this way, Jaspers continued the trend of existential elucidation typical of his discussion of the other two mechanisms, which enabled, from the methodological viewpoint of this study, the inclusion of the boundary situations within the explication of Existenz. However, it was precisely the total nature accompanying the meeting with the other in the boundary situations that brought Jaspers's discussion at this point closer to the philosophizing whose boundaries were no longer limited to the elucidation of selfhood. True, both in communication and in historicity we can identify elements that prefigured the explication of Being, but only in boundary situations did their more significant presence not enable them to be assimilated relatively easily into the Being of Existenz, and in any case the need arose to grant them a status separate from it. Finally, the boundary situations faced Existenz with two choices: to annihilate itself as an existing Being at all, or to move aside from the focus of the philosophizing and to turn to explicate the horizons revealed to it by the boundary situations. Either way, in light of the boundary situations the perception of Existenz as the focus of the philosophizing became impossible.

2. Absolute Consciousness

The maturation of Jaspers's perception of selfhood typical of this stage of his thought—after the explication of selfhood was completed and the transition mechanisms had been discussed—well demonstrated the insights achieved, but no less also stressed its limitations. Paradoxically, precisely at the peak of the explication of selfhood, Existenz was revealed as an incomplete Being facing targets it could not achieve using the instruments of consciousness at its disposal. From the perspective of Jaspers's entire philosophy we can state that the condition of Existenz, as formulated in the transition mechanisms, did not remove Jaspers's drive to make contact with totality—a drive accompanying his thought from its inception. He realized that the desired totality would not be found within the boundaries of the explication of selfhood, but rather in the horizons viewed from it but unable to be clarified within the boundaries of the philosophizing typical of it. It is no coincidence that at this stage the term "existential consciousness" was replaced with the concept "absolute consciousness," which Jaspers defined as follows:

> *Absolute consciousness*, this certainty in Being existing from the tension it has toward the uncertain source of all philosophizing, becomes an *object* for philosophizing. Instead of philosophizing only from within it, it seems as a leap beyond yourself following which there is no longer anything... The absolute consciousness cannot be thought objectively, it cannot be

> investigated like existence, it cannot be described like an experience, it is like nothing.... Absolute consciousness... can exist only from *self arrival*... [it] realizes itself knowing the danger: achieve yourself or lose [yourself], become yourself or fall apart.[3]

These words, demonstrating the complexity of Existenz's self-consciousness after the modifications achieved in the transition mechanisms had been assimilated into it, serve to describe the state of Jaspers's thought at this stage of its development, when it was on the verge of changing the central object of explication.[4] The disputing of the insights behind the constitution of Existenz made "knowing the danger" they entailed relevant to Jaspers's thought, so that the danger could be overcome and the Existenz could continue existing. The explication of selfhood, considered at this stage as a philosophical move that had achieved its objective, is repositioned by the exhortations aimed at it: "achieve yourself" and "become yourself." It seems that the desired selfhood, to which Jaspers had aimed already at the beginning, now transpired as a target that had yet to be achieved.

The concept of absolute consciousness enfolds the two facets of the situation of Existenz at this stage: first it experiences a sense of security and is even saturated by the continuing effort to constitute its selfhood. *On the level of consciousness*, the sense of security is reflected in Existenz's self-perception as not wanting to know more; *on the existentialist level* the security is reflected in its self-certainty that is no longer searching for reasons and that knows that it can continue existing even in the boundary situations, despite having no solution for the difficulties or the threat they entail;[5] *on the psychological-mental level* the security is expressed in what Jaspers called "composure" indicating a situation where people feel they can control the fear of annihilation arising from the boundary situations and achieve certainty in Being.[6] The second facet of the condition of Existenz in absolute consciousness is reflected in its ability to face the possibility of its annihilation. In this context, Jaspers described Existenz as trembling and dizzy without any grasp or support, in the destruction of all forms of objectivity,[7] feeling that the finality is sinking and that the person is becoming a "vacuum of Being."[8]

These two facets in the condition of Existenz reflected in the concept of absolute consciousness, the relative certainty and complacency on the one hand, and the feeling of standing on the edge of an abyss on the other, are merely two sides of the same coin. They do not constitute another of the contrasts with which Existenz had to deal throughout its journey of self-clarification, nor one of the antonyms revealed at different stages of the explication of selfhood and in the transition mechanisms. The presence of these two sides together creates a split in the Being of Existenz, which now seems as aiming itself to a new path of existence. In following this path, Existenz has experienced in different ways that not everything is judged by its relation toward itself. Paradoxically, at this stage

Existenz appears as standing securely and stably on both feet, enabling it to move away from its selfhood and cease seeing itself as the source and criterion for everything. Unlike the existential consciousness, which was a constituting factor for some other subjects discussed in the explication of selfhood (such as "existence," "the world," and "consciousness"), absolute consciousness itself constituted a subject for philosophizing.[9] The Existenz bearing this consciousness appears at this stage to have become capable of placing itself for discussion as if it were standing aside, distant from itself in processes it was undergoing. Even the absolute consciousness serves as a mirror for the state of the Existenz when it becomes aware of the possible existence of a Being more encompassing than the existence it is in.[10] However, the innovation is that what is reflected in this mirror is no longer the image of Existenz alone.

Let us examine three of the expressions of absolute consciousness that demonstrate the state of Existenz at this point in Jaspers's philosophy: conscience, faith, and fantasy.

A. Conscience

Jaspers described conscience as a voice not identified with Existenz's self-perception, as reflected in the discussion and its different experiences, such as the drive for communication, suffering, and guilt. Against the background of our discussion of the modifications occurring in the self-perception of Existenz, especially those reflected in the transition mechanisms, we can place conscience in the gap opened in Existenz's perception following the undermining of the solipsistic understanding of selfhood. This is how Jaspers described conscience:

> In conscience I have a *distance* from myself... between my existence and my real selfhood that has yet to be revealed to me, conscience enters as a reality, and from it what has to become a Being for me must be accepted or rejected.[11]

However, the distance of Existenz from its selfhood, enabling the phenomenon of conscience, is not an empty vacuum. The citation above shows that Existenz has some hold on it, or more precisely, it understands that this is the very place of discovering Being, though still without knowing what the nature of this Being is. Jaspers demonstrated the condition of Existenz at this stage in another context when he argued that in conscience a person stands "facing transcendence... without hearing it [but is capable of] obeying it nevertheless like a voice from another world."[12] Transcendence is perceived as being in another world to which Existenz has as yet no access, but it faces it already in the existential state of conscience. The ability of Existenz to move away from itself without requiring the other existing outside it or consciously transcending toward it, as we saw in the transition mechanisms testifies to the maturation of the internal processes that allow it to become acquainted with things beyond it but not detached from it. In conscience, Existenz discovers Being and transcendence as an other existing within itself and grants them meaning even before they become explicit elements in its consciousness. A similar approach viewing the "conscience" as an internal voice calling upon people to be themselves appears also in Martin Heidegger.[13] For a comparison, see also the concept of conscience in Jean Paul Sartre's philosophy.[14]

B. Faith

As with conscience, so in the presentation of faith within the absolute consciousness Jaspers indicated the existence of a certainty that cannot be expressed in forms of knowledge. However, more prominently than was described in conscience, in faith the ability of Existenz to surrender the security granted by the phenomena in existence is especially stressed. It seems that despite the sense of risk accompanying such a surrender, the possibility of becoming acquainted with Being and transcendence is presented at this stage as preferable to Existenz.[15] Jaspers described faith as follows:

> From a subjective point of view, faith is the way the spirit is certain of its Being, its source, and its target, without having sufficiently certain terms for this. From an objective point of view, faith is expressed in the contents that as such remain incomprehensible and in fact only get lost repeatedly.[16]

Faith is unique in that although at this stage there has not yet been any real explication of Being and transcendence, "...possible Existenz has consciousness from transcendence. Before any thought about a specific transcendence it is certain of it or prepared for it."[17] The emphasis on surrendering certainty in the phenomena accords with what Jaspers defined in conscience as the distance Existenz has from itself. Eventually, in faith as in conscience, Existenz's ability to turn away from itself in order to discover something that at this stage it has only a vague idea about is expressed. Faith is a central issue in Jaspers's writings of the third period, which is outside the boundaries of this study. See especially his works *Philosophical Faith in Light of Revelation* and *Philosophical Faith*.[18]

C. Fantasy

In fantasy, the idea of surrendering confidence in the phenomena, also typical of Jaspers's concept of faith, reaches a climax after which, it seems, Existenz is freed from the previous inhibitions that blocked it from contact with Being and with transcendence. As Jaspers put it:

> Through fantasy the eye becomes free to see Being... The contents of fantasy stand with *original certainty* before eyes whose criterion is within it. There are no tests there from reasons or purposes, [since] the moment the fantasy becomes a means its essence is denied it. In [fantasy] there is the Being from which existence is justified for me rather than the opposite.[19]

In contrast with faith, fantasy is unique in that Existenz lacks in it even the consciousness of the surrender accompanying faith. In fantasy a new type of objects of reference is created, in which "I ensure for myself the super-sensory origin of my existence,"[20] and released from the bonds of empirical reality. Jaspers did not require fantasy to be based on anything from within reality, but merely stated vaguely that "its contents become real for me."[21] The reality of these contents is determined by Existenz, and they serve for it as a source of meaning, without requiring this meaning to be accessible to consciousness or to serve as a basis for communication between Existenzes.

The penetration of absolute consciousness as a fantasy into the foundation of Being expresses another stage in the development of Jaspers's thought. After Jaspers was able to establish the perception of selfhood through wide philosophical moves, especially those aimed at achieving world orientation, he could allow himself to turn to fantasy, which in many ways embodies the opposite of world orientation.

> Fantasy allows me to experience the perfect and peace from itself. In the boundary situations everything seemed to me to be torn, impossible, or impure. In fantasy I experience the perfection of Being as beauty... While [the perfection] is not real in the sense of existence, it does not appear as a deception from the love of the absolute consciousness.[22]

From these words, Jaspers seems to be seeking to gather the shreds of the picture of reality arising from the explication of selfhood, and especially from the presentation of the boundary situations, and "stitching" them into a new picture of reality. However, considering the later development of his thinking, and especially the philosophical moves expressed in *Metaphysics*, the third volume of *Philosophy*, it is obvious that the experience of the perfect or the absolute, to which Jaspers refers in this context, was not yet an explicit experience for him, but more of an image for that basic intuition that accompanied his thought from its inception and illuminated his path. In this context, compare Jaspers's words in the introduction to *Psychology*: "The truth of the first experience was not replaced or rejected through later clarity. Substantially, the beginning is already the whole."[23]

The concluding overview of absolute consciousness from observing three of the forms whereby it finds tangible expression—conscience, faith, and fantasy—

shows that just before transcendence and Being became the main and explicit issue in his philosophizing, Jaspers returned to stressing the particular aspect of Existenz's experiences. These forms of existence do not negate the perseverance Jaspers showed in his attempts to break out of the solipsistic position, his starting point, in the later stages of the explication of selfhood, but they do demonstrate once more his basic difficulty as a philosopher in parting with one of his primal insights that had become a home to him.

It seems that what prevented the solipsistic view of selfhood from becoming the final position in Jaspers's philosophy was the introduction of the concepts of Being and transcendence into his discussion of Existenz, an introduction that was sufficient to cause a fundamental change in his perception of selfhood. These terms' becoming part of Existenz's self-perception, as will be seen later in our discussion, led to Jaspers's effort to reveal another Being, different from Existenz, a Being whose existence became apparent at the later stages of the explication of selfhood and even before the tools for its elucidation were found. Some aspects of this Being were revealed already during the process of its self-constitution and were part of it, and this has a decisive importance for the explication of Being, which will be the center of our discussion below; it can be seen as a promise that from Existenz's viewpoint the turning of the philosophizing toward the explication of Being will not occur in a vacuum.

PART THREE

THE EXPLICATION OF BEING

Eight

THE "FOUNDERING"

1. Existenz Toward Transcendence

As Existenz became acquainted with its possible boundaries of realization, as revealed in the face of communication, historicity, and the boundary situations, this created a new self-consciousness for it. It transpired that Existenz did not exist by itself, but was "directed to another Being of freedom"; it found itself "referring to a Being that is not Existenz, but its transcendence."[1] From dealing with the crisis resulting from the transition mechanisms, the understanding arose that they shared one root: the absence of a real relation toward transcendence.

> Placing itself absolutely on itself alone is for Existenz the truth of its independence of the reality of time, but this turns into despair for it. It [Existenz] knows itself that by standing completely by itself it must sink into a vacuum. To the extent that it should become real out of itself, it realizes that what is coming toward it fills it. It is no longer itself if it happens that it remains outside; it faces itself, as if it is given to itself. It verifies its possibility only if it knows itself as based on transcendence.[2]

By defining transcendence as something "coming toward it, fill[ing] it,"[3] Karl Jaspers broke through the boundaries of the discussion of Existenz to the constitution of a Being outside it. In the face of this Being, Jaspers perceived the same internal drive that motivated Existenz already in the explication of selfhood to experience different possibilities, and through them to constitute itself from a consciousness of control and freedom, as sinking into a vacuum and despair. He replaced drive with the awareness gradually forming in his thought whereby Existenz could realize its possibilities only when it recognized that it was based on transcendence. To be more precise, the relation of Existenz toward transcendence, which was at an early stage of constitution, was an outcome of its awareness that it could not exist as a complete Being with its consciousness focused solely on itself and on the existence in which it found itself. However, unlike Existenz's relation toward transcendence in the transition mechanisms, in the discussion of foundering—the central issue in this chapter—this relation was not only about this awareness, but started to become formulated as an element not depending on the meaning it represented for the self-understanding of Existenz.

The despair Existenz was experiencing at this stage denotes additional progress beyond that achieved during the discussion of the transition mechanisms. The feeling of lack accompanying them is now filled with more concrete substance. While the constituting experience in communication was defined as "the insufficiency of myself alone,"[4] the current experience is now understood as "the insufficiency of any Being that is not transcendence."[5] Hans Kunz interprets the insufficiency experienced by Existenz as related to the knowledge of its awaiting death. Against this background he interprets the relation Existenz constitutes toward transcendence as an outcome of people's difficulty in accepting the knowledge that they are destined to lose their existence, and the insufficiency they experience as related to Existenz's nature as an immanent Being.[6] This interpretation, leaving the constituting relation toward transcendence within the boundaries of the explication of selfhood, differs from the interpretation I propose, whereby the insufficiency is not primarily linked to Existenz itself, but instead to what is beyond it, or more precisely to the absence of transcendence. In the process of becoming acquainted with the Being of transcendence the final boundaries of existential freedom were also clarified. The forming awareness of the reality of transcendence naturally involved Existenz becoming aware that the sense of self-sufficiency that had accompanied it so far was based on a limited perception of reality—one that was insufficiently imbued with awareness of the finitude of its existence and itself. There exists a connection between self-consciousness and consciousness of reality—when the first is limited, this has implications also for the second. More precisely, a limited self-consciousness does not enable the formation of a complete perception of reality, which, according to Jaspers, also contains a transcendent facet.

Existenz's attempt to go beyond its selfhood by referring to transcendence reflected a more comprehensive shift in Jaspers's thought whereby the status of Existenz was altered. Instead of serving as the object of philosophizing, it now became the starting point for the constitution of a relation toward the Being existing beyond it. Existenz's aiming to transcendence not only led it along new paths beyond itself that it had known before, but also affected the insights that had been achieved regarding Existenz in the explication of selfhood. Now Jaspers was able to state that "the modes of searching for Being from possible Existenz are *ways* to transcendence, and their *clarification* is philosophical *metaphysics*."[7] The new understanding of the philosophy of Existenz as metaphysics does not prevent Existenz from continuing its self-clarification in this context, since it is the one becoming acquainted with transcendence.[8] However, it is a matter of principle that the additional layers added to its existing consciousness are derived only indirectly from the elucidation of transcendence and not from its focusing on its self-elucidation.

The new definition granted to the philosophy of Existenz was not intended to separate the explication of selfhood from the metaphysical approach—an approach that the explication of Being, at the center of the discussion in this section, was directly aimed at constituting. The very formation of transcendence as the target for explication was not only enabled thanks to the maturation of Existenz's self-consciousness, but also itself portrayed this maturity. The explication of selfhood itself transpires as an integral part of the philosophical effort to constitute a metaphysical consciousness. The new definition Jaspers gave to his thought should not be understood as a denial of the importance of Existenz in the process of elucidating transcendence, but as an expression of a change in Existenz's self-consciousness regarding its mode of existence in the world: it shifts from "existence as an Existenz" to "existence as an Existenz in the face of transcendence."

The preliminary concept Existenz has regarding transcendence is necessarily based on the contrast between them, as revealed in the explication of selfhood: transcendence was perceived as a Being in which "there is no freedom and no bondage (*Unfreiheit*)."[9] This means that on the one hand, the Being of transcendence does not rely on the freedom of Existenz to come and constitute it, but exists as it is independently, not only for Existenz. This explains the definition of transcendence as "reality without possibility,"[10] expressing the perception of transcendence itself as an existing real entity. Also, this definition stresses the contrast between transcendence and Existenz, since unlike Existenz, transcendence is not a potential Being, but an entity whose existence is independent. On the other hand, the statement that "there is no bondage (*Unfreiheit*)" shows that the Being of transcendence or Existenz's referring to it does not negate the autonomy of Existenz or make it irrelevant, even though all we know about transcendence at this stage we learned from the elucidation of Existenz's attitude toward it.

The concept "formal transcending," dealing with thought's understanding of itself as analogous,[11] reflects Existenz's self-consciousness in the face of transcendence at this stage. Existenz *still* cannot achieve a direct characterization of transcendence, beyond recognizing the very existence of a difference between this entity and its entity, but it *already* knows that everything it can know about it is obtained indirectly and never unambiguously.[12] The difficulty in distinguishing between the two types of reference of Existenz toward transcendence—the one seeing it as an entity beyond the Being of Existenz, and the more minimalist one understanding itself as analogous to it and not as directly representing this entity—will continue to accompany the explication of Being even at later stages, and perhaps can never be resolved. In any case, this duality well reflects the condition of the philosophizing at the beginning of the explication of Being: it recognizes its roots in the explication of selfhood, but at the same time aims to represent transcendence as an entity beyond the boundaries of existentialist consciousness as elucidated so far.

Since at this stage of the explication the thought about transcendence had no real basis to rely on, at this stage the thought about transcendence is defined as thought about the nothingness.[13] The nothingness is the not the object of the thought aimed at a positive reality, but an expression of the state of the thought in face of what it seeks to think about.[14] The thought experiences referring to something whose existence it does not possess the tools to confirm. To demonstrate the need for another type of thinking in the face of transcendence, Jaspers states that "about nothingness we can think only through non-thinking."[15] This means that we need thought capable of referring to something even when it has no certainty regarding its existence. However, like Martin Heidegger, who believed that "the nothingness does not remains the undefined realm against the is, ... it belongs to the entity of the is" itself, Jaspers apparently also saw the nothing as a mode of a real or positive entity and not just as a formal category of thought.[16] As he put it: "For the first time the qualified nothingness [is] as the nothing of something qualified whose meaning should be the Being of its nothing... whose correlate could be the Being in itself."[17] These words clarify the relevance of the "formal transcending" to the first stages of the explication of Being. This transcending defines simultaneously both the condition of the philosophizing on the threshold of the explication of Being and also the nature of the thought formulated in it regarding Being itself. The distance of the thought from the tangible and categorical nature becomes a positive quality of what Jaspers termed "the existential interest in Being."[18]

The Existenz directed at transcendence as a Being contrasting with it experiences a shock following which it has no way back to what it was before: "Existenz exists only in relation to transcendence or else it does not exist. In this relation it has its own insufficiency, or the annihilation (*Aufhebung*) of existence in time [it will have] its possible sufficiency."[19] However, because Existenz is responsible for the separation of the thought from its objective nature, a separation constituting the formal transcending, this prevents the possibility that the shock could lead to a more total collapse of the philosophical infrastructure originating in the explication of selfhood. The definition of Existenz at this stage as a "bond" demonstrates its centrality in the discussion at this stage, but now, unlike its self-perception during the explication of selfhood, it recognizes itself as being constituted outside itself, by transcendence.[20]

This understanding probably served later as an element in rescuing the reference to transcendence from the contrast with Existenz and the constitution of a more positive, direct approach to it. In Kantian terms, we can see this as an element for the "unthinkable" not becoming for Existenz a boundary where consciousness is no longer able to contain what it encounters, but merely a "limit" from which progress toward the constitution of direct awareness of transcendence is not necessarily denied it. The shock Existenz experienced as a result of becoming acquainted with the existence of transcendence expresses the contrast between transcendence and Existenz, and at the same time serves as a "starting point"[21] and "origin"[22] following the constitution of transcendence as a uniform Being, portraying identity between its possibility and its existing reality.[23]

Already now, even before transcendence has received any real explication, we can observe a different relation Existenz is forming toward the existence surrounding it. Existenz recognizes that there no longer exists any room to refer to existence from the consciousness of ownership and power that accompanied its attempts to realize the possibilities it identified in existence; now it transpires that only "where I push *reality without turning it into a possibility*, there I meet transcendence."[24] Jaspers's words in this context can be compared with Heidegger's discussion of technology in his later writings.[25] This background reconfirms the understanding that linked the boundaries of self-consciousness with the boundaries of the reality in which this self-consciousness is anchored. In this context it transpires that just as the perception of Existenz as sovereign over the existence surrounding it largely determined the boundaries of its horizons, so also its acquaintance with transcendence is an outcome of a different self-perception that enabled it to expand its sphere of reference. Now the absolute is transferred from the realm of Existenz to that of transcendence, and the contents of the absolute are also altered: while the absolute of Existenz was portrayed in the activity it could show toward its existence, the absolute attributed to transcendence is expressed in the fixity and thusness that create a barrier between it and what it is beyond—between transcendence and Existenz.

2. Foundering as a Philosophical Concept

The constitution of Jaspers's concept of foundering was based on the self-consciousness of Existenz as existing in light of transcendence. This consciousness causes a transformation in the Existenz's self-understanding, and as a result, in its perception of its place in existence. This is how Jaspers described the concept of foundering (*Scheitern*):

> The *foundering* is *the ultimate* (*das Letzte*); that is how the cruel realistic world orientation is proved … The knowledge sees itself placed upon the boundaries in front of antonymous in which the possibility of thought lacking any contradiction collapse; beyond and outside knowledge it floats as a thing embracing any truth that is not rational. It founders for the *world orientation* the world as existence, since it cannot be understood out of itself and in itself; this is since it does not become a self-contained Being that can be seen through, nor can the process of consciousness realize itself up to a whole. It founders *in elucidation of Existenz* the in-itself selfhood of Existenz: where I myself really exist, I do not exist only as myself.[26]

While the term "failure" indicates missing some possibilities, the concept of foundering denotes a change in the existentialist consciousness and a radical turning point in Jaspers's philosophy that has implications both for his idea of selfhood and for that of Being. While the first stages of Jaspers's perception of selfhood might be viewed as based on failures, these were local, relative, and each time some solution was found within the boundaries of the explication of selfhood. This approach was especially prominent in *Psychology*, where Jaspers proposed different alternatives of world views as a solution for the problems that had appeared in earlier world views in his discussion of "types" and "world views."[27] However, the first two volumes of *Philosophy* also showed a similar tendency, trying each time new directions of discussion that better suited the character of Existenz as Jaspers wished to constitute it. Jaspers chose to detach Existenz from the world and then found a way to reintegrate it. See the discussion in Chapter Three. Conversely, the idea of "foundering" appears to denote the impossibility of finding an escape path. The constitution of a new framework of philosophizing relying on different premises than those of *World Orientation* and *Elucidation of Existenz*, although without alienating the insights achieved there, is required. *World Orientation* and *Elucidation of Existenz* did not fail, which would have negated their value for the philosophizing aimed at transcendence, but foundered. Therefore, what is required is transcending from them in favor of a new philosophizing framework that has no existence without them as its foundation and background. This framework, to be termed the explication of Being, has to adapt itself to the new self-perception of Existenz, but especially has to enable a direct elucidation of the concepts of "Being" and "transcendence."[28]

Johannes Thyssen shared the understanding of foundering as a philosophical concept that served in Jaspers's thought as a basis for the constitution of a new framework of philosophizing. In his opinion, the failure does not primarily express Jaspers's familiar objection to positivism, idealism, and the old metaphysics that presents itself as an ontology. Thyssen states that the foundering signifies Jaspers's determined effort to constitute a positive consciousness regarding transcendence.[29] This interpretation developed for Thyssen into an almost complete separation between *Metaphysics*—the third volume of *Philosophy*—and the explication of selfhood.[30] According to Thyssen, the foundering shows that it is possible that with all the effort invested in the constitution of Existenz, it might not become a complete Being. It would not be able to form a relation toward transcendence, and would even cease to exist as such.[31] This interpretation implies that *Metaphysics* replaces *World Orientation* and *Elucidation of Existenz*, and that the idea of foundering creates a radical change in Jaspers's thought that does not allow any continuity with his earlier insights. Thyssen believed that *Metaphysics* achieved the insight whereby Existenz no longer appears in Jaspers's thought as *sui causa*.[32] However, as we have seen, this insight started to be formulated in Jaspers's thought even before the idea of the failure—already within *World*

Orientation and *Elucidation of Existenz*, and most prominently in the transition mechanisms—and in this respect it cannot be detached from the explication of selfhood, which at its early stages also revealed the boundaries of Existenz. In this respect Jaspers could, apparently, have avoided the extreme term "foundering," as suggested by Fritz-Joachim Von Rinteln, who proposed a different radical interpretation of this concept.[33] Thyssen's interpretation, which at this point granted Jaspers's philosophy a particular chaotic nature, stands in contrast to these words of Jaspers's:

> True selfhood cannot hold itself through itself alone; it can lead to its absence for itself [but] it wants not to force itself to this. As it succeeds at this more decisively, so are better clarified the boundaries where it is denied. It becomes poised for its other, [for] transcendence, when it founders in the wish for its self-sufficiency. ...*I can founder as me myself*, without the philosophical trust, the divine word, and the religious confidence helping, and despite this it appears that all the truths and the poise are there.[34]

From these words we see that foundering does *not* indicate the collapse of Existenz as a real Being in *Metaphysics*, but instead the loosening of the will for self-sufficiency. What has foundered, what has lost the meaning it received in the earlier philosophical discussion, but at the same time serves as a basis for the constitution of a new framework of philosophizing, is the solipsistic perception of selfhood. Existenz's becoming acquainted with its boundaries, through its experience of foundering, has a positive meaning precisely in the sense that it discovers that the constitution of a relation toward transcendence opens to it a wider range of meaning in its existence. A similar interpretation is that of Johannes Pfeiffer, who states that "only the foundering finitude can become a tool containing the fullness of transcendence," although this appears to be intended mainly to elucidate Jaspers's perception of faith appearing in the writings of the third period.[35] So, foundering functions, according to the interpretation proposed here, as a symbol of this meaning, and in contrast to Thyssen's opinion, Existenz continues to be relevant to the explication of Being. Kurt Salamun also presented an interpretation of the concept of foundering with an ethical orientation.[36] The condition for experiencing foundering is the presence of a positive will on its part "not to force itself," or, from the viewpoint of the philosophizing, that it should not be placed as the sole object of explication, enabling the constitution of a relation to what was beyond it. If this condition is met, the foundering indirectly testifies to the living reality of the Existenz that experiences it, since only what is itself—what is Existenz—can founder. The very experience of foundering is avoided for non-Existenzes, while failure itself is revealed as an option for the

Existenz embodied in its ability not to force itself and to open up to transcendence.

However, for Thyssen foundering is not just a philosophical concept that has implications for the relevance of the explication of selfhood to Jaspers's metaphysical approach. In his opinion, this concept also expresses the experience of extreme irrationality.[37] The perception of foundering as an expression of experiencing irrationality was shared by other interpreters. Von Rinteln formulated a similar position when he argued that presenting foundering as a central experience in the search for transcendence expressed the pessimism and prejudice Jaspers and other existentialist philosophers had regarding the spirit of objectivity and the thoughts included in it.[38] From Von Rinteln's words it transpires that such a position in principle regarding objectivity is destined to lead to an irrational position that the idea of foundering reflects.

The distinction between "irrationalism" and "a-rationalism" can help in this context assess these interpretations regarding the concept of foundering, as they reflect more widely one of the directions around which the criticism of Jaspers's philosophy and of existentialist thought in general developed. This interpretation is usually identified with William Barrett but it is also common among many researchers.[39] Irrationalism contrasts with rationalism as a world view and reacts to it by opposition, while a-rationalism is not built on the negation of the rationalist approach, although it differs from it. As we have seen in different contexts of the discussion of the perception of selfhood, although Jaspers recognized the sometimes antonymous nature of the reality in which human beings live and act, he did not tire of his effort to constitute a consciousness regarding existence that could deal with its antonymous aspect. In this respect, the concept of boundary situations, reflecting the antonymous nature of people's reality, expresses the formulation of Jaspers's attempt to introduce order and organization into the consciousness referring to it. This interpretation also applied to many key concepts appearing in Jaspers's philosophy, such as world views, Existenz, and others. This statement does not suddenly make Jaspers's approach rational, let alone grant it a rationalistic character, but it seeks to illuminate one of the crucial motivations that shaped his philosophical position.[40] This general position has direct implications for the interpretation I propose for the concept of foundering, which in any case does not attribute to it a meaning of an irrational experience, but at most locates it within the realm of a-rational experience. This means that experiencing foundering shows that we cannot expect the world in which the individual exists necessarily to react to the rational patterns on which human consciousness is based, but that it has some aspects beyond the boundaries of rationality.

Foundering, as an expression of an experience that is neither rational nor irrational, is not derived from philosophy of Existenz, but nor does it reflect an absence of possible relevance for the constitution of a metaphysical consciousness, as Thyssen believed. Positively, we can argue that the foundering revealed in the metaphysical approach as a basic datum of finitude itself demands formulation from a different viewpoint, where both positive and negative, both construction and destruction in selfhood and in the world, can find expression. In this respect, the concept of foundering reflects the basic duality in which the existential references to transcendence are anchored—it contains a negation of the selfhood as a self-sufficient autonomic Being but also affirms it as a condition for the constitution of a metaphysical relation toward transcendence. The concept of failure entails Existenz's ability to move away from itself and at the same time confirms its relevance for the explication of Being.[41]

This complex link between Existenz and the possibility of experiencing through the foundering to constitute a relation toward transcendence is concisely expressed in the argument that "transcendence must already be present, where I seek it."[42] This means that those who experience the search for what is beyond the boundaries of their existence will encounter transcendence through the relation they form toward it. However, this statement also contains the understanding that transcendence is not constituted by the very search of Existenz, but it pre-exists, and in this respect the reality of transcendence does not depend on Existenz. From Existenz's viewpoint we can state that its experience of foundering, following which it turns to what is beyond the boundaries of its existence, has a decisive value in making transcendence significant for it. Without this search, transcendence would not exist for it. As Jaspers says: "from the consciousness of foundering comes… the possibility of real activity."[43] However, it is precisely because the foundering diverts the question of world orientation as a real Being from the center of the person's consciousness and moderates the drive to elucidate selfhood that it is a grasp point for what is beyond both Existenz and the world. What foundering indicates is that any realization in the realm of the phenomena must pass. As Jaspers put it: "when Being as a phenomenon in existence reaches a high-point, then this point is simultaneously just a point that turns into loss in order to save the truth of height [*Höhe*]…"[44] Existenz's self-consciousness of the foundering enables it to state that "what is real is not yet or no longer,"[45] meaning that transcendence is marked at this point as "real" or as a source, but it has not yet been explicated. In contrast, Existenz, which so far had been perceived as "real," can no longer be considered so in the face of the modifications to the perception of selfhood, which reached their peak in the explication of the concept of foundering. Foundering as a starting point does not lose contact with the earlier moves that led to it and enabled it to be experienced, but it grants the insights apparently already achieved in previous contexts another meaning that also determines their different status within the new framework of philosophizing.

3. Freedom of Existenz and Foundering

The experience of foundering, which revealed that transcendence was the target to which Existenz aims itself, raises the question of its existential freedom. The question is simple: can selfhood stop at the upper point of the elucidation of Existenz—whatever that is—and remain there without constituting a relation toward transcendence? Can Existenz be constituted only through negative freedom, or does it only become an Existenz when it positively realizes its freedom, a freedom including the very constitution of its selfhood and its relation toward transcendence? Does Existenz even have the option of not foundering, and avoiding the formation of a relation toward transcendence, or is a person having become an Existenz obliged to constitute such a relation? It is no wonder that these general questions arise at this stage of the research, when the object of explication is replaced. Their appearance demonstrates the methodological framework in which this study is conducted, marking and illuminating the central turning points in Jaspers's process of philosophizing. The question about existential freedom becomes a key question at this stage, not only because the foundering does not negate the existence of Existenz and the world, which continue to serve as key factors in the framework of philosophizing aimed at the explication of Being, but mainly due to the changes in the status of Existenz in Jaspers's discussion, with the introduction of transcendence as a factor.

We can find a basis for dealing with this problem raised by the concept of failure in Jaspers's statement that "[since] freedom exists only through nature and against it, it must founder as freedom or as existence."[46] The vagueness of this statement leaves room for more than one interpretation. However, the interpretation Jaspers gave elsewhere to the concept of nature, which is rare in his philosophical language, can help understand the intention of this issue, which has great significance for understanding the status of Existenz within the explication of Being.[47] Nature was defined as a wholeness and as what is necessarily more than what is perceived in it. In this respect, Jaspers saw a representation of the two facets of human Being: on the one hand, nature expresses something whose internality is not accessible to people, the dark basis surrounding them, the demon in their life, and the other whose very existence is beyond their control. On the other hand, nature portrays the element of spirit and perfection existing in all things, the rationality that opens people's options for realization.[48]

Against the background of this perception of nature, we can argue that the statement that "freedom must founder" was a-priori anchored in a perception of a Being with infinite dimensions, compared with the one discussed in the explication of selfhood, which relied on the finite boundaries of existence and that lacked a relation toward a transcendent Being. Foundering does not contrast with the perception of existential freedom, as presented in *Elucidation of Existenz*, precisely because at that stage Existenz was confronted with itself and not with the possible existence of a transcendent Being that creates the very experience of foundering. The argument that Existenz must founder and form a relation toward a transcendent Being should not be viewed as an expression of a withdrawal from the perception of Existenz as a free Being, but as a more general shift taking place in Jaspers's thought that also influenced other insights related to Existenz. Finally, the interpretation of the statement that Existenz must founder "as freedom or as existence" is that finitude cannot exist as an independent entity, and Existenz, too, must recognize transcendence as an infinite space, in which it is anchored as a finite Being by its relation toward it.

The introduction of the term "nature" into the discussion of foundering redefines the boundaries of existential freedom and helps us understand the status of Existenz in light of transcendence. This is not the complete denial of Existenz's freedom—what could have led to the eventual removal of Existenz from the explication of Being. It is transcendence as a Being external to it that illuminates more correctly the image of Existenz and helps it understand itself better. Understanding the freedom of Existenz as dependent on nature[49] turns nature into Existenz's field of foundering, where it becomes acquainted both with the infinity existing beyond it and with nature. The argument that "the lack of explainability of the whole that cannot be recognized as a wholeness prevents nature turning into a Being in itself"[50] joins and complements this interpretative move. The result is preventing the identification of transcendence with nature, or more precisely, with the infinity with which Existenz becomes acquainted by reflection about nature. Also, what becomes undoubtedly impossible is the attempt to "hold Existenz as [existing] for all."[51]

Even if Existenz cannot avoid its basic struggle in existence, enabled first and foremost by the freedom it is granted, the experience of foundering makes the unbridgeable gap between it and nature in which it is destined to live into a penetrating self-consciousness.[52] This consciousness must lead, in Jaspers's opinion, to Existenz itself "crashing in existence."[53] The foundering "as freedom or existence" does not indicate the loss of freedom and of Existenz as a foundering, but instead implies a process that enabled Existenz to turn to what is beyond the space of realization that existential freedom demarcated, toward transcendence. As Jaspers phrased it: "It must take itself into the foundering, first in the activity of its daring and then in the possibility of its own foundering."[54]

However, diverting Existenz from the center of the arena of philosophizing in favor of the explication of transcendence is not enabled solely thanks to the new awareness described above. In this context we can identify in Jaspers's words two facets that contribute to the foundering occurring: on the one hand, the attitude toward transcendence is presented as an expression of the establishment of Existenz as an explicit Being described as one "whose independence [means] wanting the impossible."[55] The more it progresses decisively and is not satisfied with finite reality, the more it wants to transcend its finitude, and "therefore it must founder."[56] On the other hand, the role of Existenz as instigating the foundering is not the be-all and end-all. Jaspers showed that over-emphasizing the principle of the individuation of the individual presents Existenz in the foundering as an expression of the "wantonness of selfhood" to the point that "turning into finite would have been considered as guilt by such."[57] This perception of selfhood reflects, in Jaspers's opinion, mystical thinking in which human freedom appears to be getting lost. He argues:

> Since finitude is universal, any particular existence and not only man falls into it, it cannot actually be experienced as guilt of self-will, since this is accessible only to its own existence, where the blindness of its self-preservation exists. However, here self-will must not necessarily have the final word for Existenz, but it can be forced on... its independence. The inevitable guilt then first experiences this independence from which not only is self-will controlled, but also the measure of finitude is exceeded.[58]

With these words, Jaspers added another layer to the philosophical move in which the role of Existenz in realizing the foundering was clarified. They show that not only Existenz, but also existence as finitude is pushed from itself to founder, meaning that even finitude itself cannot exist without the existence of an infinite Being that probably supports it. In this context, Jaspers chose to stress by the term "inevitable guilt," which in *Elucidation of Existenz* was presented as part of Existenz's self-consciousness, another element. The presence of this guilt in the context of the discussion of foundering helps illuminate the forces existing beyond the Being of Existenz and acting to constitute the relation toward transcendence. Jaspers referred to the issue of inevitable guilt mainly in his discussion of boundary situations, where this guilt is one of the private boundary situations.[59] It not only continues to strengthen the consciousness of the boundaries of human Being and its subjection to forces beyond finitude and the possibilities of understanding, which are also essential for the experience of foundering, but also indicates the existence of infinite forces that influence both existence and Existenz, and epitomize transcendence for them.

Either way, whether we look at things from Existenz's point of view or from that of finitude itself, it is apparently an almost inevitable process leading to the presence of transcendence in reality—as an existential Being and as finitude at all. It is hard to assume that the deterministic hints arising from Jaspers's discussion in this context could have been unconscious, or that the contradiction between them and the essence of existential freedom was hidden from him. At this point, Jaspers stretched the line of philosophizing to the peak point, from which onwards transcendence was to become a religious position, under which the person would stand with the subjugation of accepting justice. In elucidating the attitude toward the transcendence being constituted by the experience of foundering Jaspers sought to harness to the metaphysical aspect that leads Existenz to transcendence also what appeared as a horizon viewed from existence itself and also leading to transcendence. This tendency, which was to reach its full maturation in the perception of ciphers, contributes to rescuing the relation toward transcendence from the existential nature typical of the references toward it in the transition mechanisms and the basic insights typifying the perception of selfhood that formed from examining its relation to itself.[60] See the discussion of the perception of ciphers in Chapter Ten. Although Existenz continued to play a crucial role in constituting the relation toward transcendence and was understood anew in light of this relation, for the first time in Jaspers's thought a handling of transcendence as an actual reality not dependent on the approval of the Existenz referring to it started to form.

4. Foundering as a "Cipher"

The complexity typical of Jaspers's thought is well clarified by the presentation of foundering as a "cipher"—a term that will be elucidated separately in Chapter Ten below. On the one hand, he wished to lead Existenz beyond the boundaries of its selfhood and to present transcendence as a close horizon serving for it as a target it had yet to achieve. On the other hand, Jaspers's discussion of transcendence at this stage remained within the boundaries of the relation Existenz constitutes toward it and did not include a direct elucidation of the reality of transcendence itself. This duality is reflected in the following passage:

> One cannot jump over finitude except through foundering itself. In canceling time in the metaphysical contemplation aimed at foundering, without experiencing its reality, I once again founder so decisively into finite existence. However, whoever cancels time in real foundering does not go backwards; in the inaccessibility of what remains, he requires finite existence to leave the Being of transcendence unimpeached. We cannot know why the world exists; perhaps we can experience this as a foundering, but we can no longer *say* this. In face of Being and against the dimensions of foundering, language also ceased in existence with thought. Only silence is possible in the face of the silence in existence.[61]

The perception of finite reality as a space of foundering, as a source for the constitution of transcendence, does not reflect the way this reality presents itself, but is revealed as an expression of the presence of Existenz at an early stage of the search for the meaning of existence through the attempt to transcend it. Through the idea of the cipher, Jaspers sketched the space stretched between this finitude and transcendence, as a reality that did not yet exist. This space, included in finitude but appearing to "speak" its own language, leaves transcendence as a

Being that requires mediation by Existenz, which appears at present not to have found the right words yet. The presence of transcendence within existence through the foundering is merely the other facet of its absence in the same existence and of the distance separating it from finitude. This duality is the essence of the cipher, in which transcendence appears as a "present-absent" Being: to the extent that it is present for Existenz it is absent in existence as a finitude, and to the extent that it is present in existence as a finitude and as a Being that can be interpreted, it is hidden from Existenz, which has yet to find its way toward it. The experience of foundering, through which the fullness of transcendence is condensed into the finite dimensions of the cipher, connected transcendence to finitude and to Existenz, which sees it as a source of meaning.[62] However, the Being of the cipher that represents a metaphysical presence, but does not portray this presence fully and openly, guarantees that transcendence does not develop into defined objective knowledge that with its achievement would leave Existenz behind.

In the end, the experience of foundering brought the philosophizing around Existenz to a crisis, and placed it at a point of no return—either the crisis would lead to the collapse of the philosophy of Existenz, or it would show it a new path. This path would not appear *ex nihilo*, since it was preceded by a long process where the philosophizing had made real achievements. If these achievements could survive the crisis, they would enter a new world of meanings, much wider and more encompassing—a world whose handling would require different conditions from those in whose framework the philosophizing had so far developed. This world of meanings would have to enable simultaneously both the existence of Existenz and the existence of the world as a real Being, but since after the crisis of foundering neither would be the same as before, the philosophizing after the elucidation of the concept of foundering was destined to be formulated by new criteria.

Nine

BEING AS ENCOMPASSING

The transcendence viewed through the experience of foundering still remained a Being beyond the world and Existenz. However, the task "to experience Being in foundering,"[1] with which Karl Jaspers concluded *Philosophy*, hinted to Being becoming the focus of his interest in the works published later: *Reason and Existenz*, *Philosophy of Existenz*, and *Out of Truth*.[2] It was probably due to the publication ban imposed on his writings in 1938 that Jaspers was unable to publish his book *Out of Truth* (1947) until after the end of the war. Many of the ideas appearing in this book were formulated in his writings published in the mid-nineteen-thirties, especially in *Reason and Existenz* (1935) and *Philosophy of Existenz* (1937/1938). Ernst Mayer, Jasper's brother-in-law, who followed his work closely, claimed that *Reason and Existenz* and *Philosophy of Existenz* were a preparation for *Out of Truth*.[3] Kurt Salamun and Gerhard Knauss attributed the origin of the perception of encompassing in the appendix Jaspers wrote about Immanuel Kant's theory of ideas that was appended to *Psychology*.[4] They believe this perception constitutes an interpretation of the Kantian theory of ideas.[5] Compare also Urs Richli's position, whereby the concept of the encompassing is an interpretation of Kant's theory of ideas and transcendental deduction.[6] In these writings, Jaspers addresses Being using concepts like reality (*Wirklichkeit*) and Being (*Sein*), but the central concept denoting it was encompassing (*Umgreifende*). Although crucial aspects connected to the explication of Being appeared already in *Philosophy*, the discussion of Being in his later writings marked a further advance in the development of the metaphysical consciousness in Jaspers's writings. These writings show the tendency to propose an explication precisely for what was for Kant beyond the boundaries of the philosophical discussion: Being-in-itself. Transcendence and the transcendent, extensively discussed in *Philosophy*, continue to represent in his later works some aspects of Being that are not accessible using the tools of philosophical thinking. However, in these writings, Jaspers's effort to turn philosophizing itself into a tool for the comprehensive and complete explication of Being becomes apparent.

At the center of our discussion in this chapter is Jaspers's perception of the encompassing, which reached the peak of its development in *Out of Truth*. Already the immediate meaning arising from this original term of Jaspers's shows a basic duality: the encompassing is located on the margins of another reality in relation to which it is central, but at the same time this reality is surrounded by something existing beyond it. Jaspers coined the term *Umgreifende* by combining the verb *greifen*, meaning "to grasp," and the preposition *um*, meaning "around." The English term "encompassing" attempts to preserve the meaning of the *relation* and to indicate the perception of the Being as existing beyond the consciousness referring to it. The two meanings arising from the term encompassing reveal the premises with which Jaspers approached the explication of Being. First, they indicate the basic image of Being as a reality encompassing human beings. This facet is connected to the understanding that what exists for people is not all that there is, and that people turn to what Jaspers called "*the widest extent of the possible*" to understand themselves and the reality in which they live.[7] In this context, compare Salamun's interpretation, whereby the encompassing is close to the Greek concept of *logos*.[8] Second, the duality in the encompassing denotes people's location in relation to it, meaning the perception of Being as existing beyond them. This aspect is connected to Jaspers's description of people as living and thinking within a horizon that gives them a wider knowledge. The basic phenomenon of the constant revealing of horizons beyond them raises, in Jaspers's opinion, the question of Being, which is a question regarding the nature or the power responsible for this phenomenon.[9] Third, we can view this basic unresolved duality as a reflection of the philosophical process that Jaspers himself underwent. At the beginning, selfhood was placed at the center of the philosophical discussion, but as it developed, the boundaries of selfhood and the limitations of the viewpoint focusing on it were revealed. Selfhood gradually became an issue of secondary importance, while Being was revealed as a wider and more comprehensive subject to which the philosophizing was aimed.

Jaspers expressed the status of Being within the explication of selfhood by describing Being as avoiding those who wished to perceive it as an unclosed whole "enabling a new thing always to return and come toward us as a particular Being."[10] Jaspers demonstrated the condition of a person wishing to perceive Being when he compared such a person to the Baron Munchausen trying to pull himself out of a swamp by his hair.[11] Jaspers did not perceive Being, which he wished to elucidate in his philosophy, as equaling the sum of all the existing things appearing in immanent reality, but as existing beyond them. However, he stressed that Being's ability to be portrayed also in the forms of immanent existence is what enables our contact with it.[12] The starting point that is divided—between the existential viewpoint that germinated the philosophizing directed at Being, and the aim to escape it and push the field of discussion beyond the boundaries of selfhood—will accompany the interpretation of Jaspers's perception of Being I will present below. This interpretation aims to reflect the tension arising from the basic duality in which the perception of the encompassing was anchored, and at the same time to express Jaspers's wish to overcome this duality in order to constitute a uniform perception of Being.

1. The Encompassing Between Two Viewpoints: Epistemological and Ontological

In one of his first references to the encompassing, Jaspers described it as a Being in which the things exist and through which they remain transparent.[13] This connection between reality and transparency, or between the question of Being and the question of knowledge, reflects the presence of the two viewpoints, epistemological and ontological, which were revealed as constituting elements of Jaspers's thought from its beginning. Another expression of the existence of these two viewpoints is apparent in what Jaspers presented as the basic and unresolved paradox existing in the elucidation of the concept of the encompassing: it aims to perceive Being that is not an object, knowing that the tools with which it was equipped were suited mainly for objects.[14] These words affirm the relevance of the problems already familiar to us from the explication of selfhood to the explication of Being, the need to determine the boundaries of formal reason and at the same time to grant philosophical meaning to the entity to which the philosophizing is aimed but which reason cannot represent fully. Against this background we can redefine the target of the two viewpoints whose full implications for Jaspers's perception of Being will become clear later in our discussion: the *epistemological viewpoint*, examining the operation of knowledge on the objects facing it, will save the discussion from dealing with the particular aspects of the Being of Existenz and will grant Jaspers's philosophy a more communicative nature. Jaspers devoted the third lecture in his book *Reason and Existenz* to this issue of the communication existing in each of the circles of the encompassing.[15] In parallel, the *ontological viewpoint* aims to derive from objectivity and from the phenomena an inclusive picture of Being whose reality is not derived from Existenz or from the existence in which it participates.

Within the framework of his concept of the encompassing, Jaspers did not systematically present the conditions that would make Being better understood by reason, nor the components of this Being itself. In this respect, the perception of the encompassing cannot be defined as epistemology, nor as ontology. However, we can state that both viewpoints reach their fullest development and their maximal functionality with the explication of Being. For the first time in his philosophy, Jaspers was able to develop a clear and distinct system of concepts that contributed to the clarity of his ideas and moderated the intuitive aspect that accompanied the explication of selfhood and was expressed in the vagueness that surrounded the ideas formulated there. Concepts such as "philosophical logic" and "encompassing" with its different components received definitions and separate discussions instead of being clarified indirectly, through an examination of their usage in the different contexts of discussion. One of the clearest expressions of this transformation in Jaspers's thought compared with the explication of selfhood is that the theory of the encompassing did not place as a condition for its understanding the personal involvement of the readers in the experiences elucidated in it and the fact of the readers being an Existenz themselves. An expression of this demand for involvement appears, for example, in Jaspers's statement in the introduction to *Psychology* that "this book has meaning only for those who have started to wonder."[16] This datum, and the more structured nature of the discussion in general, enable us to state that the explication of Being constitutes a more communicative stage in Jaspers's philosophy. Since such a discussion is much more accessible to criticism—both by the philosopher himself and by his readers—I argue that Jaspers's perception of Being is more philosophical than his perception of selfhood.

The clearest expression of the communicative nature typical of Jaspers's perception of Being is reflected in the manifestation of the aim to constitute a metaphysical consciousness, which up to this stage had only been implied in Jaspers's thought. For the first time in the perception of the encompassing, the constitution of a metaphysical consciousness is presented as the overt aim at which the philosophizing is aimed. Without doubt, the precondition enabling the placing of this aim at the center of the explication of Being was the awareness of the enforcing, isolating, and restricting nature of individuality[17] as expressed in some aspects of the philosophy of Existenz. This awareness allowed, and even forced, selfhood to turn from dealing exclusively with itself and to open to what was beyond it. However, the process of distancing from the solipsistic thought pattern, which originated in the constitution of the concept of Existenz, and on which the relation toward the external reality was based, was further deepened when Being was placed as the object of the philosophizing. This process had two main implications, which shaped the framework of the explication of Being. In terms of the *contents*, this was expressed in Existenz no longer being portrayed as an isolated Being nor even as a lodestone setting the boundaries of the discussion of other issues and influencing the contents Jaspers gave them. In terms of the *structure*, Jaspers's discussion was not aimed at a single object of philosophizing, and this prevented the possibility of any single object being given supremacy or even totality. The concept of the encompassing was anchored in the categorical necessity of the multiplicity of foci of reference, which were not supposed to be resolved, and could help reject even further the remnants of the solipsistic perception of selfhood and prevent the formation of an absolute perception of Being.

The encompassing that embodies a fundamental duality is based on the consciousness of the existence of an unknown boundary where individuals understand themselves as "constituting his life not from mere self-will, nor from mere obedience, but because [he faces] Being in its entirety" and everything that exists beyond them.[18] While at this stage, people perceive themselves as part of the Being they wish to elucidate, they know that it ranges far beyond them. Jaspers's philosophical self-consciousness expressed in the perception of the encompassing is not expressed only in the ability to evaluate the achievements and limitations of the way his thought had developed so far, since this evaluation appeared already in the discussion of the transition mechanisms and the foundering. In the perception of the encompassing Jaspers progressed another step by implementing these insights in the framework of a new philosophizing that was clear and transparent in its contents and concepts. The perception of the encompassing did not become a philosophical system in the rigorous sense of the word, but the transparency of the epistemological and ontological viewpoints in this context created more convenient conditions for the elucidation of the Being to which Jaspers's philosophy was aimed at this stage. Knauss argued that the perception of the encompassing is largely unsystematic and arbitrary; however, his position was an inevitable outcome of the logical viewpoint from which he examined the perception of the encompassing, which was unable to grant meaning to the tensions and contradictions inherent in it and in Jaspers's thought as a whole. A similar orientation is noticeable in Fritz Heinemann's interpretation. In contrast to the arguments of Knauss and Heinemann, I argue that the absence of a philosophical system in Jaspers's work does not reflect the weakness of this philosophy, but constitutes a positive and conscious stance of Jaspers's, whereby philosophy cannot be portrayed in a system at all.[19] On this issue, Jaspers testified to the influence of Max Weber upon him. As we saw already in the introduction, Jaspers preferred "method" to system.[20]

A. The Epistemological Viewpoint

The presence of the epistemological viewpoint in the explication of Being is reflected in Jaspers's statement that the question regarding the essence of Being is awakened in light of its discovery in a reality accessible to objective consciousness.[21] The necessity of this viewpoint arises from the requirement that whatever has for us a feature of Being should be immanent to consciousness,[22] and from the statement that "the independence from the world [present] in the relation to transcendence is real only as an activity in the world."[23] The epistemological viewpoint in which Jaspers's perception of Being was anchored reveals the necessity of Existenz to elucidate this Being. Eventually, although Being as a whole is not accessible to the tools of formal knowledge, and despite the very existence of a metaphysical Being not dependent on the consciousness referring to it, let alone exhausted by it, the activity of consciousness aimed at elucidating Being serves as a basis the transcending from which enables the conscious constitution of a metaphysical consciousness.

The presence of the epistemological viewpoint in Jaspers's perception of Being, involving, among other things, the function of formal knowledge, reveals that the metaphysical consciousness forming within the explication of Being is an inherent part of the routine of human existence in the world. In this respect, we can state that the contribution of the epistemological viewpoint to the explication of Being is similar to that of world orientation to the explication of selfhood. Just as the second anchored Existenz in the reality of the world, so in this context the human search for Being is anchored in the conscious functions people need in the different aspects of their existence. Just as the constitution of Existenz as a worldly Being in world orientation had a significant role in overcoming the solipsism and the enigmatic nature of Jaspers's early perception of selfhood, so the presence of the epistemological viewpoint in Jaspers's perception of Being distances it from mystical thinking and prevents it from becoming detached from its connection with human existence.[24]

It transpires that both the achievements that preceded the constitution of the explication aimed directly at Being—the recognition of the existence of the world as an actual Being revealed in phenomena, as formulated in *World Orientation*, and the achieving of an explicit and mature perception of Existenz in *Elucidation of Existenz*—serve as a foundation and an infrastructure for it. Jaspers's general statement that world orientation paves the way to metaphysics and gives all existing knowledge an anchor in the meaning beyond it[25] now receives its full meaning. The perception of selfhood and the recognition of the world's reality become the starting points for the explication of Being, and as such they serve as a philosophical basis on which the method of transcending aimed directly at the elucidation of Being and transcendence is applied.

My interpretation, stressing the role of consciousness in the elucidation of Being, differs from existing interpretations in the secondary literature, which see the removal of objective consciousness as a condition for the constitution of a relation toward Being in Jaspers's thought. Sebastian Samay, for instance, believes that the method of transcending, reflecting an attempt to progress beyond objectivity and intentional consciousness aimed at objects, does not enable involving the objects in the constitution of the consciousness of Being, which is not objective. In his opinion, transcendence denotes simultaneously both the supreme achievement of consciousness and its "corruption," expressed in the dissolving of objective knowledge.[26] In this context, Samay designated a decisive role to absolute consciousness. In his opinion, this consciousness is responsible for the turning to Being taking place freely and spontaneously without preconceptions. Samay offered two interpretations of the concept of "absolute consciousness": the consciousness where people are aware of their absolute freedom and also the consciousness where we have intuition about Being.[27] Samay did not discuss the relation between the two interpretations he offered, but in his interpretation in this context, he gave the first meaning of the term a more central role. Following my interpretation of this concept in the chapter concluding the transition mechanisms, I wish to argue that these two interpretations cannot be connected, since the intuition of Being simultaneously also embodies Existenz's consciousness of the limitations to which it is subject. While the absolute consciousness helps prepare the discussion for the transition to the explication of Being, once this has happened, in the philosophy of the encompassing, it fills a relatively marginal role. Jaspers's insistence on the non-objective and unknowable nature of Being and on the presentation of Being as the "original resolution" of Existenz returns, according to Samay's interpretation, the question about Being to "the question about the one searching for it," meaning to the possible Existenz.[28] Eventually, Samay believes the process of searching for Being, as expressed in the perception of the encompassing, remains subject to selfhood.[29]

The return of the question about Being to Existenz appears also in Hans Mader's interpretation. His premise is that in Jaspers's philosophy, thinking always refers to finite objects, while the search for Being expresses a wish for "the irrational for which the split [between objectivity and subjectivity] does not exist."[30] He argues that the Kantian transcendental position toward finality, as Jaspers expressed it, undergoes a continuing process of reducing the identity between thought and Being, until existence turns into a "lost symbol," and eventually the transcendental position is abandoned altogether.[31] In the absence of a real possibility of knowing Being, Jaspers's discussion, as Mader understood it, returns to the limitations of the individual's consciousness, and the person's thoughts about Being are also harnessed to the overall process of self-formation. In this process, which, according to Mader, remains within the boundaries of individual Existenz, the possibility of realizing "the announcability and it becomes merely a 'call' for those who happened to answer it" is abandoned.[32] These interpretations, linking the removal of objective consciousness from the perception of Being and the philosophy of Existenz, finally leave the perception of Being in Jaspers's philosophy implicit and vague. The entrusting of the elucidation of Being in the hands of Existenzes makes it redundant to some extent, since these already feel certainty about the reality of the transcendent Being, and an intuition regarding the existence of such a Being would, to a large extent, suffice for them. I believe that the very constitution of the framework of the explication of Being was intended to enable a systematic approach toward Being that would not be dependent on existentialist intuition. Otherwise, if we remained within the boundaries of the certainty of Existenz regarding Being, the question would arise concerning the very necessity and meaning of Jaspers's philosophical effort to coin different concepts expressing this Being (such as: the "encompassing," "cipher," "philosophical logic," and others). It is difficult not to notice the similarity between the interpretations of Samay and Mader about Jaspers's perception of Being and those who criticized the philosophy of Existenz without attributing importance to the negotiations regarding the possible contribution of the objective viewpoint. Just as Jaspers's arguments about the limitations of consciousness for the elucidation of Existenz motivated some scholars to understand Existenz as an irrationalist Being, inaccessible to scientific knowledge or understanding at all, so Jaspers's statements about the contribution of the viewpoint of consciousness to the understanding of his perception of Being were perceived as being based on irrational premises. See the discussion in Chapters Three and Four. The withdrawal from the discussion of Being to Existenz, or the subjection of the explication of Being to the framework of clarifying Existenz, as presented by Samay and more forcefully by Mader, identifies Jaspers's philosophy as a whole with the philosophy of Existenz, which is indirectly revealed as an expression of extreme individualism, self-absorbed and lacking any meaning or relation to the reality external to it.

Nowhere in his writings did Jaspers clarify the basis from which he deduced the existence of Being as a reality not restricted to the boundaries of immanence; this appears for him as a datum from which philosophizing begins. To the best of my knowledge, the only scholar who saw Jaspers's perception of Being as the fruit of experience alone and not as based on a-priori intuition, which led to the development of Jaspers's philosophy of Being, was Heinemann.[33] In this respect, the very reality of a transcendent Being or of a Being beyond the boundaries of human existence is located outside the boundaries of its philosophical explication, which is revealed as lacking a starting point. Jaspers was not even deterred from presenting the extent of decidedness of Being as an outcome of the uncompromising stance of the person seeking it. He even linked the clarity concerning Being with the person's *will* to clarify the existence of such a Being. The Being presented as a target for philosophical elucidation appears in Jaspers's work as such an inseparable part of the person searching for it[34] that the search for Being becomes identified with existence, and stopping the effort to elucidate Being is presented as an analogy of the cessation of existence itself.[35]

However, I believe that although the evidence of the existence of a transcendent Being and the drive to elucidate it serve as a basis for constituting the explication of Being, they do not constitute irrational elements in Jaspers's perception of Being. Apart from his different statements regarding the a-priori intuition about the reality of the Being, Jaspers stated that the Being under philosophical discussion is present in the concrete historicity in which people live.[36] Even if the expressions of the Being in concrete reality are themselves subject to an interpretation that could doubt them, the very statement of the presence of Being in immanent reality serves as an infrastructure for the possibility in principle to clarify Being. However, its main importance at this point is that it prevents the possibility of establishing the existence of the transcendent Being only on intuition, which does not in itself require any establishment. In this context, Jaspers argued as follows:

> It is not sufficient to live in the truth without knowledge about it; truth as truth is reliable only if it knows itself. The philosophical logic translates the consciousness of truth from unmediated to reflexive knowledge. Thus the

> reality of the consciousness of our truth makes itself certain for the first time.[37]

These words, indicating the insufficiency of evidence concerning the existence of Being for the constitution of a philosophical consciousness of Being, join Jaspers's statement that the very existence of human beings in "existence in time" (*Zeitdasein*) does not anchor them in Being, but people's consciousness and actions are what helps in this.[38] See also Jaspers's argument that the tangible reality in which we live is not in itself a reality, but only becomes such through our understanding that organizes it. This understanding gradually becomes a sort of model through which we approach the unmediated reality in which we live.[39] At this point there is a clear link with Georg Wilhelm Friedrich Hegel's approach that demanded the representation of external reality in thought, although unlike Hegel, Jaspers did not consider the two as identical. It is the requirement to achieve reflexive knowledge about Being that indicates the need for the independence of the knowledge of the Being regarding who obtained it, since only knowledge that is self-standing can serve as a basis for a philosophical discussion. It is clear that this requirement does not make this knowledge an exhaustive expression of the Being, especially not of its transcendent aspects. But the immanent expressions of the Being reflected in reflexive knowledge are able to help make the *reality of the Being* under explication independent of the consciousness referring to it, and to separate it from the *conscious process* in which people attempt to understand themselves, and tend to place their internal world and particular experiences at the center. Hence the importance of the effort directed at anchoring the philosophizing about the Being in a discursive process aware of the conscious aspects it involves, an effort that makes the discussion of consciousness an inseparable part of the explication of Being itself. Jaspers devoted the second part of his book *Out of Truth* to the issue of consciousness.[40] He also made a distinction between consciousness and mind.[41]

Here we encounter another expression of the dialectical relations between consciousness and the object of explication that was also typical of Jaspers's perception of selfhood, and that led it to move back and forth between different requirements, which instead of contradicting each other, moderated each other, and maintained the permanent presence of tension in his philosophy. It transpires that according to Jaspers, our consciousness of Being requires a tidy and self-conscious discursive process, although it cannot rely on reflexive knowledge alone. The more the reflexive process contributes to the tangible presence of Being for people, the more it can "evaporate," as he put it[42] again each time, and prevent the achievement of a uniform consciousness of Being.[43] What the thought about Being experiences reveals a basic characteristic of the Being itself. Just as this thought has many, changing facets, so, too, is Being subject to a situation that Jaspers defined as "being torn" and "being breached,"[44] which does not enable it to "close itself."[45] Jaspers used the expression "being torn" (*Zerrissenheit*) in other contexts, too: in his discussion of the concept of "world,"[46] and the concept of "existence."[47] In this respect, there is accordance between the multifaceted nature of consciousness and the multiple sources from which it feeds, and the way Being is present in the world.

For Jaspers, the basis of the essentialness and development of Being was rooted in the multiplicity of objects of reference in which the varied starting points for the elucidation of Being are anchored. Assuming a gap between the reality of Being and the thought directed at it enabled Jaspers, unlike Hegel, for instance, to present a perception of Being that was not identified with the philosophical reflection aimed at it, and to avoid constituting an absolute perception of Being. The basic nature of thought, which is unable to achieve a uniform understanding of the immanent reality characterized by multiplicity, is what served to prevent the absolutization of Being and a basis for its development in this philosophy. In this respect, thought, which served as a central tool through which Hegel wished to reveal the absolute character of Being, served in Jaspers's philosophy—that did not try to overcome what he perceived as the basic nature of thought and reality—as a means of preventing such an absolutization. In the absence of identity between thought and Being, Jaspers's philosophy lacked the demand to exhaust Being using the tools of philosophical thought. Being itself and the thoughts about it do not become identical in the reflection process, but combine together, each according to its nature, to prevent the formation of Being as absolute in consciousness.

Breaking the framework of the explication of selfhood at this stage of his thought is demonstrated by the comparison between Jaspers's handling of the question of the relation between the individual and the multiplicity in this context and in his previous writings, especially in *Psychology*. See the discussion in Chapter Two. As we have seen, in his early discussion, Jaspers wished to clarify the relations between the individual's Being, expressed in his private world view, and the multiplicity of world views, portraying the multiple possibilities in which selfhood can present itself. The solipsistic nature of the perception of subjectivity, appearing in Jaspers's early work, did not enable it to contain the dialectic between the private world view and the multiplicity of world views, and the decision in favor of the particular subjectivity was apparent. In contrast, Jaspers's aim to grant philosophical expression to broad aspects of existence, of which Existenz is only one component, allowed him to present a more complex philosophical perception, containing not only the perception of Being, but also a more mature perception of selfhood. Within his concept of the encompassing, selfhood was no longer presented as a Being in itself, nor as a Being existing alongside other Existenzes, but as existing beside other forms of existence that are not dependent on it or derived from it. However, the status of Existenz as one of the components of the perception of the encompassing did not diminish the complexity that typified it as an explicit Being in Jaspers's philosophy prior to its becoming directed at the elucidation of Being. More than the new status of selfhood in Jaspers's discussion reflected his distancing from the impulse to explicate selfhood, it expressed the ability of this selfhood to turn its attention to what was beyond it, an ability thanks to which selfhood became capable of noticing the multi-faceted nature of Being and of seeing its relative share in this Being. The attempt to characterize Being separately from the consciousness that thinks it was intended to release the explication of Being from its dependence on the framework of the explication of selfhood, although not to detach it. To be precise, the attempt to base the priority of Being in relation to thought was not intended to negate the need for an epistemological viewpoint, which, as we have seen, is essential to the explication of Being, but instead to continue establishing the distancing from the solipsistic perception of selfhood. This viewpoint, contributing to the establishment of the immanent basis in Jaspers's perception of Being, is apparent in his repeated referring to the multi-faceted nature of Being and the way that Existenz experiences this phenomenon. Although Being itself is not identical to the way it is reflected in thought, the explication of Being is built from the awareness of their common points and no less from the ability to use a particular viewpoint while being conscious that it does not exhaust the object of philosophizing to which it is aimed.

The secondary literature has granted a different interpretation to the components responsible for the constitution of a non-absolute perception of Being in Jaspers's philosophy. For instance, Richli explained it by the appearance of Being in a multiplicity of objects, so its perception is constituted from a multiplicity of objects of reference.[48] However, this factor alone could not guarantee the prevention of the absolutization of Jaspers's perception of Being, just as it did not prevent it in Hegel. I believe that, alongside the multiplicity, what helped Jaspers avoid the absolutization of Being was the condition of Existenz at the end of the process of clarifying selfhood; the awareness of the limitations of existential freedom and its withdrawal from the focus of the philosophizing. As Existenz's awareness of its limitations became established, it turned away from dealing with its selfhood and recognized itself as surrounded by a space that differed from it. The tangible expression of this awareness is in its reference to objects using consciousness, a reference that opens for consciousness spaces that had previously been hidden from it. This process, gradual in nature, leads to the formation of a more extensive consciousness that also contains the possibility of the existence of a Being that is not objective. The metaphysical consciousness regarding Being had no freedom from objects, but it does have freedom from the boundaries of Existenz. More precisely, Existenz has freedom from itself, and as a result, it forms the freedom to constitute a relation toward Being.

Consciousness of the boundaries of Existenz, presented in this interpretation as a constituting element of Jaspers's perception of Being, can also explain the different nature accompanying the presence of consciousness in the two explications. As we have seen, the entry of consciousness into the framework of the elucidation of selfhood introduced great tension into the perception of Existenz, as a result of which two directions appeared in its discussion: the separation of Existenz from the world, or its anchoring in the world. Making consciousness a component of elucidating Existenz led to a revolution in its self-perception that helped it become aware of the reality surrounding it. At this point in Jaspers's discussion there was a confrontation between two types of absoluteness competing for priority, on the assumption that the absoluteness of Existenz excludes the absoluteness of consciousness, and vice versa. In contrast, the distancing of the philosophical discussion from the absoluteness and totality typical of Jaspers's early work not only enabled placing Being at the focus of the philosophical discussion, but also opened a space for Existenz to find its place in it. It is not surprising that Jaspers's discussion regarding the role of consciousness in the explication of Being did not extend to the identification of Being with consciousness, nor was it motivated by the fear of such identification. The multiplicity that served as a starting point and an infrastructure for the elucidation of Being enabled the epistemological viewpoint not to transcend the boundaries of the viewpoint and become epistemology, and as will transpire later, it is also responsible for the ontological viewpoint not threatening the epistemological one, and even being harnessed alongside it in the philosophical effort to explicate Being.

The attempt to direct the transition from unmediated reality to the reflexive consciousness aimed at perceiving reality as a Being stresses the fundamental change between the philosophizing aimed at explicating Being and that aimed at elucidating selfhood. While the second relied on *intuition*, where selfhood was portrayed as a solipsistic Being, in the explication of Being, Jaspers wished to anchor his arguments in "philosophical logic"—a philosophical concept that largely defines the role of the epistemological viewpoint and its boundaries in the perception of the encompassing. Jaspers presented philosophical logic as *generalizing* in its penetration of the forms of thought and knowledge, as *distinguishing* the boundaries of each of its findings, as *unifying* what was revealed to it as isolated and detached, and as *opening* the horizons where reality could appear.[49] These features enable philosophical logic to deal with the basic characteristics of unmediatedness and to help Existenz deal with the opacity, crumbling, and emptiness typical of unmediated reality, which it experiences as a source of scattering and self-loss.[50] The formal element of philosophical logic allows it to organize the transition from unmediatedness to reflexivity, without directly participating in the realization in practice of these forces or being a component in people's consciousness of Being.[51]

Philosophical logic, penetrating the concrete expressions of Being in existence without fully identifying Being with them, is revealed as an *organon of reason*. Jaspers defined reason, which rescues thought from its tendency to remain within the boundaries of the objects at which it is directed, as a "transobjective" force directing thought to formulate a unity from its materials[52] and as "mysticism for mind."[53] These qualities of reason granted it its status as a "bond" of the forms of the encompassing—meaning that it *connects* the forms of the encompassing that represent the different modes of Being in the world[54] and *guarantees communication* between the different appearings of Being revealed by philosophical logic.[55] In this respect, reason transpires as the force *urging* each of the expressions of Being to go beyond its boundaries and to join the others in order to express the presence of Being more fully. Finally, being an organon of reason, philosophical logic enables the realization of reason in different areas of life—a realization meaning the identification of the multi-faceted presence of Being and the connection of these facets into one Being.[56] See also Jaspers's statement that just as Existenz knows its boundaries through the clarification of Existenz, so is the part of reason in the explication of Being clarified by philosophical logic.[57] This statement reveals the parallel between the relationship existing between philosophical logic and reason, and the clarification of Existenz and Existenz itself: while philosophical logic and the clarification of Existenz served as tools for discovering the possibilities contained in the object of the philosophizing—Being and Existenz—reason and Existenz represent the drive to bring these possibilities to transparency. Jaspers argued that this ratio also exists between formal logic and general consciousness, between world orientation and the world, and between metaphysics and transcendence.[58]

The qualities of philosophical logic, which enabled it to illuminate the range of possibilities of accessing Being without involving itself in any of them, led some interpreters to see it as an *instrument* through which the individual's consciousness of Being is formulated. James Collins, for example, defined it as an unclosed method, and Samay believed that it expressed a discursive-phenomenological facet of Jaspers's perception of Being.[59] Collins' interpretation of Jaspers's perception of the encompassing relies mainly on a single statement appearing in his discussion of philosophical logic.[60] These interpreters stressed the existence of a formal facet without contents in philosophical logic, expressing a degree of awareness of a turning point in Jaspers reflected in a more structured and systematic form of philosophizing. But this awareness was not shared by other interpreters. Heinemann, for instance, believed that Jaspers's philosophical logic reflects the contradiction between the principle of flow, the lack of system, and the personal facet, which generally typify Jaspers's philosophy of Existenz, and his later attempt to create logical systemization in the theory of the encompassing.

However, according to Heinemann, Jaspers's philosophical logic is ruled by subjective thought that has no connection with the concept of logic as we understand it.[61] Heinemann believed that just as Jaspers avoided being systematic, he also distanced his approach from the presentation of real contents. This situation is the outcome of his understanding of Jaspers's philosophy as "dethroning" objectivity and subjectivity,[62] because it could not accept the final status of contents at all.[63] Heinemann denied Jaspers's philosophy both contents and system. This interpretation is similar in its extremeness perhaps only to that of Otto Friedrich Bollnow. See the discussion of his approach in Chapter Four. It appears to be connected to the anti-Existentialist mood typical of philosophical research in Germany after the Second World War. In this spirit, Heinemann presented Jaspers's philosophy from before the war as "impossible to implement practically" (an approach similar to that of Werner Schneiders),[64] while what was included in the writings Jaspers termed "the philosophy of reason"—meaning all the writings of the third period, defined in this study as "socio-political"—as having potential for realization.[65] Compare Heinemann's and Bollnow's interpretations to those of those scholars belonging to the alternative tendency to Jaspers.[66] For Heinemann, Jaspers's philosophy of the encompassing constitutes a direct continuation of his philosophy of Existenz, and both were characterized by the lack of system and order. These interpretations of the perception of Being reflect the general approach to the question of Jaspers's entire philosophy. Understanding Jaspers's entire oeuvre as "philosophy of Existenz," which in practice does not recognize the developments that took place within this philosophy, contributed to blurring the uniqueness of the perception of the encompassing and to reducing it to the tendencies typical of Jaspers's early work. In contrast, understanding the development in Jaspers's philosophy enables the distinguishing of the changes that occurred there in general, including the development of the perception of Being at its later stages of development.

In any case, the profound differences between the nature of the philosophizing aimed at the elucidation of selfhood and that directed at the explication of Being do not allow us, in my opinion, to accept the interpretations of the perception of the encompassing described above. The presence of philosophical logic in the elucidation of the perception of the encompassing is understood in the interpretation offered here to Jaspers's perception of Being as expressing a real turning point both in the contents with which Jaspers dealt and in the method of his handling them, a method that became more systematic. In addition, the presentation of philosophical logic as a "formal principle of consciousness" through which the methodical viewpoint from which reality should be approached is formulated does reflect the transition to a more systematic and organized philosophical discourse. However, we should clarify that this facet of philosophical logic does not exhaust the full meaning it was granted in Jaspers's perception of Being. Alongside its definition as a function determining the ways in which we can know, accept what is accessible to consciousness, and "hold myself internally" within consciousness,[67] Jaspers described philosophical logic as "performing simple thoughts related to the *element of all reality*."[68] Through observation of the reality around the person, these thoughts penetrate the depth of our human Being and demonstrate to the person something of the uniform character of Being. Jaspers stressed that only from experiencing the search for the uniform and complete element existing beyond the expressions of immanent reality is the person allowed other forms of thought,[69] including those involved in objective thinking. The penetration of philosophical logic into what Jaspers termed "the element of the entire reality" exceeds its role for consciousness as clarifying the range of possibilities of contact with Being; it touches the metaphysical infrastructure that serves as a source for these possibilities, and as such serves also as an element for the varied forms of human consciousness. The contact with this infrastructure exposes the source from which the selfhood of Existenz originates, and in this respect philosophical logic enables what has been called in this context "freedom of becoming yourself."[70] However, this fact is perceived here as secondary in relation to this source not being the sole property of a specific Existenz, but from it the different forms of the presence of Being are enabled.

The effort to reveal using philosophical logic the origins of Existenz's consciousness of Being[71] permits making contact with the unknowable depth on which it relies; a depth that was hidden from it during the processes of clarifying its selfhood, which were characterized by its tendency to isolate itself from what was around it. Philosophical logic is revealed in this interpretation as containing two levels: the conscious and the metaphysical. The conscious level portrays the general facet of the thought that has a communicative nature, following which the distinction between Existenzes and non-Existenzes is diminished. The metaphysical level revealed through the method of transcending is aimed in this context at the thought elucidating the absolute unity existing beyond the boundaries of human Being, a Being revealed as a result as anchored in a wider space. From a horizontal viewpoint this space is perceived as encompassing it, and from a vertical viewpoint it is revealed as the depth supporting its presence in the world. Jaspers was able, through the concept of philosophical logic, one of the pillars of his perception of the encompassing, to expose two facets of his perception of Being. The first affirms that Existenz is essential to the perception of Being and indicates that it is not in itself a self-bearing wholeness,[72] while the second portrays an element independent of Existenz. In this way he guarantees that Being is not identified with the consciousness directed at elucidating it. Against the background of the discussion of philosophical logic, we can state that the definition of the perception of the encompassing as "turning thought" that can "draw us out" of the objective knowledge to which we are accustomed and to direct us to know the boundaries where Being exists for us[73] sums up the role of the epistemological viewpoint within the explication of Being. This viewpoint makes "*thinkable that the unthinkable exists.*"[74]

B. The Ontological Viewpoint

The ontological viewpoint in Jaspers's perception of Being is intended to rescue the philosophizing from sinking into a multiplicity of objects and foci of reference, in order to achieve a more uniform and complete understanding of Being. From this viewpoint, the multi-facetedness of Being is perceived as an expression of its "collapsing," and the contrasts arising from it are to "be annihilated." In this context, the multiplicity appears not only as a reflection of the variety of Being and as a tangible expression of the "dismantled" state in which it is revealed to human beings, but it is also presented as a source of dissatisfaction.[75] However, Jaspers stated that it is precisely from this experience that people become acquainted with the "hidden depth" within them, which they experience only in moments of exaltation. This depth, which was lost in the philosophizing that sank into the world, arouses the drive to penetrate the foundations on which Being relies,[76] represented in the different modes of the encompassing. Now the unity that serves as a source for the different expressions of Being becomes a target to which the philosophizing aims itself.[77]

The philosophizing, defined at this stage as the "search for reality," was also described as "pushing while thinking to the place where *thought would become an experience of reality in itself*."[78] This reality does not exist within the boundaries of reality alone or only for Existenz, but is described as present in its absence for those who experience longing for a reality they do not know and which is not their reality.[79] The search for reality far from the familiar boundaries of human experience is based on becoming acquainted with the limitations of consciousness and Existenz as tools for discovering the desired reality: consciousness made the world into a phenomenon and limited the reality to a mere perspective, while Existenz, stressing the realization within the boundaries of possibility, detracted from the realistic meaning of existence as a whole thing.[80] Eventually, individuals are left with a constant yearning in their heart for more than consciousness and Existenz can give them[81]—two facets of their being that were the focus of the philosophizing for a while. We cannot dismiss the contribution of the epistemological viewpoint, which helped break out of the existentialist thinking patterns that were typical of Jaspers during the elucidation of selfhood, and also established the place and role of consciousness and Existenz within the explication of Being. However, against the background of the new familiarity with the limitations of consciousness and Existenz, the quest for reality is revealed as an expression of the search for absoluteness and completeness to be placed as a permanent and constant element against the transient and worthless aspects of human Being.

The placing of reality at the center of the philosophical elucidation directed at Being is based on an opposite premise than the one typical of the Cartesian approach, which deduced reality from thought. Ernst Mayer presented another interpretation to the stage of transition from *Philosophy* to *From Truth*. In his opinion, Jaspers's focus of interest in *Philosophy* was the reality (*Wirklichkeit*) of Existenz and of transcendence, while *From Truth* did not deal with the reality of Being but instead with its truth.[82] However, according to the proposed interpretation, Jaspers did not develop his perceptions about Existenz and transcendence in a single philosophical move, but in a complex process that underwent profound modifications. The reality of Existenz was at the center of discussion in *Elucidation of Existenz*, and only in *Metaphysics* did Jaspers turn to elucidate the reality of transcendence and Being at all, after Existenz had been diverted from the center of the philosophizing. The reality at whose elucidation Jaspers was aiming at this stage of his philosophy was defined as prior to the person's thoughts, opposing them and subjugating them.[83] Breaking the bridge linking reality and thought, and defining the desired reality as the "source" and "target" of our lives[84] hedged the philosophy of Existenz in from both sides: both withdrawing from it to a more primal reality than that of the Existenz, expressing only one of the possibilities existing within it, and at the same time transcending it in favor of a more encompassing Being that included it as a possibility alongside other possibilities. Whereas the epistemological viewpoint revealed the multifacetedness of the Being revealed in human reality, the ontological viewpoint relied on its ability to escape the oppression forced upon it by the order of objects in the world, of which it is itself a part.[85]

The description of thought as "concentrating on one connecting thing"[86] or as searching for "the one in everything, the final goal, the primal basis, the wholeness of the world, [and] God,"[87] expressed the intuitive basis in the observation called here the ontological viewpoint. Jaspers called this aspect "internal awareness" of Being, and compared it with the thought behind the ritual action that was customary in the past, through which people ensured real reality for themselves.[88] In this context, this awareness served as a sort of measure of the proximity or distance a person has from Being, and achieving this awareness decides whether a person experiences Being or nothingness.[89] The role of the epistemological viewpoint in shaping the philosophizing aimed at elucidating Being largely determined the nature of the intuition on which the awareness of Being was based: on the one hand, it was not opposed to the contemplative thought Jaspers presented as part of this thinking itself,[90] but on the other hand, it was clarified from the discussion above as prior to it. A different argument is presented by Kurt Hoffman, who saw awareness of Being as a sort of bridge enabling us to think of something not objective from objectivity.[91]

What Jaspers defined in this context as searching for "reality" was not essentially alien to the general trend of the renewal in metaphysics that was typical of philosophical work in that period. The "hunger for Being," as Herbert Schnädelbach put it, was the basis for the birth of a new ontology in this period. This ontology sought, on the one hand, to deal with the decisive influence of the empirical sciences that imposed methodic rules on the philosophical discourse, and in reply to propose its own rules and method. On the other hand, despite the basic obligation to the form of scientific discourse, this ontology sought to free itself from the restrictions typical of positivistic approaches that presented a theory of knowledge using logic, and as a substitute for them, to offer a perception of Being with real contents.[92] These ontological approaches did not always succeed in avoiding what they opposed; however, the awareness of the motives at their basis created tension within the philosophical discourse of the period. Schnädelbach showed that precisely what served as a basis for the criticism of philosophers at this time was expressed in the philosophies they created themselves.[93]

Against the background of the discussion of the expressions of the epistemological and ontological viewpoints, we can state that Jaspers's perception of Being was intended to deal with this double challenge. On the one hand, Jaspers wished to avoid constituting a perception of Being that would deal with the question of existence as the "question of is where it is," as Nicolai Hartmann defined it.[94] According to Hartmann, the process of consciousness does not determine the existence of reality, but only reveals the way reality is formed at the particularity to which it is subject.

However, even though he stressed the role of reflection and selfhood in general in the constituting of the perception of Being, Jaspers did not wish to examine it only from the perspective of the person experiencing it as Martin Heidegger did in *Being and Time*. The premise on which Jaspers based his perception of Being was that Being does not exist only within the boundaries of immanence, and it cannot be exhausted solely within the boundaries of human existence. The philosophy of Hartmann and the early Heidegger represent two extremes in the philosophical discourse of the period when Jaspers was formulating his main ideas, and his perception did not serve as a middle approach in relation to them, but instead aimed to disprove the foundations on which they were based. Against the positivistic approach, which Jaspers never tired of criticizing, it was crucial for him to stress, especially at the stage when he himself took significant steps to establish Being in his approach, that Existenz was not removed from the arena of philosophizing. Jaspers believed that the implementation of the positivistic approach regarding Being—and in this context, Hartmann was chosen as a representative of a sort of "ideal type" of this approach, but from his point of view, Heinrich Rickert, Edmund Husserl, and others could also have served as its representatives—could destroy philosophy. This position reflects in his opinion surrender to the world view claiming that in the modern era philosophy has lost the objects it traditionally dealt with to science, which in his opinion inevitably turned philosophy into science's miserable slave.[95] As such, philosophy became a framework where the history of science is told, and the interest in philosophy could be aesthetical at best. Some relevant approaches include those of Heinrich Rickert,[96] and Edmund Husserl in his essay "Philosophy as Rigorous Science."[97] Jaspers himself testified to the influence of these approaches on shaping his positions.[98] Despite this, I have chosen to refer to Hartmann's approach in this section due to the strong connection between his ontological approach and metaphysics, and especially in order to detach the discussion from the ethical implications it had especially in Rickert's theory, which is beyond the framework of this discussion. The question of the relations between science and philosophy was one of the issues Jaspers never ceased dealing with throughout his creative years, and it has also received extensive attention in the secondary literature.[99]

Jaspers's inclusion of Existenz in the arena of philosophizing stems, first and foremost, from the philosophizing being based on the "decision of the will for Being."[100] It expresses the human freedom that realizes itself in its facing a reality wider than the boundaries of its existence, or even a transcendent one.[101] Also, the desire for reality on which the appeal to Being is defined as "a search for the reality of our Being in the selfhood of our independent essence"[102] and as resulting from the hidden depth existing within us and returning us to the foundations.[103] From the viewpoint of the encompassing, Jaspers asserted that "*Existenz* is one of the words denoting reality," and as such, the philosophy of Existenz is perceived as the "pattern of the one original philosophy" whose purpose is to observe "*reality in its origin and to perceive it by means of the ways in which I deal with myself...*"[104] These citations show that Existenz continues to constitute a significant part of the process of the search for reality.

However, the new framework in which Existenz is anchored does not only define the space surrounding it, but also penetrates the perception of Existenz and alters it significantly. As a result, henceforth Existenz is perceived as one of the modes of the encompassing. Even if the presence of Existenz in the discussion is reduced, and it is given a new meaning that enables reality to be placed at the focus of the philosophical discussion, the approach to reality as the target of the philosophizing and the basis from which we live does not negate the relevance of Existenz within the process of the explication of Being. Against this background, we should understand Jaspers's approach as expressing his rejection in principle of the two meanings granted to philosophy in the positivistic world view: both as a field of knowledge where the forces of consciousness are used without placing them as the topic of the philosophizing, and also as a framework where there is no room for the person's world as an individual. From Jaspers's point of view, the positivistic approach toward being could be reduced to the concept of "general consciousness," a concept that for Jaspers constituted only one component of the perception of the encompassing, which like its other components lacked an independent status within it. Jaspers stated that the roots of the position subjecting philosophy to the methods of scientific knowledge were in René Descartes's philosophy.[105]

The opposite pole regarding Jaspers's position is represented by Heidegger's perception of Being, which, unlike that of Hartmann, grants a significant role to human beings. Unlike Heidegger, who presented the person as existing in two basic conditions (authentic and inauthentic), and who determined that the question of existence arises only from authenticity, for Jaspers the interest in existence is at the basis of human existence and becomes a general human feature. Like Heidegger, Jaspers did not think that this question occupied people at every moment of their life. However, the very possibility that a person could live an entire life without dealing with the "question of existence," as arises from the Heideggerian dichotomy between authentic and inauthentic existence, was unreal for Jaspers. From his point of view, people can reach an insight or visualization (*Vergegenwärtigung*) of Being or alternatively miss it all their life, but in any case a degree of dealing with it will be part of their existence in the world. "The question about the essence of Being," as Jaspers phrased it, could illuminate the question of the role of the philosopher and of philosophy in an individual's world, which is one of the crucial issues in this philosophy. In this context, Jaspers expressed a Socratic position, seeing the philosopher and philosophy as an integral part of human existence, and presenting philosophy as the property of the individual as existing in the world.[106] This position of Jaspers's, whereby the interest in Being penetrates all layers of human existence, forced him to shape Being in such a way as to enable it to permeate every corner of human existence and at the same time to include aspects not restricted only to the viewpoint a person has regarding it. This is the idea behind the perception of Being as encompassing: a perception containing everything related to humanity, but also having "margins" beyond the boundary of human Being. This idea is demonstrated in Jaspers's scheme of the map of Being, in which its two poles remain open: the upper one where transcendence is located, and the lower one, where wisdom is located.[107] This understanding also arises from the interpretation Jaspers himself gave in the chapter "*Deutung der Figur*."[108]

Beyond this difference in principle, Jaspers opposed the total status granted to human beings (*Dasein*) in Heidegger's approach in *Being and Time*, whereby the mode of people's existence in the world portrays the ontological structure of Being, and people are granted a decisive role in determining the boundaries of the discussion of Being. In contrast, Jaspers wished at this stage to anchor his discussion of Being beyond the area of the person's existential framework and believed that its solution could be found in transcending these horizons, meaning in transcendence, which is first and foremost everything beyond human Being, without which the most crucial source of meaning for the individual is denied. Whereas for Heidegger there was no person without the world, for Jaspers there was no person without transcendence, and from the person's viewpoint the question of Being must be discussed.

Compared with the two viewpoints presented above, we can state that Jaspers's question of Being reflects a critical position regarding his period, and also contains his criticism of the modern Being that places the person at the center as a ruler of all areas of life. Jaspers aimed to present a figure of a person searching for the meaning of individual existence as the model of philosophy, and this is why he was opposed to the positivistic position in science that removed human beings from its domain. At the same time, he wished to go beyond the narrow framework of the person's existential range of meaning in the world and to turn to the wide horizons of transcendence, since he believed that individuals could achieve meaning for their existence by constituting a relationship toward transcendence. Clarifying his position in principle on the question of Being with relation to the philosophical world where it operated can demonstrate the totality to which his philosophy as a whole was directed. Totality in its Jasperian form is not based on the action of hypostasis performing itself upon one element and applying it to the entire system—whether in its positivistic form, as represented by Hartmann, or in its Heideggerian guise. Against these two extreme positions, Jaspers wished to propose a wide framework where both people's existential element and world of experiences, and also the metaphysical element of transcendence, which is first and foremost all that is "not man," can find their place.

The ontological level and the epistemological level revealed in our discussion above are harnessed together, at this stage of the development of metaphysical consciousness, to the task of elucidating Being as a certainty outside Existenz. However, the transcending of the boundaries of Existenz by the introduction of these two levels into the discussion is conducted differently. The epistemological viewpoint contributes to making the discussion of Being accessible to all people, or at least to all those who have aimed to achieve certainty of its existence, and not only to the closed community of Existenzes. The ability of thought to exceed the world of objects to the reality beyond it does not diminish the communicability of this thought, since the very transcendence toward a transcendent Being occurs within the boundaries of human thought. In this respect, the epistemological viewpoint in the perception of Being serves both the basic requirements Jaspers had set himself: first, that the answer to the essence of Being should be achieved through following the sources from which self-consciousness is filled,[109] and second, that the metaphysical thought should remain anchored in the world's immanence.[110]

The ontological viewpoint, in contrast, represents the aim of the metaphysical consciousness to break through to beyond the realm of human Being, to what exists not only due to its reference to humans and immanence in general. It is the perception of Being as transcending human immanence that is revealed by following the presence of this viewpoint, as a source of meaning for humans. This insight is expressed for Existenz in the experience of the disappearance of the pattern nature of consciousness in the face of the possibility of transcendence as an absolute Being.[111] Being—whose presence in existence, consciousness, and Existenz had been revealed by the epistemological viewpoint—appears in light of the ontological viewpoint to accord with its description by Jaspers as "an absolute opposed to finitude" that cannot be present in such a consciousness.[112]

The need to establish the relationship between these two viewpoints is inevitable, but at the same time, the different considerations that could lead to this do not enable an unambiguous statement on this issue to be reached. Regarding the matter of determining the priority of one viewpoint over the other, the logic whereby establishment within the boundaries of human Being should occur before it breaks out of them requires the location of the epistemological viewpoint as prior to the ontological one. However, the epistemological viewpoint can be seen as a tool for elucidating the ontological observation, which is mainly an expression of an intuition that cannot be derived from following the way people deal with their world through consciousness. In this respect, the epistemological viewpoint can be seen as later than the ontological one, and as denoting the possibilities it contains. Breaking through the boundaries of human Being through the ontological viewpoint is based on the clarity existing in the background and as prior to it, or, alternately, the clarity provided by the epistemological viewpoint to the perception of Being also contributes to the establishment of the intuition on which the search for Being relies.

Regarding the qualitative value of the epistemological and ontological viewpoints, the question arises whether the communicability (*Mitteilbarkeit*) of the perception of reality in relation to people and their environment is more crucial than the very contact with the absoluteness of Being, or whether this contact maintains its reality and quality even when it does not entail the possibility of mediating and transmitting the certainty accompanying it. To some degree we can state that at this stage, after Jaspers moved away from the basic insights typical of the explication of selfhood, he no longer had the option of ignoring the requirement for the clarification of the philosophical contents forming within the explication of Being. In this respect, the ontological viewpoint is subjugated to the epistemological one, without which the communicability of the explication of Being is damaged. However, we can see the very presence of the intuition about the existence of the transcendent Being as raising the requirement for clarity, and also as a basis for the constituting of the epistemological viewpoint. In this situation the instrumentality of the epistemological viewpoint is stressed in relation to the ontological one, which is itself at the center of the explication of Being.

These different examinations, each of which has its own logic, do not accord with each other. It transpires that a precise decision regarding the priority and qualitative preference of one of the viewpoints over the other is impossible. As in the previous philosophical moves, here, too, the effort to demarcate the boundaries of the philosophizing, typical of this philosophy at all its stages and in this context, too,[113] does not allow the separation of the different forces acting in the discussion, but mainly helps identify them and clarify the relations between them. The inevitable tension between these two viewpoints does not stem from what Samay defined as an essential contradiction between the need for clarity and the requirement for transcendence, but instead from the fact that they cannot be separated.[114] This is because the more clarity increases, the more urgent the requirement for transcendence becomes, and it cannot be formed into a requirement without clarity about the world from which the person wishes to transcend. Samay apparently settled the contradiction by arguing that the tension between these two requirements is what creates the open spaces in which thought can move freely and from which authentic Being can speak to us. He did not clarify the nature of these open spaces and to what extent they were free of the limitations of formal knowledge. However, Jaspers's effort to make positive statements regarding the framework in which Being was elucidated leaves no doubt regarding the importance attributed in this context to consciousness, which was perceived in his philosophy as a framework with quite clear boundaries. The interpretation offered here, seeing the two viewpoints—epistemological and ontological—as a basis on which Jaspers's perception of Being relied, avoids making clear decision in favor of one viewpoint or the other, and instead follows their influence on forming the philosophizing as an organic and complete move. As we will see below, the Being revealed from the study of these two viewpoints grasps immanence through consciousness, but at the same time the ontological viewpoint does not allow it to be exhausted by the boundaries of immanence alone.

2. The Two Facets of Being as the Encompassing: The Immanent and the Transcendent

Jaspers presented the different components of the encompassing in a table that will serve for the discussion below:[115]

	The encompassing that is us	The encompassing that is Being itself
The immanent	Existence Consciousness in general Spirit	The world
The transcendent	Existenz	Transcendence
	Wisdom	

A first glance at the table shows that most of its components—the "modes" (*Weisen*) as Jaspers put it—were not new in his philosophy, but in this context they were examined as expressions of a more comprehensive Being.[116] The two viewpoints, the ontological and the epistemological, will be clarified in the interpretation I will present below as the depth structure of the perception of the encompassing. Following the tension these two viewpoints introduced into Jaspers's perception of the encompassing shows that they served as a central tool in implementing the method of transcending that had accompanied Jaspers's thought from its beginning. Just as in the explication of selfhood this method helped Jaspers constantly expand the area of the discussion, so in the current context it helped view the object of the philosophizing from a wider and more inclusive perspective. However, in the framework of the explication of Being the method of transcending had a different influence on the two frameworks of philosophizing.

As we may recall, the boundaries of the framework of the explication of selfhood became rigid as additional facets of selfhood were revealed, and it became the touchstone that determined the meaning granted to additional issues that arose during the discussion. The solipsistic perception of selfhood was more typical of Jaspers's early philosophy, before the central insights about selfhood were formulated in the philosophy of Existenz. However, as we saw in the chapters dealing with the constitution of the Being of Existenz, the solipsistic image of selfhood remained as a background infrastructure even when awareness of the limitations it imposed on the explication of selfhood was formed.

In contrast, within the framework of the explication of Being, the method of transcending not only expanded the boundaries of the discussion of one central object; it also enabled elucidating additional objects along with it without seeing in this a threat to the possibility of granting full meaning to Being itself. In this context we can state that the method of transcending contributed to softening the rigidity of the philosophizing and opened to it new horizons of metaphysical meanings; these eventually influenced the perceptions formulated previously in Jaspers writings, first and foremost selfhood. Within the explication of Being, the method of transcending contributed to the splitting of the discussion into multiple objects and at the same time to the directing of the philosophizing from the multiplicity to the encompassing unity. These changes undoubtedly reflected the maturation of Jaspers's philosophical thought, but at the same time also the uniqueness of Being as the widest possible object to which the philosophical explication could be directed.

The discussion below will not focus on a conceptual clarification of each of the modes of the encompassing, but on a functional analysis of the way in which the two viewpoints, epistemological and ontological, served as means of adapting the method of transcending to the framework of the explication of Being. A wide observation of Jaspers's philosophy from the genealogical perspective indicates three stages of transcending in Jaspers's perception of the encompassing, in each of which the epistemological and ontological viewpoints reveal new facets. These stages are *not* equivalent to the three stages of the development of the encompassing that Jaspers presented.[117] In addition, these stages express integration between the basic insights achieved in the explication of selfhood, perceived here as an a-priori infrastructure for the perception of the encompassing, and the immanent components of the encompassing itself.

At the first stage of the implementation of the method of transcending, the two viewpoints discussed above reveal two types of encompassing that together constitute the complete picture of Being. The epistemological viewpoint indicates the "encompassing that is us," constituting a framework in which the different forms of presence of Being exist for us,[118] while the ontological viewpoint reveals what Jaspers defined as "the encompassing that is Being itself." Jaspers described this Being as including in it everything through which and in which we exist.[119] The different components revealed in each of these two types of encompassing are not joined at this stage into a uniform Being, although this exists as a wholeness beyond its different expressions. These types of encompassing reveal our split experience of Being.[120] In this respect, the explication of Being, revealing more than one viewpoint, reflects the nature of the basic experience of Being.

"The encompassing that is us" reflects the essence of our thinking that is directed at different aspects of people's Being: existence, consciousness in general, spirit, and Existenz. As we have seen, these aspects did not first appear in the perception of the encompassing, but instead already in the explication of selfhood. However, in this context, the perspective of the encompassing, enabling them to be seen as part of Being, was added to the meaning they received in the previous contexts. Alongside the references to existence as expressing different aspects related to the direct experience of phenomena, Jaspers saw existence at this stage also as an expression of the unmediated presence of Being itself, "the presence of an enclosed whole," a mode of encompassing that also contains the possibility of nothingness as a jump beyond it.[121] Existence itself can serve as a starting point for experiencing a reality that does not exist within the boundaries of the phenomena. More precisely, experiencing such a reality is perceived from the viewpoint of the phenomena as nothingness. A similar principle is also reflected in the definition granted in this context to the concept of "consciousness in general." Alongside his familiar definition of this concept as the framework in which consciousness turns its different experiences into objects (objectivizes them) and produces knowledge from them, "consciousness in general" is described as an instrument through which we can open to the possibility of an other that we do not know and that we cannot turn into knowledge.[122] The boundary of objective consciousness, that marked the end of the space of knowability, beyond which was nothing, transpires from the overall perspective of the encompassing as a potential source for the exposure of Being. A similar interpretation is also possible regarding the other modes of the "encompassing that is us," both spirit and Existenz. The presence of the epistemological viewpoint is apparent already in the multiplicity of modes included in the "encompassing that is us." Existence, "consciousness in general," and "spirit," which received a new explication within the framework of the encompassing, represent in their separateness the link each of the modes of the encompassing has to Being as a whole that exists beyond them. In this spirit, Jaspers described these components as beginnings that turn Being into something that we can experience.[123] Even Existenz is placed within the framework of the encompassing in one section along with other concepts, whose presence, in Jaspers's early thought, was considered as threatening the status of Existenz in the philosophizing and even its very existence. Henceforth Existenz is presented as one of a range of modes through which Being is accessed. The epistemological viewpoint transpires not only as a tool through which the connection with the framework of elucidating selfhood is preserved, while reinterpreting the previous philosophical concepts in a manner that enables them to be harnessed to the framework of the explication of Being. It also reveals an even more basic datum, whereby there is not just one way of elucidating Being, and so none of the modes can claim priority over the others.

The "encompassing that is Being itself" begins with the question that arises from establishing the different aspects revealed in the "encompassing that is us": do the different modes through which Being might be accessed represent and exhaust it, or perhaps it exists beyond them?[124] The ontological viewpoint, on which the "encompassing that is Being itself" is based, diverts the emphasis from the facet of accessibility that typified the epistemological viewpoint to the discussion of the nature of Being as such. Jaspers described Being as the "other" indicated by the "encompassing that is us,"[125] and as stemming from our interpreting drive that does not let us rest and settle in a perceivable realm.[126] Unlike the different modes included in the "encompassing that is us," which resulted from people's different ways of experiencing the world, the independence of the "encompassing that is Being itself" is stressed in relation to the framework of human existence. This encompassing is felt by people as the "self-declaration" of the other, whose existence is independent, unlike that typical of the "encompassing that is us."[127]

These features of Being do not enable the epistemological viewpoint to become a single tool through which Being is elucidated, but raise the need for the existence of the ontological viewpoint that aims to clarify the character of Being beyond the ways human beings can access it. The ontological viewpoint, representing the search for uniformity of Being, is also expressed in the few modes included in the "encompassing that is Being" revealed by it. The modes appearing in the "encompassing that is Being itself"—"world" and "transcendence"—are inclusive and general, and even within the framework of the elucidation of selfhood these two concepts represented an independent facet regarding the character of Existenz, which saw them as "other."[128] The explication of the "world" and "transcendence" as part of Jaspers's perception of Being appears to be less dependent on the interpretation that presents them as expressions of Being. The "world," and even more so "transcendence," is almost identical to the complete Being as Jaspers saw it. An extended discussion of the question of the relation between the concepts of "Being" and "transcendence" will be presented below in Chapter Eleven.

The constitution of the two types of encompassing, from previous components that had appeared in the clarification of selfhood, expresses another fundamental fact regarding the perception of the encompassing, meaning its being the outcome of a transcending from the explication of selfhood. From the genealogical perspective of Jaspers's philosophy we can argue that this transcending was enabled thanks to his liberation from the perception of Existenz as the widest framework into which all topics of philosophizing are drawn, in favor of a more flexible position where the discussion of Existenz is included as a component of a wider discussion. The transcending is mainly reflected in the transition from a single object of philosophizing to multiple objects or from Existenz to the different modes of the encompassing. However, a deeper observation shows that the framework of the whole encompassing reflects a unifying vision in relation to which Existenz and also existence, consciousness in general, and the other modes of the encompassing are revealed as details within the whole Being known as the "encompassing."

At the second stage of implementing the method of transcending, after these two viewpoints have helped split the discussion on Being into two types of encompassing, in both types of encompassing the same observation continues to be applied, fed by the two viewpoints: the epistemological, revealing the components constituting the "encompassing that is us," and the ontological, revealing those included in the "encompassing that is Being itself." The epistemological viewpoint also indicates the immanent facet of the two types of encompassing, while the ontological viewpoint indicates their transcendent facet. The transition from the immanent layer to the transcendent layer leads to a reduction in the modes of the encompassing. In the "encompassing that is us," this is expressed in the transition from existence, "consciousness in general," and "spirit" to Existenz, while in the "encompassing that is Being itself," the transition is from the "world" to "transcendence." The singular nature of "Existenz," the "world," and "transcendence" standing in transcendent relation to the multiplicity of immanent modes in the "encompassing that it us" is not external to this encompassing, but reveals the unifying power of the reflexivity aimed at its elucidation. Jaspers argued that "all three modes of the encompassing that I am are inevitably conditions for Existenz in itself achieving appearance and becoming real."[129] The different components of the Being of Existenz—existence, consciousness in general, and spirit—receive their meaning as modes of the "encompassing that is us" only when they are perceived within the context of wholeness by the Existenz transcendent to them, without which they are "baseless."[130] This means that immanence, portrayed first and foremost by the multiplicity of modes of the encompassing, enables their accessibility to elucidation from the epistemological viewpoint. However, Existenz, responsible for revealing the unity encompassing the multiplicity, is transcendent in relation to immanence not only in its not being present in any of the three immanent modes of the "encompassing that is us." Its very separateness indicates the presence of a transcendent facet in Existenz itself that urges it to transcend the boundaries of immanence. Therefore Existenz is placed under the same category defining "transcendence," meaning the transcendent element of the encompassing. This interpretation of the status of Existenz among the other modes of the encompassing helps clarify Jaspers's description of Existenz as wishing to achieve clarity and transparency regarding itself and constituting "a source of the real Being."[131] The definition of Existenz as a source is not identical to its perception as a "source" that was elucidated as an infrastructure for the constitution of the transition mechanisms.[132] See also the discussion of this idea in the chapter Introduction to the Transition Mechanisms. The use of the concept "source" regarding Existenz in this context demonstrates the overcoming of the rigid boundaries of the solipsistic perception of selfhood—a development that enabled Jaspers to perceive Existenz as capable of serving as a source for exposing a different and more encompassing entity.

A similar interpretation may also be offered for the "encompassing that is Being itself." The epistemological viewpoint, which sees in the world a framework of multiplicity, perceives it within the context of the encompassing as a portrayal of Being itself. In contrast, the ontological viewpoint, naturally turning to a more encompassing unity, indicates transcendence as representing Being in itself. To be precise, transcendence lacks its meaning as such without the framework of the world as a multiplicity, transcending from which enabled it itself. However, transcendence does not only represent the unifying framework of the multiplicity in the world, since already in the concept of the "world" the three immanent components of the "encompassing that is us" are unified. Transcendence indicates the existence of a unity beyond the world and is the name of this unity.

The presence of the immanent layer and the transcendent layer expresses a process of internal transcending within the two encompassings. This transcending is based on its predecessor, but at the same time deepens it by penetrating the internal components of each of the modes of the encompassing and defines its status within the whole framework of the encompassing. Whereas the first transcending was a constituting step of the perception of Being as encompassing, the second transcending reveals the relativity typical of all the modes of the encompassing, whose meaning is determined according to the viewpoint directed at them. Placing Existenz alongside existence, consciousness in general, and spirit in the "encompassing that is us" is an outcome of the epistemological viewpoint, while from the ontological viewpoint the very same Existenz is revealed as transcendent. In parallel, a similar process takes place in the "encompassing that is Being itself." Jaspers argued that our consciousness of Being changes through transcendence: on the one hand, the world ceases to be merely a world and is perceived as representing transcendence, while we feel it itself only through the world from which it faces us.[133] The world represents a unity that is transcendent in relation to the three immanent modes of the "encompassing that is us," but at the same time it represents in relation to the transcendence in the "encompassing that is Being itself" an immanent layer characterized by multiplicity, and as such serves as a foundation for the epistemological observation.

This move reveals the structural similarity characterizing the two types of encompassing, each divided into an immanent facet and a transcendent facet, and demonstrates the relativity of the immanent and transcendent categories in the context in which they are discussed. This understanding, that immanence receives this meaning in light of transcendence, which in itself lacks any meaning without immanence, does not enable the separation of the two encompassings from each other. The conclusion arising from the relative understanding of the modes of the encompassing, whereby they draw their meaning from the mutual contexts formed between them, is that the intuition about the existence of the transcendent Being has no meaning without the process of elucidating all of people's varied forms of experience in the world, represented by the different modes of the encompassing.

At the third stage of implementing the method of transcending, after the two viewpoints have been applied and the whole framework of the encompassing has been formed, as presented in the table above, the question arises whether it does represent Being itself, or whether this is a continuing process, and the more the explication movement continues, the more analogs of this Being will be discovered. The centrality of the method of transcending in Jaspers's philosophy makes the question of the boundaries of the philosophizing inevitable especially when the presentation of the framework of the discussion appears to have been completed, and apparently there is no possibility or need to move another step forward. In this respect we can see this stage of the explication as an expression of a stop in the process of revealing the different facets of Being and as an attempt to evaluate what has been presented in the philosophical discussion so far. Jaspers, in turn, left the question open. On the one hand, his discussion of Being is based on the different modes appearing in the table of the encompassing presented above, and even in his other writings no new components were added to it. After analyzing the different components included in the encompassing, Jaspers presented a scheme that expressed figuratively the location and meaning of the modes.[134] This situation could serve as a basis for the argument that Being itself is portrayed in the particular modes of the encompassing that Jaspers elucidated. On the other hand, Jaspers himself stated that the table represents only one of the possibilities of approaching Being, only examples of possible analogies of Being, while the encompassing is "not closed in itself."[135] In addition, the book *Out of Truth* was presented as the first volume of *Philosophical Logic*, and Jaspers planned a sequel that was never realized. However, we should note that in the books written afterwards dealing with Being, the framework of the encompassing as plotted in *Out of Truth* continued to serve as the infrastructure of the discussion, which shows that Jaspers himself did not uncover additional components that appeared to him to be part of Being.[136] The encompassing not being closed means that there are countless possibilities for representing analogies of Being, but none of them could represent it itself, but only different modes of experiencing it.

Despite this, we can find indirect expression of the handling of the question of the boundaries of the whole thought of the encompassing in Jaspers's dealing with the problem of the multiplicity of modes of the encompassing compared with the image of Being as something complete and uniform. Jaspers's arguments regarding this problem simultaneously enable two different directions of interpretation. One stresses the analog nature of the theory of the encompassing in relation to Being. This interpretative direction allows the viewing of the framework of the encompassing as an analogy of Being itself, and of the different modes as means that help constitute this relation toward Being that itself remains concealed. In contrast, the other interpretative direction perceives the encompassing as a representation of Being itself. I will describe these two interpretative directions below.

(1) The basis of the interpretation seeing the encompassing as an analogy of Being itself is Jaspers's statement that even the philosophizing based on transcending cannot clarify the one outside the multiplicity.[137] The multiplicity of the modes of the encompassing is merely an expression of the "branching of presence" of Being in our thought, and it loses this meaning when we isolate the parts from the whole encompassing them, or when we mistakenly identify the relations between them as relations of mutual negation.[138] Knauss and Samay saw the encompassing as representing the ways a person accesses Being and not as an explication of Being itself.[139] The fact that Being is revealed as being split, and that the distinction between the different modes of the encompassing relies on categories taken from the immanent world in which we live,[140] is perceived as evidence for the failure of thought to represent Being within itself,[141] or as expressing the gap between the perception of the encompassing and the reality of Being itself. However, Jaspers's words show that it is from the situation of the multiplicity of modes of the encompassing that the need arises to determine the relations between them and the "one fundamental relation" connecting the different modes. This view of the multiplicity of the modes of the encompassing softens the rigidity of the objective form of reference, which perceives its objects

through distinctions that isolate them from each other, and makes more flexible the reflection directed at Being. In the inability to decide between the parts of the multiplicity and to identify Being itself with any particular expression of it, the understanding of the Being as a "relational Being" is formed.[142] Eventually, thinking about the relations existing between the modes of the encompassing does not provide people with organized knowledge about them and cannot represent Being inside it and face the person with what Jaspers called "absolute thusness."[143] However, the very awareness of the inaccessibility of Being and the inability to clarify the one Being outside the multiplicity of analogies human beings constitute toward it leads to the perception of the modes of the encompassing as means that people's spirit creates in order to enable them to think about Being.[144] These modes serve as anchors of thought, or as Jaspers put it, as "beginnings"[145] for the philosophizing aiming itself at Being. Jaspers attributed this statement to the immanent modes of the "encompassing that is us," but it is also suitable for the other modes. Thinking about Being that is aware of its analogous nature, meaning that it knows that it cannot reveal Being itself, fills two roles simultaneously: it demonstrates Being for the person through its different modes, constituting a sort of attempt to concretize it, and at the same time in this way it hides Being itself from people. Either way, both in its action as demonstrating Being and in its action as hiding it, Being itself remains outside the reach of analogous thinking.

Awareness of the inability of analogous thinking to represent Being inside itself and to expose its presence in its different expressions in immanent reality did not diminish the original philosophical drive that motivated Jaspers to decipher the "primary mystery" of the one Being.[146] This drive remained intact, as a constant target and task directing the philosophizing. This completed the move of determining the status and weight of the modes of the encompassing within the general system of the perception of Being: they do not become in people's consciousness what Jaspers called, using Weber's term, "ideal types" of Being.[147] The modes of the encompassing do not reveal Being fully and perfectly, but should be seen as "thread ends" serving as a grasp point in the continuing task to constitute a uniform consciousness of Being, defined in this spirit as a "fabric."[148]

Viewing the perception of the encompassing as analogous to Being preserves the basic gap between the character of Being as an object of philosophizing and Being itself, as an eternal goal to which human consciousness aims.[149] In this, the Kantian thinking, stressing the limitations of the transcending of thought from the world of phenomena, is also noticeable. Just as Kant's philosophy granted the subject a central role in constituting the phenomena and in marking the boundaries of the thought revolving around them, so the interpretation seeing the encompassing as an analogy of Being grants Existenz a central role. In this context, Existenz was described as "a source from which all the modes of the encompassing receive their vitality and for which it simultaneously becomes an interlocutor," and as such, "for it transcendence becomes real for the first time."[150] The advantage of Existenz over the other modes of the encompassing has a far-reaching impact on the interpretation I propose for Jaspers's perception of Being. First and foremost, it emphasizes the relativity of the epistemological and ontological viewpoints, revealed as two key axes in the development of the perception of the encompassing. Accordingly, the different modes of the encompassing are perceived at different stages of the explication Existenz conducts of Being: in the "encompassing that is us," the components that Existenz has already elucidated in the framework of elucidating selfhood appear, while in the "encompassing that is Being itself" there is a new integration of them that reflects progress toward the constitution of a uniform consciousness regarding Being. The two central encompassings reflect at one and the same time different degrees of distancing on the part of Existenz from itself and approaching Being. In any case, in neither of them is it able to uncover real discoveries about Being itself, let alone the uniform image of Being, which was and remains beyond the boundaries of the existential consciousness.

The relative understanding of the two types of encompassing enables us not to negate the role of the ontological viewpoint in the first two stages of transcending. Although this viewpoint was unable to represent Being itself or even to form a uniform consciousness regarding it, it did help uncover the "world" and "transcendence"—two much more inclusive modes compared to those in the "encompassing that is us." In this context, the importance of the third transcending lies in its contribution to the understanding of the ontological viewpoint as relative. This means that ruling out the possibility of representing Being in thought does not present the ontological viewpoint as an empty vessel; its main importance is in helping expose the infrastructure common to some of the images of Being taken from thinking about immanence, and as a result, reducing the multiplicity typical of the "encompassing that is us" into just two modes included in the "encompassing that is Being itself." At the same time, this interpretative move projects upon the epistemological viewpoint and illuminates it, too, with a relative light. However, while the relativity of the ontological viewpoint disputes its ability to represent Being itself, not to mention the possibility of constituting a uniform consciousness regarding Being, the relativity of the epistemological viewpoint enables the unifying of the different expressions of Being into a relatively limited number of modes, included in the immanent section of the "encompassing that is us" and the "encompassing that is Being itself," meaning "existence," "consciousness in general," "spirit," and "world." The relativity of both the epistemological viewpoint and the ontological viewpoint indicates the distance of the philosophizing based on these two viewpoints from Being itself. However, the more they reflect this distance, the more they contribute—each in its way—to combining all the varied expressions of Being and to the reduction of the number of modes of the encompassing. While they do not help bring the philosophizing aimed at Being to its destination, they do help reveal more analogies of it.

The relativity of the two viewpoints confronts the framework of the explication of Being with a basic antonym Jaspers indicated in this context: every discovery about Being must enter some pattern, metaphor, or symbol in our consciousness, without which we lose our grasp on Being,[151] although according to the analogical approach this is insufficient for its complete representation. The expressions of Being also become its covers. The method of transcending, through which our thought wished to become liberated from its tendency to be fixated in some thought patterns, reaches the end of its boundary at this point. Jaspers called the fixation of thought in fixed patterns that restrict it "solidifying" (*Verfestigung*).[152] It helps open the space of reference of Existenz to beyond the boundaries of its selfhood, and as a result people can understand the different aspects they encounter in existence as possible analogies of Being, even if direct and uniform consciousness regarding this Being is still beyond them. The boundaries of the method of transcending in relation to the constituting of a uniform and complete consciousness of Being do not indicate only the basic continuity accompanying the three transcending moves presented as an infrastructure for the development of the theory of the encompassing, but also indicate a basic continuity between the explication of selfhood and that of Being. While this interpretation does not assimilate the perception of the encompassing into the clarification of Existenz, as the scholars whose interpretations were presented above did, it does present the explication of Being and the philosophizing in general as a constant process of widening and expansion—a process where on the one hand, selfhood serves as a basis and an anchor, while on the other hand it appears as experiencing a constant opening up to what exists beyond it.

(2) The interpretation seeing the perception of the encompassing as representing real discoveries from Being itself relies on a basic intuition regarding the existence of a uniform Being and seeing it as a basis on which the whole perception of the encompassing is constructed. The internal persuasion characterizing intuition served Jaspers as a basis for the argument that the split between object and subject, typical of his experience of Being, does not represent Being, which is the source of this split, but that its wholeness remains beyond it.[153] Compare also the argument that "anything, what has become an object for us, be it the greatest, still always exists for us within something else, it is not everything."[154] Even the statement that Being is "itself the first [question]" that arises in people in the different situations in which they participate,[155] indicates the existence of a hidden depth existing within individual and felt at moments of elation, when they feel that they are penetrating the elements of existence and rising above the routine sinking into the world.[156] Jaspers was not deterred from characterizing these moments as "remembering,"[157] and in this term he wished to

indicate the existence of awareness of the wholeness of Being—an awareness serving as a basis for our ability to refer to it in more partial contexts using consciousness, which in itself cannot contain the unity of Being. In another place, Jaspers wrote that from the encompassing "something happens that man calls unsatisfyingly 'feeling,' but [in fact] this is something that is more than a feeling, [this is] the ability of my deepest Being to be expressed."[158] These statements reflect different attempts by Jaspers to give tangible expression to the presence of intuition regarding the existence of a uniform Being, constituting a basic infrastructure enabling the explication of the different expressions of Being itself and perhaps even of its unity as such. Jaspers presented the relation between intuition and its expression in the perception of the encompassing as the relation between the prelogical and the logical. Salamun commented in this context on the influence of Friedrich Wilhelm Joseph Schelling and Plotinus on the perception of Being as an original unity that people can experience in moments of spiritual elation.[159] Jaspers knew Schelling as a philosopher who tried to overcome the split between object and subject, and reach an encompassing Being.[160] From this point of view, "the conscious realization of the modes of the encompassing does still not develop logic in the narrow sense," meaning that it is not a reflection on the validity of objective knowledge and its forms, but it operates as a clarification of the prelogical, serving as a basis and a precondition for logic itself. The encompassing as such represents an insight that does not ignore the requirement of thought for objectivity, but imagines the "fragility" of objective distinctions[161] and prevents the "loss of Being within knowledge."[162]

The difficulty in establishing the interpretation that sees the encompassing as a representation of Being itself is especially prominent in comparison with the interpretation viewing it as an analogy of Being itself. While the second found support and many direct references in Jaspers's words, the first depends on a few indirect arguments, and the impression is formed that the interpretation seeing the encompassing as a representation of Being itself is more forced and problematic. However, this situation is a direct outcome of the basic character of the argument around which each of the interpretations forms. An analogy diverts the philosophizing into the realm of phenomena that can naturally be presented discursively, with the split into a multiplicity of images and realizations perceived as part of the analogous nature of the thinking itself instead of as a flaw. In contrast, the interpretation seeing the encompassing as a representation of Being itself is based on an intuition that as such cannot be given an exhaustive expression in language, which can only expose partial expressions of it. This intuition constitutes a sort of psychic-conscious position of which people become capable only after knowing themselves. This means that the thought seeking to clarify or reflect the intuition as such is aware of its limitations and of the basic fact that the more it concentrates on the intuition's different expressions, the more it moves away from it as a whole. Contrastingly, when the intuition is supported by few phrases and references, this is not considered as a disadvantage, and in any case cannot deny its existence.

The basic difficulty entailed in the interpretation seeing the encompassing as an expression of Being itself can be demonstrated by determining the relation between Jaspers's ideas and Kantian thought. Alongside the connections between the interpretation seeing the encompassing as an analogy of Being and Kant's concept of phenomena, we can indicate proximity between the position seeing the encompassing as a representation of Being itself and Kant's concept of the "thing-in-itself." However, while the approach seeing the encompassing as an analogy of Being itself reflected Jaspers's reliance on Kant's thought, the perception of the encompassing as an expression of Being itself does not stand in direct relation to Kant, but can be seen as providing an answer to what is lacking in his philosophy. Schneiders hints at this interpretative direction in his criticism of Mader's position presented above, when he asks "Should Jaspers's encompassing be understood as a development of the Kantian theory of ideas, or perhaps this is an interpretation of the very same idea?"[163] Such an interpretation of Jaspers's concept of the encompassing is presented by Janos Kelemen. He argues that Jaspers, like other interpreters of Kant, believed that the concept "the thing-in-itself" presents an impossible position: through this concept Kant wished to define objectivity as if Kant were outside the space in which it exists, when he existed within this space. Kelemen even argues that Jaspers's concept of the encompassing proposes a solution to this contradiction, whereby we should not understand Kant's concept of "the thing-in-itself" in discursive terms, but instead it should be seen as "nomina," meaning that through the encompassing the "thing-in-itself" is interpreted as a category not containing a component of experience, but thinkable by pure reason and not by objective consciousness. As a result, the "thing-in-itself" is interpreted not as a possible or impossible category, but as a boundary concept of consciousness, which cannot explicate it.[164] In Jaspers's interpretation of Kant's concept of the "thing-in-itself," as presented by Kelemen, he was able to require the existence of a Being transcending the boundaries of experience without presenting an absolute perception of it or presenting an equivalent foundation for it.[165] A comprehensive evaluation of Jaspers's interpretation of Kant's philosophy would exceed the boundaries of the current discussion.[166] However, his understanding of the concept of the encompassing as referring in some way to the Being that breaks through the boundaries of the phenomena—as arises from Kelemen's interpretation—can be harnessed to the interpretative move presenting the perception of the encompassing as an attempt to explicate Being itself. The interpretation that views the encompassing as a representation of the unity of Being or at least of parts of it sharpens the distinction between the third stage of the transcending and the previous stages. In the first two stages of the transcending, the encompassing expressed different levels of reflection on the expressions of Being present in the world of phenomena. In contrast, in the third stage the thinking about Being transcends the boundaries of consciousness. In this transcending, reason, which Jaspers defined as "a bond of the modes of the encompassing,"[167] may help the person imagine the existence of a uniform Being that at the beginning was merely an intuition. As a result, not only is the significant difference stressed between the two viewpoints, which in the perception of the encompassing as an analogy were perceived as relative, but the supremacy and primacy of the ontological viewpoint over the epistemological one is revealed, to the extent of removing the epistemological viewpoint from filling a significant role in the realization of the third transcending of Being itself. This interpretation, indicating the different status of the three stages of the transcending, does not enable us to argue that the elucidation of the "Being that is us" contributes less to the constituting of a uniform consciousness regarding Being in comparison with the elucidation aimed at the "encompassing that is Being itself." This is because the third stage of transcending is enabled only after the different modes of the encompassing have been explicated and the first two stages of transcending have been implemented. However, the basic continuity of the explication of selfhood and that of Being, as arising from the interpretation of the encompassing as an analogy, is not characteristic of this interpretation, which stresses the distinct status of the third transcending. This transcending, which pushed the epistemological viewpoint into the margins of the explication, also stresses the difference between the two explications and the distancing of the thinking of Being from the boundaries of the elucidation of selfhood. While in the explication that viewed the encompassing as an analogy of Being the philosophizing was characterized by constant expansion, in the interpretation seeing it as a representation of Being we can notice the existence of a tendency aiming to gather together the philosophical insights it had accumulated—a tendency aimed at identifying the element common to several of the expressions of Being, and perhaps even to formulate a uniform consciousness of Being by observing them.

The development of the interpretation in two separate tracks—from the identifying of a basic duality in the term encompassing, through the discovery of the two viewpoints on which the perception of the encompassing is founded, and up to the splitting of the third transcending into two different perceptions of the encompassing as a whole—reflects the attempt to follow the stages of the constituting of the theory of the encompassing as Jaspers himself presented it. The consistent duality, which has evidence throughout Jaspers's text and that at no stage of the explication lost its hold, receives its final support from his words that the philosophy of the encompassing does not have one single starting point. He says that the possible existence of such a starting point would apparently indicate the wish for intellectual control over Being that is so extremely contrary to the thinking of the encompassing that the existence of such a wish would harm the very possibility of realizing it.[168] In this spirit we can also understand the basic condition of indecisiveness reached by the interpretation presented above: on the one hand, it raised the possibility in principle of exposing systematic aspects in the philosophy of the encompassing and following them throughout its length, but on the other hand, no aspect or interpretative line was found to be preferable to the other, but instead the relativity of the different aspects and their dependence on each other was demonstrated. This interpretation largely suits Jaspers's description of what he called "the foundation of the thinking of Being":

> There is no system of Being, no system of existence, no system of the thinkable, no known whole. The thinking from the encompassing requires with its conducting the consciousness of its transcending nature and thus of the parable nature of all the objects appearing within it. Only through knowledge of this parable nature do they stay real.[169]

These words show that Jaspers's interest in constituting the perception of the encompassing was mainly in establishing the independence of Being in relation to the thought that thinks it. The awareness of the absence of a system in Being is what preserves the person wishing to elucidate Being from the danger of reductionism—a mistake that Jaspers saw as the inevitable outcome of philosophical positions that presented themselves as a complete system. Samay's interpretation of the encompassing fits into this context. Samay argued that transcendental metaphysics is a tool that preserves the fragmentary nature of Being, which does not crystallize into a system, but sees its "non-objective" and "unknowable" nature as expressing Being itself.[170] However, in my opinion, Samay tended to overemphasize, both in his interpretation of the encompassing and in other contexts, the role of objectivity, and therefore missed the intuitive aspects that are fundamental to Jaspers's philosophy.[171]

3. Periechontology

The duality revealed by following the stages of the development of the perception of the encompassing finds its uniform expression in the term "periechontology" (*Periechontologie*),[172] meaning the philosophizing aimed at the encompassing. It is no coincidence that this term first appeared only after Jaspers finished clarifying the different modes of the encompassing. Jaspers used the Greek verb *periechon*, meaning to encompass, and gave it a nominal form, and periechontology is philosophy or thought dealing with the encompassing (*Umgreifendes*).[173] In this term, Jaspers wished to present a new philosophical framework for elucidating Being, which would serve as an alternative to the ontological approach to Being. Jaspers's objection in principle to ontology as the "theory of the is" stemmed first and foremost from its basic scientific presumption to offer a "system of Being," following which Being was perceived as an order of objects or as an expression of what he termed "unities of meaning." Jaspers believed that the linkage of ontologies to the framework of objective thinking made them identify Being with "what is," and as a result Being was limited to the realm of immanence. The analysis of the different meanings of existence, which is the heart of the practice of the ontological position regarding Being as Jaspers understood it, expressed the avoidance of treating Being as a wholeness existing beyond the private entities and constituting their source. As a substitute for this activity, the ontologies he criticized "overcome the undefinablity of the primary" or else it "becomes an object and an issue,"[174] and as a result, philosophy becomes a "*dilution of Being*... or *a fixation* for a *defined* and categorical Being that has become known."[175] The aim of achieving a complete perception of Being is replaced with the ontological approaches, which Jaspers saw as whole systems creating a barrier between Being and the thought that thinks it.

Unlike ontology, periechontology is focused on the expressions, "spaces," as Jaspers put it, where Being exists and where we find ourselves. The different modes of the encompassing should not be seen as a basis for the presentation of defined statements regarding Being or as tangible expressions of its structure, but while they are clarified, Being continues to be considered as "*prior* to all the defined entities or as *absorbing* and granting meaning that in itself cannot turn into an object."[176] While we cannot perceive the encompassing in such a satisfying way, so that we could deduce from it Being in its entirety, the advantage of the perception of the encompassing is in its being anchored in advance in the assumption that such a Being does exist. From the perspective of the encompassing we can state that "what exists is not for us like the encompassing that we know, but is like the presence of the here and now in their depth [that reaches] the source."[177] The expressions of Being, revealed through the perception of the encompassing, constitute part of a whole, surrounding encompassing that exists beyond them. Even the perception of the encompassing as an analogy presumes the very existence of such a Being, although the analogical position itself is permeated by the consciousness that it is not able to represent it or parts of it. It is completely clear that the more periechontology connects the consciousness of people's Being to the boundaries of their experience and helps them understand themselves as part of Being, the farther it is from providing them with a feeling of controlling it. Periechontology is anchored in the framework of the encompassing and the philosophical possibilities it contains: as an analogical perception of Being, or as a representation of Being.

The possibility in principle that periechontology could not grant a full or even partial representation of Being led several interpreters to understand periechontology as lacking real positive contents. For instance, this is the opinion of Heinemann, who defined Jaspers's philosophy in general and the encompassing in particular as "an adventure of radical openness," which by aiming at openness and inclusiveness avoids positive decisions regarding the issues under discussion.[178] In this spirit, Mader also defined the encompassing as "a horizonless horizon" (*horizontloser Horizont.*)[179] The use of the term horizon for clarifying the encompassing was made by Jaspers himself.[180] In this context, see also Samay's comment regarding the image of the concept of the encompassing as a horizon.[181] Heinemann's interpretation, placing the experience of radical doubt from the negation of final and objective categories at the center of Jaspers's philosophy, led him to define Jaspers's approach as "a sort of reverse Hegelianism, since while for Hegel the absolute was a result, for Jaspers it was a non-result,"[182] and to present Jaspers himself as a "floating philosopher."[183] Richli's interpretation, too, reflects the same impression that appeared in Heinemann's, whereby Jaspers does not make real statements regarding Being. In his opinion, the commitment of periechontology not to see the contents produced by the mind and objective thinking as part of the perception of Being introduced into periechontology a basic contradiction, following which "it cannot express what it has to say."[184] This image of Jaspers's perception of Being results, in Richli's opinion, from the very method of transcending, which is by definition "movement into the whole," and he believes it is no wonder that Jaspers did not present any perception of the whole itself. In his opinion, transcending or "the power of going out is simultaneously the consciousness of the helplessness" of itself, and this is identical to the consciousness of the transcendence of Being. Eventually transcending does not lead Jaspers, according to Richli's interpretation, to "another world," but only enables him to experience the openness and enigmatic Being of the world.[185] It is from a positive consciousness that he interprets Being made inevitably relative to the interpretative position he holds regarding it.[186]

The basis of the interpretations of Richli and Heinemann, more generally reflecting the understanding of the encompassing as part of the object-subject split and as an attempt to overcome it, Jaspers's perception of Being was identified with the very practice of transcending.[187] This identification denies Jaspers's perception everything that could be seen as the fruit of this transcending, meaning real arguments regarding Being. This interpretation leaves Jaspers's arguments about Being within the boundaries of immanence. The inevitable result of these interpretations, which placed the very act of philosophizing at the center of this thought, was the inclusion of Jaspers's perception of the encompassing within the philosophy of Existenz. The interpretations of Richli and Heinemann do not express Jaspers's insights regarding the boundaries of Being and Existenz, insights that had started to be formulated already in *World Orientation*, even before the perception of the encompassing had appeared in his writings. Nor do they demonstrate how much Jaspers's perception of Existenz decisively influenced the understanding of his entire philosophy even when Being instead of Existenz had been set as the object of the philosophizing.

However, unlike these interpretations, I believe that Jaspers's discussion of Being reflects a real turning point in his philosophy, and can no longer be seen as part of the philosophy of Existenz. Jaspers's perception of Being expresses his desire for real contents of Being itself, which became revealed as the original target of Existenz. Especially in his statements regarding the "encompassing that is us" we can see a process of renewed observation of different aspects that had appeared within the explication of Existenz from the perspective of the encompassing that revealed them as expressions of Being. In this respect, what was earlier defined as the epistemological viewpoint, in which the role of Existenz and of consciousness in elucidating the encompassing was clarified, served as a framework in which the contents of Being were discovered.

At the same time, the periechontology that Jaspers wished to constitute is not limited to these contents alone. Using what was called the ontological viewpoint, the intuitive aspects behind Jaspers's attempt to constitute a uniform consciousness regarding Being were revealed. While the epistemological viewpoint revealed the materials on which the philosophizing could act and organize itself, the ontological viewpoint expressed the "form" that is their essence. Just as form is what gives matter its shape and essence, so the ontological observation is responsible for the contents accumulated during the philosophizing process being perceived as expressions of Being or at least as an analogy of it, and are not limited to the direct immanent meaning arising from them. In this respect, the ontological viewpoint can be seen as a barrier against the materialization and mystification of the expressions of Being, and as a central tool through which Jaspers released the contents he dealt with from the "structurality" that characterizes them in the ontological systems he criticized.[188] Jaspers was able to include within the framework of the periechontology two elements, neither of which could stand alone: an *experiential element* related in essence to the finite reality in which people live and act, and an *intuitive element* thanks to which the experience of the finite reality becomes "a pattern of a different thought,"[189] meaning: experiencing Being itself that Jaspers described as follows:

> The unity of the modes of the encompassing is an indisputable basic certainty of our philosophizing. But the question about this unity does not find its answer in the Being-construction that can describe the one Being through the modes of the encompassing, but in pushing the question above any premature insufficient unity to the one that no philosophy can indicate except as a possibility that becomes perceptible on the boundary that can only be perceived by the historistic Existenz and not by any knowledge of the one.[190]

So periechontology clarifies the boundaries of the realization of the wish to constitute a uniform consciousness regarding Being, but absolutely does not give up the attempt to constitute a positive consciousness regarding Being itself. From the viewpoint of the method of transcending (*Transzendieren*), transcendence is perceived as one of the modes of the encompassing, and so the real constitution of a uniform perception of Being is always perceived as "premature realization," meaning that it must remain as a task for the future. However, since the uniformity of Being is a basic certainty that cannot be disputed, it exists as a Being beyond it (*Transzendenz*), and never remains within the boundaries of immanence alone. As the practice of transcending went deeper within the framework of the encompassing, Jaspers concluded that "[there is] a higher Being than the one that is us ourselves; the fact that we can think it from within and beyond our limitations contains a hint of its real Being."[191] So, periechontology combined the consciousness of entities as a multiplicity and the consciousness of the entity itself that is transcendence, which Jaspers defined as "the encompassing of all encompassings."[192]

Ten

THE CIPHERS OF TRANSCENDENCE

1. From the Foundering and the Encompassing to the Concept of Cipher

The experience of the foundering, which deepened the awareness of the boundaries of Existenz, refined Karl Jaspers's awareness that Existenz cannot exist without constituting a real relation toward a Being external to it and more encompassing than it. While this experience undermined the basic insights achieved in the explication of selfhood, it did not make Existenz irrelevant, nor did it lead to its becoming closed within its boundaries, but instead opened to it new horizons that served as a target for clarification and experience. The two insights achieved through the elucidation of the foundering—placing Being as the central target of the philosophization, and making finitude, instead of Existenz, the starting point for elucidating the Being beyond Existenz—altered the basic understanding of immanence compared with the one typical of the discussion within the elucidation of selfhood. Immanence was no longer perceived as the opposite pole to Existenz, or as hiding the real and the original from philosophy. Quite the opposite, at this stage the understanding formed in Jaspers's thought that it is immanence that holds the key to elucidating Being itself—an understanding following which immanence became the symbol or cipher (*Chiffre*) of transcendence.[1] Jaspers usually used the terms symbol and cipher synonymously. Immanence, as the concrete reality of the world and as the real consciousness of human beings regarding this world and themselves, is now perceived as a possible source for elucidating transcendence due to the metaphysical depth it contains.

The connection between the experience of the foundering and the new perception of immanence as a cipher of transcendence, and the more general distancing from the existential viewpoint, arises from the following passage:

> … The foundering is the covering ground of the entire cipher-Being. Seeing the cipher as the reality of Being originates first and foremost in the experience of foundering. From it, all the ciphers that are not rejected receive their final approval. What I allow to sink into annihilation, I can receive back as a cipher.[2]

As we have seen, the experience of the foundering indicated two possible ways: the negative one, which Jaspers defined as "despair," returned the discussion to Existenz, apparently recognizing that Being and transcendence were blocked to it.

Alongside it appeared an option that against the background of the discussion of the encompassing can be seen as preferable to the previous one. This possibility, bearing a more positive nature, makes the foundering the starting point for clarifying transcendence, and indicates that what "must be doubted before the uninterpretable foundering" is perceived from the viewpoint of the cipher as capable of elucidation and as a basis for "the source of the life that experiences... Being."[3] What in the foundering was blocked from understanding becomes in the perception of ciphers a source for the understanding of Being. In this respect we can state that the perception of immanence as a cipher of transcendence realizes the constructive possibility that arose from the foundering. It turns Being, which had been a source of dissatisfaction for Existenz in the experiences included in the transition mechanisms and blocked for interpretation in the foundering, into a target that the philosophical elucidation approaches with faith that it can succeed.

However, the perception of the encompassing, explained in the previous chapter, also reflected an attempt to propose an elucidation of Being and transcendence, and this raises the question regarding the necessity of the concept of the cipher for the framework of the explication of Being. This question is even more important since the framework of the perception of immanence as a cipher of transcendence contained no direct explication of this immanence, but it relied on the premise that it is an existing entity—a premise appearing from *World Orientation* onwards. Different scholars of Jaspers's thought have already dealt with this question. Johannes Thyssen asks whether Existenz's experience of transcendence as self-insufficiency, through the absolute consciousness, is not enough. His answer is that beyond and because of the existential experience of finitude, the need arises for transcendence to be represented in the finite reality that is split into object and subject. The concept of the cipher, which Thyssen defined as a "semi-objective" form portraying the existential attitude toward empirical reality, enables, in his opinion, the representation of transcendence in finality without turning it into an object.[4]

Xavier Tilliette discussed the question of the necessity of ciphers in Jaspers's philosophy from another direction by asking whether ciphers were destined to lose their importance in light of periechontology and philosophical logic as rational elements on which the discussion of Being was based.[5] In his opinion, the ciphers enable the inception of the method of transcending, and they exist precisely for those who were unable to divert themselves from the path of objective consciousness, but especially for Existenz, which is the only one that hears the "voices" of the ciphers and determines the criterion according to which their truth is determined.[6] He believes that Existenz experiences these "voices" as "shining lights" showing the way to transcendence, and only thanks to them does it not move blindly in circles around itself.[7] On the basis of the premise that "the scheme of Existenz in its structures and situations is the formal skeleton of the experience of cipher," Tilliette concluded that this experience "must be revealed as an image and a backwards look of the clarification of Existenz."[8] Even though Tilliette located the question of the necessity of the ciphers within the explication of Being, his interpretation anchored their meaning within the boundaries of the elucidation of Existenz.

However, unlike Thyssen, who asked about the necessity of the ciphers from the viewpoint of Existenz, and Tilliette, who returned them to the boundaries of the explication of Existenz, I believe that the ciphers are both the question and the answer to the framework of the explication of Being. The concepts cipher and encompassing were responses to the need for extra-existential elucidation of Being, since Existenz itself has certainty regarding the existence of a transcendent experience. More precisely, the need for extra-existential elucidation also belongs to Existenz, but this does not link the attempt to realize it with the explication of selfhood, but instead with that aimed at Being. It is within the framework of the explication of Being that the necessity of symbols is clear: they enable the accessibility of transcendence itself.

> Everything must be capable of becoming a cipher. Were there no cipher [there would be] no transcendence....
> The very fact that there is a cipher is identical for us to there being transcendence ... Instead of asking why there is existence, the question appears before us why there is a cipher. The answer to this: for existential consciousness it is the only form where transcendence rises, a sign that for Existenz transcendence is hidden, but had not disappeared.[9]

The concept of the cipher appeared in Jaspers's writings even before he presented the perception of the encompassing, but both of them relied on the same premises and served as means of dealing with the same philosophical problems: the basic tension between the ontological element and the epistemological element, and the attempt to elucidate immanence as part of the process of explicating Being. The cipher first appeared in *Philosophy*, while the encompassing first appeared in *Reason and Existenz*. The concept of the cipher appeared alongside the concept of the encompassing almost throughout the book *Out of Truth*.[10] Using the concepts of encompassing and cipher, Jaspers wished to lay down a path that would enable the transition from the discussion of Existenz to the elucidation of Being and transcendence and to guarantee that immanence would be essential in the explication of Being.

Despite these two terms being located genealogically at the same stage of Jaspers's development, they do not overlap each other, but each of them includes different contents that were suited in a different way to dealing with the fundamental philosophical problems characteristic of the explication of Being. The argument at the center of the discussion in this chapter is that through the concept of the cipher, Jaspers was able to establish the status of immanence and

Existenz within the explication of Being, beyond what he was able to do within the encompassing. While in the perception of the encompassing immanence served as a framework gathering within it aspects that appeared separately within the explication of selfhood and representing an opposite facet to Existenz, the concept of the cipher clarified the place of immanence as an integral part of the explication of Being. In the perception of immanence as a cipher of transcendence, Jaspers largely overcame the duality typical of the encompassing that was split into "the encompassing that is us" and "the encompassing that is Being itself." While the split made it possible to see immanence as merely a preparation for the explication of Being and not as an actual part of it, the cipher, which always originates in immanence,[11] leaves no such doubt. The cipher is just a path of the viewpoint toward immanence—an attempt to see immanence as an expression of Being—and should not be viewed as part of another reality existing beyond the one we witness in the tangible world. In this respect the cipher, the mental creation of Existenz, which constitutes a metaphysical relation toward immanence, does not leave room for an interpretation attributing to Existenz a merely marginal role in the explication of Being. While Existenz itself is one of the modes of the encompassing, its location in the "encompassing that is us" could apparently have the understanding that it had no place in the "encompassing that is Being itself." The perception of ciphers presented below can also be seen as a framework for examining the relation between the two basic encompassings from a new angle.

2. Foreshadowing Aspects of the Cipher in *Psychology*

As we have seen, the framework of object-subject relations served as a starting point in the mental-conscious experience of constituting a world view.[12] Beyond the philosophical aspects relating to selfhood as having this experience that were discussed in Chapter Two, Jaspers's ideas, as appearing in *Psychology*, can also be seen as the start of a philosophical move that only matured within the perception of ciphers. The basis of the comparison between the process of constituting a world view and the perception of ciphers results from selfhood constituting a new perception of reality in the experience of both points of views they entail. As the experience of constituting a world view perceives the "experience flow" of subjectivity as fully anchored in immanence, Jaspers defined it as creating new contents through which it changes itself.[13] The world view does not serve only as a tool for handling the different experiences of reality, since in the process of such handling the person forms another understanding of the experiences and of the reality in which they occur. Similarly, the experience leading to the perception of reality as a cipher of transcendence—a perception at the center of our discussion in this chapter—changes the person's perception of reality, which is no longer perceived as merely immanent. Knowingly or unknowingly, Jaspers already drew the line leading from *Psychology* to the concept of cipher when he wrote:

> From these boundaries, enclosing all the complete spheres of the split between object and subject as a mystical thing in which the spirit cannot escape… an inexpressible and insubstantial light is shed that always urges for the achievement of a form within this split. This becomes a symbol, a parable that has infinite desire for clarity. This desire, which is spiritual in essence, immediately ceases to be merely such a desire.[14]

In this passage, Jaspers explicitly indicated the clarifying potential of the object-subject relations entailed in the experience from which the world view results. Perhaps these words can also be seen as a hint of the possibility that beyond this clarity metaphysical horizons will be reflected that transcend the boundaries of the perception of reality in which the world view is anchored. The argument that *Psychology* contains aspects that foreshadow the concept of cipher is not based only on the passage cited above, but also on wide philosophical moves characteristic of Jaspers's thought in *Psychology*. This refers especially to Jaspers's prominent effort to present thought frameworks where the character of the subjective Being that constituted them and the perception of reality that guides it could be clarified. Jaspers discussed in detail "approaches," "world pictures," and "spirit types."[15] As we may recall, the understanding that the subject-object relations framework is expressed in different forms reflected in the different world views guided Jaspers in *Psychology* in his search for systematic thought[16] that would enable proposing an explication of the human soul. While the soul was already perceived from the beginning as incapable of being exhaustively elucidated, Jaspers argued that "the devotion existing in all finite matter enables us to somehow find an organizing viewpoint."[17] The phenomenological observation of the phenomenon of multiplicity of world views can provide us with some grasp points to serve as a basis for elucidating the human soul as a Being that cannot be exhausted by observing the different world views. The advantages of the phenomenological viewpoint regarding the multiplicity of world views, by their very nature distant from the observer's individual viewpoint, are clear: it enables the critical observation of selfhood, it may help uncover the infrastructure shared by the world views as such, and even creates *openness* toward the experiences of other people. Also, the process of exposing the structural characteristics accompanying the experiences involved in world views may help it see these experiences as reality and to use them as grasp points in reality.

The contribution of these advantages, typical of people's experience of constituting a world view, to Jaspers's developmental stage when he was writing *Psychology* becomes more tangible in light of this being Jaspers's first work after leaving the practice and science of psychiatry. Unlike pathology, whose expressions from Jaspers's point of view could always surprise without maintaining a degree of regularity, he perceived the "normality" indicated by the word "psychology" as capable of prediction and methodical elucidation. He expected to be able to expose systematic aspects of the constitution of world views, especially the experience of the range of normality. The specific patterns discussed in *Psychology*—the "approaches," "world pictures," and "spirit types"—served him at this period as framework for the formulation of the perception of selfhood that he called at that time "subjectivity."

Just as the discussion of the systematic aspects typical of world views revealed the objective foundations on which the explication of selfhood relied at the time, so the discussion of immanence that became the cipher of transcendence clarified the objective foundations on which Jaspers based the philosophizing aimed at elucidating Being. Like the advantages of systematic thought for the elucidation of selfhood in *Psychology*, the perception of ciphers made the metaphysical consciousness that was formulated in this context open and critical, and gave it a grasp point in the concrete reality where Existenz finds its existence. As a result, people's metaphysical consciousness is portrayed as relying on reality itself and not as a fantasy whose boundaries spread into the non-obligatory realm of human imagination.[18]

In a way, the need of metaphysical consciousness for defined thought patterns was filled already in the perception of the encompassing, where Jaspers indicated seven modes whose elucidation, and the clarification of the relations between which, could serve as a means for constituting consciousness regarding Being itself. The seven modes of the encompassing and their division by Jaspers are represented in a table in Chapter Nine, in the section The Two Facets of Being as the Encompassing. The seven ways are: "existence," "consciousness in general," "spirit," "Existenz," "world," "transcendence," and "reason." But the concept of the cipher provides a better answer to the need for the philosophizing of thought patterns that would serve as a receptacle for the insights being formulated regarding Being and transcendence. While the encompassing contains a defined number of patterns that to a great extent determined the boundaries of metaphysical consciousness, cipher, as we will see later, turns any object in reality into a potential pattern in which metaphysical consciousness can be formulated. In this respect, immanence, which has become a cipher of transcendence, contains an infinity of thought patterns in which the perception of Being itself can be formulated.

The perception of world views and the cipher as thought patterns organizing the philosophical insights in relation to the context in which they were clarified stresses the functional facet of these two key concepts. This argument, which does not diminish the importance of the contents aspects that Jaspers developed while clarifying the concepts of world view and cipher, demonstrates his effort to anchor his discussion in concepts that would grant clarity to his complex philosophical ideas and make them accessible to a wider critical discussion. However, it is against the background of this argument that the question inevitably arises, why the works appearing between *Psychology* and the appearance of the concept of the cipher abandoned the trend to present thought patterns or even to define terms that would help organize the philosophical discussion more systematically. This question could similarly be asked regarding the appearance of the concept of the encompassing, but it still arises more sharply here, in light of my interpretation whereby the cipher provides a better answer to the need for more defined thought frameworks. The answer to this question is linked to the most fundamental infrastructure on which the two frameworks of the philosophizing where the concepts of the world views and the cipher were developed, namely the explication of selfhood and the explication of Being.

I believe that the prominent absence of an organized system of concepts results from the solipsistic image of selfhood, which influenced the framework of the philosophizing aimed at its elucidation; even when this image became a conscious element, and the limitations it imposed upon the possibility of achieving a complete understanding of Existenz were gradually exposed, its presence was felt in Jaspers's thought. This image, which served the need to stress the unique character of Existenz, could not accord with the constitution of stable thought patterns that could grant the framework of the explication of selfhood a more consistent and systematic nature. Jaspers did not completely abandon this value, and as we have seen he had to deal with what he called "repeating analogical patterns" in the different world views[19] in order to be able to present a "catalog" or "relative scheme" of world views.[20] However, the power of the solipsistic image of selfhood was more dominant, especially in his early writings, including *Psychology*, which found expression in Jaspers's effort to propose an explication of world views from a private viewpoint and as an individual experience.[21]

In some respects, the tension created by the joint presence of these two viewpoints in *Psychology*—the viewpoint regarding the multiplicity of world views and the one aimed at elucidating the individual world view—was resolved with the constitution of the philosophy of Existenz, where the tendency that made selfhood unique in its surroundings and isolated it even from other people, themselves Existenzes, dominated. Even when the idea of communication appeared, the impressions of this tension, which was not completely resolved at any stage in the development of this philosophy, remained. Even the placing of Being at the center of the philosophical discussion did not propose a more general and systematic viewpoint regarding human beings, but made selfhood into the background for the explication of Being. Jaspers's philosophy included no perception of selfhood that overcame the difficulties raised by its solipsistic image; these difficulties contributed to the constitution of a new framework of philosophizing in Jaspers's thought, where they no longer had the same weight as in the framework of the explication of selfhood. In any case, the weakening of solipsism, which also involved overcoming the need to grant selfhood an absolute status in the philosophical discussion, enabled the constitution of the concepts of the encompassing and the cipher within the framework of the explication of Being. These concepts, which were not mainly intended to help the explication of selfhood, and that dealt with the metaphysical aspects of existence that were not exhausted by the meaning they had for Existenz, reflected distancing not only from the solipsistic selfhood, but also from the drive to elucidate Existenz. These processes, enabling the very constitution of more structured thought frameworks, explain why at this stage of the development of his philosophy Jaspers was able to realize things whose importance he had probably already recognized already at the start of his journey.

3. Immanence as a Cipher of Transcendence

The interpretation of the perception of the encompassing presented in the previous chapter apparently left Existenz in an impossible situation. On the one hand, its awareness was heightened of the gap between Being itself or transcendence and the way it was perceived in its thought; an awareness that also indicated the limitations of the method of transcending in serving as a sole tool for the explication of Being.[22] On the other hand, the understanding that the very existence of Being for individuals depends on their ability to experience it is a datum that encourages Existenz not to accept the abyss between it and the direct understanding of Being itself, and the possibility that such an abyss could become the last datum of human existence. The possibility that awareness of the boundaries of the method of transcending could develop into acceptance of the gap between human consciousness and Being itself constitutes a real threat both to Existenz's self-understanding and to the framework of the philosophizing as laid out so far. This is because the transcending on which the most basic infrastructure of Jaspers's thought was established is no mere method or viewpoint; it has become a mechanism through which the framework of the philosophizing was determined and the aims of the philosophizing itself were set. Surrendering the method of transcending at this stage due to the exposure of its limitations could have raised serious doubts regarding the value of the philosophical insights achieved using this method. There would have been no less far-reaching implications for the acceptance of the existence of the abyss between the person and Being itself. Such acceptance is first and foremost contrary to the basic intuition regarding the real existence of the transcendent Being, an intuition that fed Jaspers's metaphysical drive, and thanks to which the philosophizing was able to continue its constant development. This acceptance could have immediately turned the boundary situations into the final datum in Jaspers's philosophy and undermined the foundation on which the metaphysical consciousness was based, aimed primarily at constituting a positive consciousness regarding Being itself.

These insights and the awareness of their far-reaching implications for Jaspers's thought were at the basis of the constitution of the term "immanent transcendence,"[23] a term that was probably intended to satisfy two requirements that apparently do not accord with each other: the attempt to experience Being and at the same time to preserve the transcendent aspect in its perception. These two facets reveal two philosophical commitments of Jaspers's, which only the maturation of his philosophy enabled him to present explicitly: the commitment to immanence as a reality with its existence and as a source that could enable Existenz to experience it. As he put it: "only immanent transcendence grants Existenz weight in the world."[24] Also, the unconditional commitment to the process of searching for the transcendent Being, with clear knowledge that it is not fully accessible to an individual.

This dual commitment was expressed in denying the pantheist position, locating itself only in immanence, and in denying the ascetic position, which, in its approach to transcendence, abandons the world as a reality with its value. Jaspers viewed these two approaches, to which he believed rational thought led, as a "decline."[25] He clarified that what immanent transcendence indicates is that immanence has a role in powers that cannot be perceived using the tools of immanent consciousness, but at the same time, these powers can be expressed, or as he put it, "speak," in the immanent reality itself.[26]

The need for the way of Being embodied in immanent transcendence originates in the recognition that the entity as "Being in itself" is not present in the world in full as real reality or as a Being external to this world, but in what Jaspers defined as "unity without identity."[27] This means that people cannot give full expression to the way transcendence is present in immanence, because Being's reality is not identical to the way in which it is reflected in human consciousness. However, consciousness is responsible for us not accepting the abyss between us and transcendence, which could have turned it into "other in itself" for us and into its sinking for us.[28] The relation that people constitute toward the transcendent Being is what makes it significant for them, without negating their egos as Existenzes or the unbridgeable gap between it and human consciousness as such. This relation is precisely the experience of Being.

From the viewpoint of Existenz we can state that the meaning of the expression "immanent transcendence" is that immanence and transcendence are not alien to Existenz or to each other. The ongoing effort to determine the boundaries of the Being of Existenz and of the world and the constantly continuing acquaintance with the reality of transcendence are revealed as fruitful. Henceforth, Existenz is revealed not only as capable of constituting a relation toward realities different from it without this undermining its self-consciousness, but also as ripe for recognizing the separateness of what is different from it without facing it with a sense of alienation. It understands itself as connected to immanence and transcendence, although it knows it is not identical to them.

From the viewpoint of immanence, the term "immanent transcendence" indicates the perception of immanence as a cipher of transcendence. The change in the way immanence is understood deeply undermines the foundations of the approach that identifies Being with the empirical and the finite.[29] The understanding that the defined and fixed logical categories of reality cannot be implemented in the elucidation of transcendence[30] leads to the disappearance of the perception of immanence that was anchored in them.[31] Jaspers's need to return and express in this context, too, his familiar criticism of the positivistic world view[32] does not indicate that his perception of Being was founded on the principle of denying the reality of the world, but instead shows his awareness of the need to redefine the boundaries of the philosophizing aimed at Being. Just as in the framework of the explication of selfhood, the distancing of the objective viewpoint did not lead to the denial of the reality of the world, so here the denial of the understanding of reality as empirical did not serve as a basis for the perception of Being as existing outside the boundaries of the world as a self-existing reality. In this respect, the extreme phrasing that presented immanence as opposed to empiricism serves only as a first stage in the discussion, which will not be aimed at detaching the experience of Being from the empirical aspects of immanence, but will harness them to its explication.

The perception of immanence as a cipher of transcendence was anchored in the new understanding of objectivity, whereby it "contains the transcendence revealed in it."[33] The definition of ciphers as ciphers of transcendence appears throughout *Philosophy* in different forms.[34] The booklet *Ciphers of Transcendence* collects Jaspers's lectures on this issue at Basel University in 1961.[35] Jaspers's discussion in this booklet contains no innovation regarding his approach as it appeared in *Metaphysics* and in *Out of Truth*. The publication of this booklet, like other publications on specific issues from his whole philosophy, was characteristic of the third period of Jaspers's work, when he sought to present his philosophical thinking more simply or even in a popular form (see the division of Jaspers's work into periods in the Introduction). In this respect, metaphysical consciousness based on the perception of immanence as a cipher of transcendence does not create a new reality, but reveals a hidden facet of objectivity itself. The concept of the cipher does not deny the reality of the world, but shows immanence to be essential for the constitution of a philosophical consciousness of Being. The perception of ciphers preserves the original meaning granted to the perception of immanence as empiricism, and exists alongside it as such. In Jaspers's words, the perception of ciphers "is simultaneously *across the width of any objectivity*,"[36] or "taking place simultaneously across the width of reality in a depth dimension where man must sink himself but from which he cannot emerge without immediately losing it [this reality] completely."[37] The deep affirmation of the world embodied in the perception of immanence as a cipher does not allow the ciphers to be viewed as a Being isolated from the real reality in which an individual participates, or alternatively, as an internality without any external expression in reality.[38] The argument that the ciphers "exist in historistic sense of fulfillment [which is] like an unignorable depth"[39] connects their hidden internal facet with their exposure in the existential reality of human beings.[40] Understanding immanence as a cipher makes transcendence into something that a person can experience, and the reality of the present from which the perception of Being is constituted can also be seen as an element in the reality of transcendence itself.

Immanence, which no longer required proof of its very reality, became in the perception of ciphers more than mere immanence. Jaspers's original metaphysical intuition, which served as a substrate for the understanding that did not identify the existence of Existenz with empirical reality, was, in this context, too, at the basis of the perception that did not identify what was considered to be immanent reality with what existed in it but was concealed.[41] This perception did not enable the attribution of a total status to such immanence, but constantly directed toward what appeared close and accessible to human beings. Thinking about transcendence, which does not release people seeking the meaning of their existence, makes the objects represent what could never become an object: Being itself.[42] Compare also Jaspers's description of the process of converting objective and tangible reality into ciphers as part of the elucidation of Existenz.[43]

Eventually, the viewpoint of the cipher, expanding the boundaries of the meaning immanence could be granted, does not apply only to what appears as an object. It redefines life in general, perceived as a result as a totality expressing Being in different ways.[44] Under its inspiration, people reveal the metaphysical depth hidden in ordinary things and routine events,[45] in nature,[46] in history,[47] in art,[48] and in all the forms of human beings' grasp of existence where their search for meaning and significance is expressed.[49] This process is so deep that alongside the immanence that world orientation sees as empirical, the viewpoint of the cipher places "another mythical reality."[50] This mythical reality is not separate from immanence, since existence, which the viewpoint of consciousness sees as empirical, and the cipher are two aspects of one world.[51] The perception of the cipher is anchored in the understanding that in the reality in which we live there is a remnant that cannot be assimilated into anything else of the real,[52] a remnant concealed in the same factuality that world orientation wishes to report. Compare also the argument that Being is not a second reality.[53] This clarification, which moderates the potential for error that exists in the definition of this reality as a "mythical reality," enables us to state that the ontological picture behind world orientation does not contradict the one on which the perception of immanence as a cipher of transcendence is based. Support for this clarification can also be found in Jaspers's discussion of the differences between the conscious relation toward objective reality and the one expressed in reading the cipher. In this discussion,

Jaspers withdraws more explicitly from the definition of the cipher reality as a "mythical reality."

Jaspers described a sort of interrelationship between the viewpoint of world orientation and the viewpoint of the cipher: on the one hand, any knowledge that world orientation obtains makes the certainty of the cipher's viewpoint more decisive.[54] World orientation, defined as a "ladder rung," grants the person, thanks to its rational element, protection from the false perception of ciphers,[55] without which metaphysics would become fantasy. On the other hand, metaphysical consciousness, originating in the cipher's viewpoint, may serve as an incentive and a drive for deepening the scientific investigation, though the concept of cipher should not be seen as a justification or proof of any reality. In this spirit, Jaspers described "the search for transcendence… simultaneously as a relentless wish for knowledge of the real, conducted as an unsatisfied study of the world."[56] He went even further, arguing that the categories of thought are shaped only by the metaphysical drives,[57] and that the realization of the world orientation was tested by its ability to enable those involved in it to detach themselves from total views of the world and to direct themselves to transcendence.[58]

Against the background of this description of the relationship between the perception of the ciphers and the nature of the experience of world orientation, we can understand more accurately the argument whereby the viewpoint of the cipher exists "across the width of objectivity." World orientation constitutes a significant layer of the Being of the cipher since already there the person discovers that reality is not exhausted by what can be studied empirically. The experience that leads to the turning of "the facts of world orientation into possible ciphers"[59] expresses the peak of Jaspers's attempt to establish the role of immanence in the metaphysical consciousness revealed as deeply connected to the world reality that it seeks to transcend. Not only does the perception of immanence as a cipher of transcendence not negate the essentiality of the framework of world orientation for establishing metaphysical consciousness, it even enables a person to achieve consciousness about Being without detaching him from immanence as such. It shows that the same immanence that from one viewpoint serves as a source for the achievement of world orientation can also grant its owner, through another viewpoint, orientation in Being.

At the same time, Jaspers's commitment to elucidating transcendence as Being in itself did not enable him to be satisfied with clarifying "immanent transcendence," clarifying Being only from the viewpoint of immanence. The definition of the cipher as "Being which *transcendence* brings to presence without [it] having to turn Being into object-Being" and as "a gift from the source of Being"[60] indicates the existence of a force driving transcendence to discover itself in immanence. This philosophical drive constitutes a sort of continuation of Jaspers's effort to guarantee the presence of the metaphysical Being from different directions. Like the explication of the foundering, where Jaspers wished to show that not only Existenz but also existence itself was driven from itself to founder,[61] so also in the context of elucidating the cipher he aimed to show that there were different forces working for the presence of the metaphysical entity in human reality: immanence due to the metaphysical depth it contains, and transcendence that is driven by itself to be revealed in immanence.

Transcendence embodied in reality in the form of the ciphers[62] appears as an element a-priori to immanence, thanks to which the second was able to become the medium where transcendence was revealed. The argument that "in penetrating the world we fall into transcendence,"[63] as a "prototype,"[64] reflects the perception of transcendence as prior in presence to immanence. In this respect, the very presence of transcendence does not depend on being revealed through the viewpoint of the cipher. According to Jaspers, this viewpoint reflects the "response" to the already existing reality of transcendence.[65] The cipher's viewpoint is a-posteriori, and is enabled only thanks to the a-priori presence of transcendence, characterized by the power that motivates it to realize its immanence.

Compared with the detailed explication proposed for the immanent part of the expression "immanent transcendence," the elucidation Jaspers offered the transcendent part was partial and vague. This situation is not surprising, and is even similar to the difficulty in establishing the interpretation presented regarding the perception of the encompassing, whereby in the third transcending the philosophizing achieves a presentation of Being in itself. In these two contexts, it transpired that immanence by its very nature is capable of being more fully elucidated compared with transcendence, the main arguments about which rely mainly on the intuition that the boundaries of its explication constitute an essential part of it. However, precisely due to this difficulty, Jaspers's efforts to make some positive determinations regarding transcendence are especially noticeable. Although these statements are not easily defended, this does not call into doubt Jaspers's conviction regarding the existence of a power in transcendence itself. This power leads it to be revealed in immanence, with the ciphers serving as a medium where this power expresses itself.

The concept "immanent transcendence," linking transcendence and immanence—with transcendence making itself present while the metaphysical depth of immanence turning into a medium through which transcendence is revealed—transpires as a framework for the clarification of the objective part of the explication of Being, or more precisely of the extra-existential part of it. Unlike scientific objectivity, which scientists define in accordance with the research framework they set themselves, objectivity that was defined at the beginning of the discussion as "extra-existential" is revealed as a reality independent of people's relation toward it. Jaspers distinguished in the following passage between these two types of objectivity:

> *Reality-Being* for empirical knowledge exists as a Being only in contexts and dependence types through which it is understood. Genesis and causality show if and how something indeed exists there. They are not the existence [of this thing] in itself, but everything [in them] exists in relations. In contrast, the *symbol-Being* as a cipher of transcendence is not in a relation, but exists directly only for those people for whom it is transparent.[66]

From these words we can understand that beyond the permanence and the stability typical of objectivity as such, including objectivity in science, the extra-existential objectivity expresses the idea that the very reality of Being and transcendence is not a speculative matter, or as Jaspers put it: "is not in a relation." The dependence existing here applies to individuals, since without constituting a relation toward Being and transcendence they would not have a metaphysical consciousness granting meaning to Being and transcendence, while the reality of Being and transcendence themselves exists without any connection to any consciousness that could affirm them.

The need to establish the perception of Being outside the boundaries of Existenz, in order to grant it an objective aspect, also arose in the explication of selfhood, which also required world orientation—a framework that granted the perception of Existenz a sort of objective anchor, or more precisely an extra-existential one. Jaspers, who himself dealt with the importance of objectivity in the discussion of Being and Existenz,[67] was probably concerned that this philosophical move could accidentally lead to Existenz and the world becoming objects, and clarified that this was not the case.[68] However, what is noticeable in this context is the difference in the way Jaspers presented the role of objectivity in the two contexts. In the discussion of selfhood, the anchoring of Existenz in objectivity was the conclusion of a tortuous philosophical move that, among other things, examined the possibility of detaching Existenz from the world.[69] In contrast, in the discussion of ciphers objectivity was perceived as a datum on which the explication of Being was based, instead of as a problem that should be overcome. The new attitude toward objectivity in this context is a continuation of the earlier philosophical move, which appeared already in *World Orientation* and even benefited from it.

Against this background, we can state that the objectivity in which the discussion of Being was anchored was not perceived as an opposite pole to subjectivity, whose duty was to decipher the symbols and reveal the metaphysical element contained therein as ciphers of transcendence. Separating the discussion of objectivity from the subjectivity that sustains it, intended for methodological purposes, stresses at this stage of the discussion that the area of ciphers applies to whatever represents itself tangibly or could appear as such.[70] Jaspers's words about symbols in the fourth edition of *General Psychopathology* do not appear even in abbreviated form or in hints in the first edition of this work, but in my opinion they constitute part of his philosophical approach that is reflected in the expanded edition of this book. See the discussion on the relation between the two editions in Chapter One. The obvious conclusion from the discussion of the term "immanent transcendence" is that the cipher does not represent a new type of objectivity. The entirety of the concept of the cipher is in the new meaning granted to objectivity that Jaspers sometimes called "metaphysical objectivity,"[71] a meaning following which immanence was revealed as a source for a wider meaning. As he put it: "ciphers are not new objects, but newly filled objects."[72]

4. The Concept of Cipher and Consciousness

The anchoring of the explication of Being in immanence as a tangible reality, known for its accessibility to the tools of formal consciousness, required Jaspers to discuss the role of consciousness regarding the cipher Being, too. Jaspers's argument in principle in this context was that "consciousness in general, in all its valid forms... [is] the *skeleton* of existence, without which there is no understanding and no continuity of certainty."[73] This means that consciousness defines, at least in a preliminary way, the general framework in whose boundary the cipher's viewpoint functions. In his words:

> Sinking into symbols is not a mythical sinking, which in the lack of objectivity of transcendence enters a union lacking any objects and thus is also uncommunicative. In fact, *in hearing the language of the symbol, the phenomenon of transcendence is articulated for Existenz in the split existing between object and subject* in the medium of clear consciousness.[74]

Immanence, which appears in consciousness as a split between object and subject, and that when acted upon by consciousness acquires clarity and a degree of communicativity, has some weight in Existenz's becoming acquainted with transcendence. This expresses the presence of the epistemological viewpoint in the perception of immanence as a cipher of transcendence, a viewpoint that gives the certainty of the Being of transcendence a general aspect and that releases it from dependence on the necessarily particular relation Existenz shows it. Alan M. Olson proposed a different interpretation of the perception of ciphers when he stated that the source of the split between objectivity and subjectivity does not necessarily depend on objective consciousness, but on the ontological element, meaning the uniform Being of transcendence.[75] At the same time, consciousness bases the role of immanence in metaphysical consciousness; more precisely, the necessity of consciousness for the perception of immanence as a cipher of transcendence affirms metaphysical consciousness as being anchored in the same immanence accessible to the tools of consciousness. Unlike what Jaspers termed "mythical sinking," the action of consciousness occurs according to clear rules that are not derived from the needs or personality of the conscious person. The importance of the discussion of consciousness within the framework of the perception of ciphers stems from its contribution to delineating the boundaries in principle within which the metaphysical consciousness relying on the concept of cipher may move.

The discussion about the meaning of formal consciousness in the context of the perception of ciphers complements the philosophical move aimed at establishing the status of immanence in constituting metaphysical consciousness. While the concept "immanent transcendence" exposed the existential facet of immanence, the connection between objective consciousness and the cipher's viewpoint clarifies the conscious facet of this immanence. The viewpoint seeing immanence as a cipher of transcendence exceeds the boundaries of objectivity and grants it, as we have seen, a much wider significance than that granted it by formal consciousness. As Jaspers said: "The clarification through the symbol walks a path that is above objectivity."[76] Jaspers stressed that the same consciousness in which the individual "participates impersonally," enabling "unambiguous understanding," is the basis of our trust in order, and "dread takes us if its collapse appears real."[77] Consciousness, as an extra-existential anchor of Being, may guarantee the stability of metaphysical consciousness and its linking to the immanent reality where people live and act. The meeting that takes place at this point between the existential motives in the metaphysical search and the character of immanence at the basis of this search reveals the nature of the metaphysical consciousness Jaspers wished to constitute: it does not rely on the occurrence of a "total conversion" of the existence and consciousness in which people live, but instead all its depth depends on its ability to expose hidden aspects embodied in the two facets—existential and conscious—of immanence. For further discussion, see Jacques Waardenburg's argument that the creation of symbols always passes through some existential discomfort, and that thanks to the symbolic expression internal and external reality become bearable.[78]

This insight can correctly illuminate the essence of the reorientation that Jaspers's philosophy underwent. This reorientation not only placed the explication of Being as the desired object of the philosophizing and opened new horizons for it, but also reflected a release from the commitment to one exclusive viewpoint, like the one accompanying the elucidation of selfhood. This release not only enabled a relieving of the tension between different components of the discussion—such as "consciousness," "existence," and "Existenz"—typical of his earlier thought, but also enriched Jaspers's philosophical discourse, which became increasingly complex. In contrast with the tension typical of the framework of the explication of selfhood, between the wish to establish the superiority of Existenz and the aim of expanding the boundaries of the philosophizing, the framework of the explication of Being expressed Jaspers's tendency to use as many viewpoints as possible in order to constitute metaphysical consciousness, revealed as multi-faceted.

However, although the "essentiality of the universal legality [of consciousness] is a support and a comfort,"[79] in the complex process of constituting metaphysical consciousness, the correct dimensions of consciousness within the framework of the explication of Being transpire from the following passage:

> If everything threatens to erode into coincidence then in the law I have a place where I can take hold of solid ground. If Being sinks for me, I perceive all of existence in this law. But then this law is a cipher, and like any cipher it is ambiguous... I can grasp it, but not final[ly] and absolute[ly]. As with any cipher, I must go deep in this one, without ever finding a ground. I no longer see it when I perceive validity as merely objective.[80]

Only after the clarification of objectivity by consciousness has been exhausted does objectivity itself become a cipher of transcendence. Objectivity transpires as the first and overt layer of understanding, but its perception as a cipher reflects the hidden meaning it contains, that the awareness of the insufficiency of objectivity constitutes a condition for its exposure. It is clear that in order for something—an object, a word, a way of speaking, or a way of behaving—to symbolize something else, other than itself, it must first have its meaning, and only then can it serve as an indicator of another meaning. Similarly, the cipher also requires the background existence of the objective understanding of immanence as the first layer of meaning, which in itself would constitute a transcending or addition thereof. The philosophical move in which Jaspers sought to combine on the one hand the epistemological viewpoint of consciousness in its perception of immanence as a cipher of transcendence, and on the other hand to try to limit this viewpoint so that it would not exhaust the perception of ciphers—or more precisely so that the second would not be subjugated to the viewpoint of consciousness—receives its concise expression in the following passage, which also summarizes this interpretative move:

> Order, rules, and laws of everything, precisely those that appear to cancel any symbolism and to enforce the uncompromising separation between reality and illusion, themselves become a cipher: *the fact that existence is like this, that it contains order, and that this order exists, is the cipher of its transcendence.*[81]

It transpires that only after the place of world orientation and of consciousness was guaranteed within the framework of the philosophical discussion around Being did Jaspers wish to stress that not all the viewpoints have an equal status in the process of constituting metaphysical consciousness; that their coming together in order to achieve a shared goal does not remove the differences between them. The concept of cipher shows that "the object does not become through change a construct by a methodic view of a single science, but it becomes transparent through philosophy."[82] This statement, distinguishing the way consciousness handles immanence and the viewpoint of the cipher, can indicate some crucial aspects of the concept of cipher: first, consciousness cannot deal with all the facets of immanence, but only with those accessible to the tools of objective thinking, from which knowledge can be produced. In a way, this activity of consciousness can be seen as distancing from immanent reality, because it cannot represent the aspects existing in it that are not accessible to the rules of objectivity. In contrast, the cipher making this immanent reality transparent expresses an attempt to cling to it enabled by the very ability of consciousness to "breaking away from sensuality as such."[83] This ability is what enables immanence itself, and not another reality, to be seen as an expression of Being. While for consciousness the objects constitute the only object of reference, with everything remaining outside the objective patterns considered as non-existent, the perception of ciphers, which does not neglect those aspects to which consciousness refers, transpires as exhausting the fullness of immanence. However, the exhaustion of immanence is not revealed only by clinging to it, but as the ability to experience also what is reflected in it but whose reality does not match its own, meaning transcendence.

The release from the bonds of consciousness enables a different way of experiencing immanence, anchored in the distinction between two types of symbolism: "*interpretable symbolism*" and "observable symbolism."[84] The first disintegrates immanence in order to rebuild it according to the rules of objectivity, and places a barrier between indicator and indicated, meaning between immanence and transcendence. The second, in contrast, maintains the integrity of immanence and of the human being as an organic part of it without contradicting the basic effort to which the perception of ciphers is aimed, meaning the creation of continuity from immanence to transcendence. Even if the observation behind the cipher's viewpoint does not reflect complete passivity, its relation toward immanence lacks the same emphasis on activity and sovereignty on the individual's behalf that is typical of consciousness' relationship toward immanent reality. Similarly, Jaspers differentiated elsewhere between "penetration" of the cipher, which is a tool for its clarification, and "interpretation," which stresses the control a person has over his object of reference.[85]

Sebastian Samay's interpretation emphasized another facet of this distinction between these two types of symbolism, but accords with the interpretation offered here. In his opinion, the first symbolism sees its objects as an absolute thing, and treats them the way "consciousness in general" treats its objects. The object of this symbolism ceases to be perceived as a symbol and is perceived, following this treatment, as reality itself.[86] In contrast, the other symbolism does not achieve an unambiguous understanding of its objects.[87] He defines this symbolism as poetic, since it penetrates the metaphysical depth contained in objects.[88] Samay's interpretation also shows, although in a different way, that immanence that becomes a symbol of transcendence does not lose its connection to immanence as such.

At this point we can indicate the traces of the method of transcending, on which Jaspers's entire philosophical thought was constituted. Beyond the general contribution to expanding the scope of the philosophizing familiar from previous contexts we have discussed, in this context this method aided the escape from the rigid categories of consciousness,[89] and undermined the logical and rational structure of arguments about reality[90]—an undermining following which Jaspers defined the objects in reality as "floating."[91] However, unlike in previous contexts, where this method led to the expansion of the scope of discussion by means of transferring its focus elsewhere, in this context of the cipher, the expansion was achieved by "penetrating the world"[92] and "deep study" of the symbol it created.[93] The implementation of the method of transcending within the framework of the perception of ciphers expresses the main philosophical message Jaspers wished to express through it, whereby individuals do not have to go far from their position in the world and seek the meaning of their life elsewhere, since it is right within their reach.

The change in the way the method of transcending is expressed reflects the status of Existenz at this stage of the explication. Following his discussion of consciousness within the framework of the perception of the cipher, Jaspers stated that "real Being should be perceived only in the loosening of the possible Existenz,"[94] meaning that Existenz is liberated from the drive that had controlled it in the framework of the explication of selfhood. After discussing philosophy's need for objects, he stated that the cipher's viewpoint grants objectivity symbolic validity, when "their content becomes feelable."[95] Compared with the consciousness of conquest and achievement that fills the conscious person, Jaspers noted that "in the cipher *I delay*,"[96] and chose to emphasize the sense of magic,[97] the experience of wonder and of facing a reality filled with secrets.[98] These descriptions of the Existenz becoming aware of the symbolic aspects of immanence enable the characterizing of the cipher's viewpoint as what Peter Wust termed "second naiveté," meaning a renewed turn toward absolute Being, with awareness of the scientific and philosophical criticism of the world and of the intention to repair the rift caused by this awareness. This concept was developed in Wust's book *Naivität und Pietät* (*Naiveté and Piety*) (1925),[99] although its early elements can be found in his first book, *Die Auferstehung der Metaphysik* (*The Rebirth of Metaphysics*) (1921),[100] and in articles published between these two books.[101] Alternatively, Existenz can be defined in this context as existing in what Olson called, following Paul Ricoeur, as "post-critical naiveté," meaning openness to the wonder from a view to what the symbol and the myth can imply.[102] In this context, Olson mentions Jaspers as expressing the need for openness to the wonderful through symbols, and he also refers to the argument Jaspers had with Bultman, as published in Jaspers's work *Demythologization*. Like the "second naiveté," and the "post-critical naiveté," the cipher's viewpoint, too, does not detach itself from people's basic aim of understanding the world around them using the tools at their disposal, and it cannot be defined as a skeptical position. Quite the opposite, the cipher's viewpoint on the one hand reflects Jaspers's attempt to find a way to preserve the spirit of intuitive certainty regarding the existence of a transcendent Being, while on the other hand expresses his certainty that the philosophical medium where its explication is carried out can help in this task.

However, while the cipher's viewpoint, which was defined above as "the loosening of the possible Existenz" aiming at the "observable objects" and preserving the wholeness of immanence, Jaspers clarified that it by no means constitutes an aesthetic viewpoint. Several scholars have discussed the influence of Friedrich Wilhelm Joseph Schelling and Immanuel Kant's "Nature's cipher" on Jaspers's perception of ciphers.[103] In my opinion, Kant's emphasis on the aesthetic aspects is not equivalent to Jaspers's explicitly anti-aesthetic position.[104] Unlike the cipher, indicating the presence of transcendence in the world, in his opinion the symbols become non-binding aesthetic contents in which no reality is present.[105] Compared with the aesthetic observation, which from Jaspers's point of view was perceived as meaningless for self-Being, the thought that perceives the world as filled with the presence of transcendence was defined as creative thought.[106] Defining the relation of the cipher's viewpoint to immanence as "a possibility of *appropriation*"[107] reveals unambiguously the observers' commitment to what is revealed to them from the ciphers. The appropriating position that adopts something from what already exists establishes the connection of the perception of ciphers to immanence, and at the same time stresses the difference between the method of observation depicted in this perception and both the aesthetic viewpoint and the viewpoint of formal consciousness. Eventually the release from the specificity of the categories of objective consciousness and from people's conscious relation toward reality[108] leads to the diminishing of the area of tangency between the cipher's viewpoint and that of consciousness to the point of the cipher being defined as "a vague fantasy of consciousness."[109] Although the all-inclusive horizons of transcendence to which the symbolic observation was aimed enabled the different viewpoints to coexist, they also demanded the "surplus meaning" over what the consciousness of immanence could grant and the concept of cipher could indicate.

5. Metaphysical Consciousness as a Language

The connection between the perception of ciphers and the framework of the explication of Being was achieved through the anchoring of this perception in two elements independent of Existenz: the metaphysical potential embodied in immanence and transcendence's drive to immanentize itself. However, these elements are insufficient to exhaust the philosophical depth contained in the viewpoint seeing immanence as a cipher of transcendence. Although it is clear that before the appearance of the concept of cipher Jaspers's words referred to clear processes that reflected the diversion of Existenz from the focus of the philosophical discussion, he stated:

> If we go in metaphysics *directly* from absolute objectivity up to transcendence as a cipher, then there is no possibility of grasping it. [This means] that we should search for contact with *its existential roots*.[110]

Existenz transpires from this passage as a necessary condition for the constitution of a relation toward transcendence through the cipher's viewpoint.[111] In order to establish this argument, Jaspers sought to indicate a significant connection between the cipher's viewpoint and the most explicit characteristics of Existenz. He wrote that "the ciphers in the historistic sense of fulfillment are as an unignorable depth."[112] The cipher's viewpoint, which reveals new facets of the reality in which Existenz exists, reflects Existenz's ability to detach itself from its form of existence and to examine other possibilities. In this respect, the ciphers can be considered a metaphoric expression of the undeciphered existence possibilities that were available to Existenz but hidden in the absence of a more profound examination of immanence. This interpretation accords with Jaspers's statement that the connection between ciphers and the historicity of Existenz does not allow Existenz to observe the order of the cipher world "from above,"[113] but instead to see them as a space where its possibilities for realization lie.[114]

The dual relation of the ciphers—both to the immanence where they are anchored with Existenz, and to the transcendence they indicate—is reflected in the two different ways Existenz faces them. As we have seen, Existenz was described as delaying and as loosening in the face of the Being of transcendence arising from the ciphers. This description, aimed at preventing the identification of transcendence with immanence in a way that could have turned it into a sort of knowledge, differs from the description of Existenz's stance toward the immanence in which it identifies the ciphers of transcendence:

> *As a tangible thing* objectivity is an existential *possibility*: the possibility of *appropriation* is what turns in the world into an object—as empirical

> reality, as rational validity, as nature and history, and as handed down cipher text.[115]

The direct contact the cipher's viewpoint has with Existenz's mode of existence served as a basis for granting legitimacy to the activity Existenz shows regarding them. Precisely because Existenz does not experience the immanence in which the ciphers are anchored as a reality external to it, but as "its own world," it sees itself as free to appropriate from among the ciphers taken from immanence the possibilities they contain for it, and not to face them with the distance typical of its stance toward transcendence. Against this background, the definition of the concept of cipher as the possibility of "appropriation" receives its full meaning. On the one hand, it indicates the rooting of metaphysical consciousness in immanence, and on the other hand, since this consciousness revolves around the transcendence beyond the boundaries of immanence as such, it also indicates the distance between metaphysics and immanence—a distance that requires Existenz to show activity that could bring it closer to transcendence, although transcendence remains distant from Existenz.

The implications stemming from anchoring the concept of cipher in the existential infrastructure are clear: this infrastructure does not allow immanence to lead to the constitution of a uniform metaphysical consciousness in different people, since beyond the differences between people, immanence reveals itself in different and varied facets.[116] As he put it: "empirical existence, which through the expression [of Being] is supposed to be perceived and ascertained, does not therefore exist *per se*,"[117] and the ciphers "enable a variety of viewpoints."[118] The given gap between transcendence as Being in itself and immanent reality is joined, through the existential infrastructure, by another gap stemming from the differences between human viewpoints about immanent reality.

The barrier against constituting a uniform consciousness regarding transcendence through the ciphers does not stem only from the individual differences between people. Even for the same person it does not always happen on the same level, since it depends on the "person's elation ability" that changes over time. In this respect, the ciphers indicate, in their undeciphered form, the person's development potential, and so Jaspers saw the ciphers as reflecting the real human Being,[119] and argued that they "open themselves for me in accordance with my essence."[120] The conclusion resulting from the existential infrastructure of the ciphers—both the multiplicity of viewpoints of different people regarding the same reality and as a function of the frequently changing state of the individual—is unambiguous. The metaphysical grasp in the cipher text is not finally valid, but is subject to people's state when they turn to transcendence, which in turn grants itself to those seeking it in a different way each time.[121]

Olson's interpretation, seeking to distinguish between Jaspers's perception of ciphers and that of the church's dogmatic theology, illuminates from a different angle the essentiality of Existenz in becoming acquainted with the symbolic aspects of immanence. According to Olson, Jaspers's perception of ciphers stresses the centrality of the individual experiencing the constitution of the symbol and activity involved in interpreting it, compared with Christian theology, which grants a different weight to the individual and to the symbolic aspects of religion. In his opinion, the fear that pandeism or the tendency to reduce faith into the external means by which it is obtained would eventually lead to the viewing of these means as having purely subjective, and also mutable, validity, was behind the Catholic church's emphasis on the objective truth of the symbols themselves in relation to the individual religious experience.[122] Olson bases his words on Bernard Joseph Francis Lonergan's work.[123] Stephen A. Erickson discussed the difference between Jaspers's religious approach and that of Søren Kierkegaard as the difference between a non-voluntarist position and a voluntarist position.[124] Olson's interpretation, revealing the religious aspects of the experience of constituting the Being of the cipher, accords with his discussion of the role of subjectivity in revealing the metaphysical depth contained in immanent reality, although it is clear that Jaspers's perception of the ciphers cannot be seen as a basis for his identification with the dogmatic theology of the church, which was in any case not discussed in his writings of this period. Jaspers's book *Der philosophische Glaube* (*Philosophical Faith in Light of Revelation*) (1963) contains a more direct dialog with Christian faith.[125]

The centrality of Existenz in the constitution of the approach seeing immanence as a cipher of transcendence and the individualistic facet accompanying this experience remind us of the rhetoric typical of the framework of the elucidation of Existenz. Jaspers's reference to these aspects at this stage of his philosophy has a different meaning than the one familiar from the explication of selfhood. As we recall, in the second, controlled by the drive to solipsism, the uniqueness of Existenz was perceived as an essential tool for its elucidation, and the isolation of Existenz from the world and from other Existenzes was an essential condition for its constitution as an explicit Being. In contrast, in light of the cipher's viewpoint, the unique character of Existenz helps elucidate the eternality of the ciphers themselves. In this context, Jaspers differentiated between the multiplicity of meanings that is a result of the "interpretable symbolism" and the multiplicity of meanings that is a product of the "observable symbolism." The first one relies on a fixed starting point aimed at achieving the interpretation as a final target. In contrast, the existentialist viewpoint behind the other symbolism observes its objects as possibilities for appropriation. No less than the reference revealing the presence of transcendence in immanence expresses the quality of Existenz, it also testifies to the anchor ciphers have in infinity itself.[126] Even the fact that "*infinite multiplicity of meanings of all the ciphers* shows itself in the reality of time as its essence"[127] does not enable the isolation of the ciphers, since each symbol gives rise to a new symbol.[128] In the framework of the elucidation of selfhood, the singularity of Existenz served as a tool for emphasizing its particular uniqueness, which largely isolated it from its surroundings, but in the framework of the perception of ciphers, this singularity functions as a tool for elucidating Being as an extra-existential and infinite entity existing beyond Existenz.

In addition to the multiplicity of meanings granted to the ciphers not enabling them to be isolated from the historistic universe of Existenz[129]—Jaspers puts it as thinking "out of the ciphers" and not "about them"[130]—it does not allow a valid and complete understanding of them.[131] This situation requires the definition of ciphers as a relativized Being-consciousness,[132] and so they are perceived as an absolute barrier against the constitution of a dogmatic metaphysical system[133] characterized by the institutionalization and canonization of the symbols. Waardenburg distinguished between "free symbols," which have not been canonized, and "established symbols," characteristic of organized religions and institutions.[134] Jaspers, who was aware of the "price" that must be paid by a metaphysical approach rooted in the world of a person as an individual, indicated the danger of instability[135] and the constantly threatening doubt.[136] It is no wonder that he stated that "it would not be possible for there to be any research of a symbol, but only the perception of symbols and creation of symbols."[137] The poor formality and the weak generality characterizing the symbols not only do not enable the world to be known through them,[138] and do not provide any knowledge about it,[139] but even make the undeciphered possibilities for existence in the world into the last datum of human Being. Therefore, Jaspers argued that seeing immanence as a cipher of transcendence charges individuals with finding for themselves the justification of the metaphysical consciousness they form. This point makes more prominent the difference between metaphysical consciousness based on symbolic observation, which tries to deal with the gap between itself and transcendence as an absolute Being, and the myths that are usually understood as having a relative meaning that leaves the gap between transcendence itself and its description intact without seeing the overcoming of this gap as a worthy challenge.[140]

In some respects, the discussion about the role of subjectivity in the constitution of the cipher-Being demonstrates the difficulties entailed in elucidating Being itself and also those entailed in the constitution of metaphysical consciousness regarding this Being. Hermann-Josef Seideneck, who stressed these aspects of Jaspers's thought, stated that what apparently appeared to be blunt concepts reflects the doubt of the philosophical thought. This general argument about Jaspers's thought is especially stressed in relation to the ciphers, which in Seideneck's opinion mainly reflect the experience of Being through the doubt that moves between the possibilities at Existenz's disposal and the reality of Being in itself.[141] While the ciphers reflect, in his words, "daring to doubt," they also exist on the same impassable boundary that only faith and communication between different religions through theological thought, instead of philosophy, can overcome.[142]

The interpretation emphasizing the element of doubt entailed in the symbolic viewpoint of reality has some support in the text, but doubt in this context has only a role similar in principle to that of "restraint" (*epoché*) in Edmund Husserl's thought. This means that the presence of doubt is required as an inevitable component in Jaspers's perception of Being, which sought to rid itself of absolute aspects that could grant the metaphysical consciousness that was formulated in his thought a dogmatic nature or present it as a religious commitment. But despite the importance of Existenz in determining the character of the developing metaphysical consciousness and in creating the connection with the philosophy of Existenz in the background, the existential infrastructure remained, in which doubt is anchored as a background understanding, and did not take over the elucidation of the concept of cipher. According to the basic principles that most generally typify the framework of the explication of Being, we can find in Jaspers's words a real expression of his attempt to qualify the existential aspects that arose in his discussion of the concept of cipher. After presenting the ciphers as an existential possibility, Jaspers wrote:

> Only on the basis of Existenz's ground does objectivity become a present reality, if it cancels the mere possibility of identifying with the existential selfhood.[143]

These words affirm the premise of the perception of ciphers, that immanence contains a metaphysical depth or what was called here a "present reality," and establishes the meaning of appropriation in the framework of this perception. Unlike the appropriation ability in the elucidation of selfhood, expressed in the translation of different contents and experiences into the language of existential selfhood, the meaning of appropriation expressed in the symbolic observation of immanent reality is almost the opposite. The Existenz that constitutes the cipher's viewpoint and appropriates the possibilities it recognizes in immanence does not subject the objective contents it encounters to its needs, nor does it aim to identify itself with the possibilities it has chosen to appropriate. Existenz's ability to appropriate to itself possibilities from the symbolic observation of reality depends on negating the very possibility of identifying its selfhood with what it chooses to appropriate.

The different meaning granted in this context to the concept of appropriation, containing one of the explicit meanings of Existenz, is part of a wide philosophical move characterizing the explication of Being, where there is a deep transformation of the basic insights achieved in the elucidation of selfhood. In this spirit, Jaspers argued that denying the factuality of transcendence can be considered a human freedom, but that the possible Existenz that knows its boundaries cannot deny the reality of transcendence.[144] While the framework of the elucidation of selfhood expressed the freedom of Existenz in its ability to constitute itself, in the explication of Being, Existenz is presented as not observing transcendence as a possibility at its disposal, meaning a Being that teaches it something about itself, but as becoming "identical to the certainty of the Being of transcendence."[145] The maturation of Existenz's self-consciousness is reflected in the certainty it has of the Being of transcendence. Eventually, to the extent that Existenz can have any certainty about its Being, this certainty is related to its ability to experience the presence of transcendence.[146]

Although the presence of Existenz makes the difference between seeing immanence as merely empirical and perceiving immanence as a cipher of transcendence, the existential viewpoint does not exhaust the full meaning of the concept of cipher. This is because the metaphysical interpretation granted to immanence does not function as a mechanism for confirming the real existence of the Being of transcendence, but is intended to grant an explicit expression to the intuition regarding the existence of an extra-immanent Being. The cipher's viewpoint is intended to answer the requirement in principle that transcendence should be accessible to the tools of human consciousness. Jaspers wrote:

> ... to the extent that Existenz appears to itself in existence, so what is exists for it only as patterns of consciousness; therefore even what is transcendence receives for the Existenz connected to existence the form of objectivity.[147]

Following the philosophical move that clarified the connection between the viewpoint of consciousness regarding reality and the perception of that reality as a cipher of transcendence, these words also express the need to make metaphysical consciousness more communicative. What rescues the experience of ciphers from being the individual's private experience and turns it into part of philosophical metaphysics stems from the existence of a process of "systematic analysis of absolute objectivity" and of turning the objectivity perceived as a cipher into a "meant concept."[148] Even if this process does not completely remove the doubt inevitably accompanying the symbolic observation portrayed in the perception of ciphers, it reflects handling it using the tools of philosophical explication. Objective consciousness is part of the process of forming the metaphysical relation toward immanent reality, which guarantees that the metaphysical consciousness formed does not rise up against its maker, detach it from itself, and become a dogmatic religious commitment or a mystical experience. However, especially in the face of the doubt, which is an essential component of metaphysical consciousness, the product of a person's self-constitution—doubt that the objective part of the perception of Being is supposed to answer—the reliability of Jaspers's commitment to preserving the centrality of Existenz within the perception of immanence as a cipher of transcendence is noticeable. The innovation in this commitment Jaspers showed toward Existenz stems from it not being intended only for purposes of its self-understanding, but also preserved when the philosophizing directs itself toward the transcendent Being.

Jaspers's effort to grant the idea of the cipher an aspect of generality by elucidating it separately from the framework of the explication of selfhood, but without alienating it from the Being of Existenz, reaches its peak with its definition as a language of transcendence.[149] Just as every language is based on some rules, and familiarity with them and internalization of them enable communication, so the language of the cipher, too, relies on accessibility to the general aspects of immanence as empirical reality. Like all languages, the language of the cipher has no existence as such, but only by being understood by particular people. The definition of immanence itself as a cipher text[150] emphasizes the dependence of the cipher language on people who can decipher it. While the general facet on which the understanding of ciphers is based is responsible for their perception as a language of transcendence instead of as a language of Existenz, the need for the cipher language to be comprehensible ensures the essentiality of Existenz as the one that indicates in practice that immanence is a cipher of transcendence.

In order to define the nature and uniqueness of the cipher language compared with other expressions of human Being, which themselves constitute a language, Jaspers differentiated between three languages. Olson argued that these three levels of the cipher language are close, if not entirely identical, to the three movements of absolute spirit in Georg Wilhelm Friedrich Hegel.[151]

The first language represents the experience of the unmediated presence of transcendence in the absolute consciousness of Existenz. Although Jaspers perceives the experience in the widest sense as a source for certainty regarding transcendence and as an answer to the need for its presence in historistic reality, he stressed in this context, "*The metaphysical experience lacks any verifiability* that could have turned it into a valid thing for every person." Whether the individual sees it as knowledge or it remains merely a subjective feeling, the experience of transcendence through the first language is destined to turn into a deception.[152] Compared with Jaspers's presentation of absolute consciousness in *Elucidation of Existenz*, which still emphasized the dealing with the question of selfhood,[153] here Jaspers stressed its role as mediating between Existenz and transcendence—although this facet was already present in its earlier appearance. See the discussion in the chapter summing up the transition mechanisms following Chapter Seven. In this respect, the role of absolute consciousness in the context of the discussion of ciphers can be seen as an expression of its development and as affirmation of the interpretation offered here whereby selfhood is moved aside from the center of the philosophical discussion with the transition to the explication of Being.

The inability to conduct communication on the basis of the first language and its insufficiency even for the person trying to use it serve, apparently, as a basis for the constitution of the second language, where the metaphysical consciousness is embodied. Unlike the first language, anchored in the historicity of the individual's present, the second language is based on the premise that transcendence takes place in contrast to the real present as empirical reality.[154] The constituting experience of this language is not "the fault in reality, but the lack of transcendence"[155] that should be accessible to a person's world of metaphors and thoughts. So it is not surprising that the form in which this language is expressed is that of myths. The commitment of the second language to making transcendence accessible to the objective forms of expression, as portrayed in the formation of myths, constitutes an opposite pole to the first language, free of these needs and mainly committed to the individual existential experiencing of the metaphysical experience.

Between these two languages, Jaspers placed the third language, the cipher language. He defined it as a mediating language,[156] and the transcendental thoughts arising in it as speculations:

> They are not knowledge of an object, nor appealing to freedom through reflection that elucidates Existenz, nor a categorical transcending that does not perceive anything but liberates, nor even an interpretation of existential relations to the transcendent, but [they are] contemplative self-sinking for purposes of contact with transcendence through a formulated, deep, and self-understanding cipher text that brings transcendence before the spirit as metaphysical objectivity.[157]

The cipher language transpires from this passage as connecting what appeared separately in the two previous languages. On the one hand, it recognizes that it is the product of the individual's self-search, and so it does not blur its being an expression of human creativity, as happens in the second language. On the other hand, awareness of its being based on speculation, meaning "a thought that in thinking pushes beyond the thinkable,"[158] sets the boundary between it and the first language. Unlike the first language, transcendence is not perceived in the cipher language as an expression of mere existential relations or as exhaustible as reflection about sensory understanding revolving around objects in reality.[159] Existenz understands itself as aimed at the Being existing beyond the familiar boundaries of immanence, though it knows that only through the symbolic function of language can this Being become accessible to it. As Jaspers said: "the symbol does not only clarify, it makes *real* what would otherwise be as nothing."[160]

The definition of the cipher as a "language" that summarizes all the features of the cipher-Being also meets the real needs of Jaspers's philosophy at this stage of its development. First, language serves as a clear framework of rules and semantic boundaries, and this accords with Jaspers's need to provide the metaphysical experience with a more general and communicative facet, and even explains the extensive dealing with the "objective" aspects entailed in the concept of cipher. Second, like language, the concept of cipher is also a human creation and so is dependent for its very existence on a human Being to create it. Therefore, even if Jaspers assumed that the very reality of immanent reality contained metaphysical depth not exhausted in the existential relation toward it, he made the possibility of revealing it dependent on people interested in transcendence as a source of the meaning of their existence. In this respect, the parallel between the symbol as a way of people's relating to what is beyond them and language, which also refers to a reality not identical to it, stresses the human creativity expressed in the very constitution of the relation and in the contents formed thereby. Third, just as language reports a reality in accordance with the rules and meanings typifying it, so also the cipher reports the existence of a transcendent Being within the boundaries of symbolic observation, though from awareness that "there is no simple parallel between the sensory fullness and the fullness of the contents of the Being."[161] The definition of the cipher as a language leaves intact the awareness of the unbridgeable gap between the human Being constituting the metaphysical relation and the object to which it is intended. This affirms that analogous nature of the cipher's viewpoint, expressed in this context in recognition that the "meeting" with Being in a "real and whole" way is impossible.[162]

Jaspers's commitment to proposing a positive elucidation to the "Being in itself" led him to argue that precisely because it is the language of a fable, the cipher language does not lead to the loss of transcendence. As he phrased it: "truth is lost if it changes when it becomes an identical and general Being for everyone, and becomes lacking the indirectness of language."[163] The special emphasis granted to the element of indirectness in the cipher language, becoming a criterion of the truth of the metaphysical experience, reveals that the comparison between the cipher and language was not primarily intended to stress the semantic aspects, constituting an inseparable part of the symbolic view of reality. The quality of indirectness defines the relation between the cipher as a concept and transcendence as a Being: the cipher expresses the human creativity revealed in the process of searching for the meaning of existence. Transcendence, however, is a reality that one can become acquainted with indirectly—though its differentiation from human reality turns it into a source for meaning in life. The indirectness typical of the cipher language as a way in which we can become acquainted with transcendence ensures a meeting point between the metaphysical search and transcendence itself. It also explains and even justifies the variety of forms of the metaphysical consciousness based on the cipher's viewpoint that can always "*communicate itself in a different way*."[164] The definition of the cipher's viewpoint as a language, the exposure of the metaphysical elements in immanence, and the image of subjectivity being driven to search for the meaning of existence in the worlds existing beyond it can serve as a basis and inspiration for dealing with Jaspers's ideas also from the hermeneutic perspective, an approach that is currently in its early stages in research. The infrastructure for this direction to interpreting Jaspers's philosophy exists already in Olson and Ricoeur.[165] The scope of the current study does not permit such a discussion of Jaspers's thought, but we can state that unlike other philosophers such as Hans-Georg Gadamer, Heidegger, Ricoeur, and Ernst Cassirer, who offered a "theory of interpretation" or a basis for one, such a basis does not exist in Jaspers's philosophy, and even the cipher language described above has a mainly intuitive nature.

In the context of the ciphers, as in other subjects, Jaspers expressed his tendency to deal with the conditions enabling the development of real philosophy, or more precisely, to clarify the conditions that do not prevent it, while avoiding a general description of the correct practice of philosophizing. Jaspers conveyed the unique nature of the knowledge to which his philosophy was directed in his definition of the term "fundamental knowledge."

> We call fundamental knowledge the knowledge where the person *discovers himself by* all his defined knowledge being dependent upon him, or [the knowledge] that is *a premise* for any other knowledge. [This knowledge] is also called a-priori. As such it is the general a-priori of consciousness in general in the categories of the mind, the a-priori of the spirit in the ideas, the a-priori of existence in practical motives and response patterns; this is the *historistic* a-priori of the tradition of human Being that experiences its world as a one-time pattern, as a realization of the general that has meaning and weight not as general but as infinite.[166]

Although these words of Jaspers's were not written in the context of the discussion of ciphers, they can be seen as an explicit disclosure of the usually hidden intentions and motives of his ideas, and perhaps even as a general phrasing of the wider ethos guiding his philosophical work. In this context, the a-priori and one-time nature of "fundamental knowledge" can explain the intuitive aspect characterizing the language of ciphers, which cannot serve as a basis for the constitution of metaphysics in the full sense, even if it illuminates an aspect of the experience of constituting a metaphysical relation toward reality. Olson argues that Jaspers did not exhaust the hermeneutic potential contained in his ideas, and even states that Jaspers was wrong not to call his philosophy of transcendence hermeneutical.[167] In his opinion, Jaspers's objection to dealing with formal questions of logic and epistemology was an inseparable part of his interpretative approach as such.[168] Thyssen argued that meeting transcendence through the ciphers is meeting contents.[169] Unlike the arguments of Olson and Thyssen, I believe that Jaspers's familiar objection to system or any formalization of philosophy that would present itself as a wholeness that exhausts itself could serve as part of the explanation for him not using these elements and developing an interpretative theory on their basis. It is possible that the decisive influence of Heidegger's philosophy in *Being and Time*, which was already a real fact in the philosophical discourse in which Jaspers operated, largely determined the basic understanding of hermeneutics as ontology. Jaspers's objection to ontology, which was part of his objection to positivism as a whole, probably did not enable him to define his thought as hermeneutics or even to indicate the possible implications of his ideas for this realm of thought. Finally, the primary importance of the comparison between the cipher's viewpoint and language rests in it clarifying the basic idea on which the explication of Being relied, that the human need to express metaphysical experiences using the tools of consciousness does not serve as a final test for the reality of the Being of transcendence to which this experience is aimed.

6. The Concept of Cipher as Mediating between the Elucidation of Selfhood and the Explication of Being

The distinction between the three languages of metaphysical tangibility, which served as a basis for the definition of the uniqueness of the cipher language, helped sharpen crucial aspects contained within the concept of the cipher. However, an additional examination of these three languages as one complex reveals that they reflect milestones in the process of the development of Jaspers's thought. From this genealogical viewpoint, the cipher language reflects a new integration of early insights related to the framework of the elucidation of selfhood and represented by the first two languages. Samay offers another interpretation to these three languages. In his opinion, the first language reflects "the immediate language of Being," the second reflects the person's answer to the language of transcendence, and the third reflects the translation of the experience of Being appearing in the first two languages into a speculative language. In Samay's opinion, these three languages reflect a hierarchy aimed at making the ciphers into a more communicative Being.[170]

Perhaps this statement about the cipher language reveals some awareness on Jaspers's part of the developing nature of his philosophy, and perhaps the distinction between the three languages was merely a methodical tool aimed mainly at clarifying the concept of cipher. In any case, unique nature of the cipher language as revealed from its comparison with the two other languages may serve as a basis for a reexamination of the connection between the processes of the explication of Being and the early philosophical insights that were formulated in the framework of the elucidation of selfhood.

As we recall, the first language represented the experience with the unmediated presence of transcendence of absolute consciousness of Existenz. Jaspers's statement in this context that "the experience of the first language immediately requires *the self giving its utmost of possible Existenz,*" and more generally the definition of Existenz as "the place where the cipher text is read,"[171] indicate the centrality of Existenz in it. However, although Jaspers himself discussed the existential infrastructure contained in the cipher's viewpoint that is located in the third language, the character of the Existenz related to the cipher is not equivalent to the one constituting the first language. Unlike the existential aspects in which the concept of cipher is anchored, representing the selfhood that has matured and as a result found in itself the power to turn to elucidating the Being existing beyond it, the Existenz that constitutes the first language is connected to some aspects of Jaspers's early perception of selfhood.

This argument is based, first and foremost, on the definition of the first cipher language as "un*verifiable*," a definition that indicates the uncommunicative nature of the experience of transcendence in this language.[172] Additional support for this is found in that statement that "I affirm [the reading of the cipher text] through my selfhood, without having another measure from this selfhood for knowing the transcendence of ciphers."[173] Finally, the reference repeated in the following citation to the idea of possibility and the element of struggle, which filled a central role in the elucidation of selfhood, also supports the impression about the presence of the early perception of selfhood in the first language. As Jaspers put it:

> I do indeed have consciousness of the real Being only in the Being of transcendence; only here there is peace for me. However, I always find myself again on the unquiet island of struggle, I remain alone, and appear to get lost; I lose myself if I no longer feel Being … in my philosophizing I remain suspended between adjusting and my possibility for my reality to be given.[174]

Jaspers's repeated confrontation with the thought patterns typical of his early perception of selfhood is apparently no coincidence. The statement that "the reality of transcendence is still decided only in the first language"[175] indicates that the elements of the explication of Being are anchored already in the early perception of selfhood. In this respect, "something" from the first language is present in the cipher language. So the selfhood that constitutes the cipher language must be capable, as part of its self-understanding, of comprehending the language of the early selfhood as a sort of "ancient writing" of its own.

Like the first language, we can also identify in the second language of metaphysical tangibility the presence of early philosophical ideas Jaspers had handled in the explication of selfhood. The general element typical of Christian myths within the second language may serve as a basis for the communication, or "mediation" in Jaspers's word, of the metaphysical experiences it contains.[176] A basic similarity exists between the process of creating myths as Jaspers described it in this context and his perception of the process of the objectivization of the scientific viewpoint. Even the role Jaspers attributed to the scientific viewpoint in the elucidation of selfhood is not different from the one he granted myths when discussing the concept of the cipher. Just as the act of scientific objectivization defines the boundaries of the reality that it created and sets the general criteria for its reality, so the observation seeing immanence as a cipher of transcendence determines the boundaries of the reality on which metaphysical consciousness is based. Just as the act of scientific objectivization grants the scientist a sense of connection to the objective reality, and a real grasp of it, so the myths grant the metaphysical experience a sense of a grasp of something real. Recognizing the advantages of the positivistic viewpoint and the contribution of formal consciousness to the clarification of the concept of cipher does not enable the simple rejection of the way of dealing proposed in the second language. In the following passage Jaspers sketched the philosophical move originating in the elucidation of Existenz, continuing in the second language and ending in a detailed justification for its rejection:

> The objectivity of the metaphysical tradition attracts at first the forming Existenz, even before it disassembles itself again in the formed Existenz. As a historical thing, objectivity has stable sides; it can be significant only in raising the question whether Existenz reaches its selfhood alone. ... The pretension to become familiar is realized even before it could be sought. Against [this pretension], the experience of Existenz turns with the world orientation that expands itself and can bring itself not to believe in anything as empirical and finite. If this positivism collapses, within the boundaries that it perceived, [then] for the first time only the stable and authoritative objectivity can be perceived anew. Fused into the movement of the existential ascertaining of transcendence, this [objectivity perceived anew] serves as a function where the substantial ground becomes present. This is because the objectivity of transcendence in the ciphers of the second language cannot be exhaustive at any moment either from principle or ad hoc, but it is only acquired historistically.[177]

The connection arising from these words between the rejection of the second language that crystallized the metaphysical consciousness in the framework of myths, and the objection Jaspers raised during the elucidation of selfhood toward the positivistic world view is clear. The eternality of the Being embodied in selfhood and in the cipher is perceived as contradicting the very possibility that it could be exhausted using the tools of finitude. Just as positivism cannot propose a complete elucidation of the experience of constituting selfhood and of the reality viewed from it, so the myths do not embody the metaphysical reality that the concept of cipher is intended to indicate.

Jaspers's choice represented in the second language, to establish his objection to metaphysical objectivization precisely on the basis of existential considerations related to the processes of its historistic formation, constitutes a continuation of the philosophical move that appeared already in the first language. In these two languages we can notice the attempt to deal with the ways of forming metaphysical consciousness in light of the central aspects that had appeared in the elucidation of selfhood. Although the idea of historicity has been interpreted in this book as a transition mechanism reflecting a transcending of the framework of the explication of selfhood, Jaspers's criticism of positivism, as raised in the presentation of the second language, does not allow us to ignore the prominent connection this language has with the questions guiding the discussion of the early perception of selfhood.

The ongoing dialog Jaspers conducted with these early insights, which had become the constituting elements of the framework of the explication of selfhood in his philosophy, demonstrates the continuity between the different issues he discussed over the long years of his work. While the third language where the cipher's viewpoint is located is not satisfied with the one-time experience of Existenz as expressed in the first language, nor does it turn to the other extreme that organizes the metaphysical experience within the fenced boundaries of the myths that fill the second language. However, the third language is revealed from the interpretation presented above as anchored in the early philosophical processes represented in the two first languages. So the cipher language shows, on the one hand, recognition of the self-sinking ability of Existenz that typified the elucidation of selfhood, though unlike the first language this ability was directed toward the transcendent Being. On the other hand, the cipher language reflects Jaspers's attempt to satisfy the philosophical need for defined thought patterns at some level—though unlike the second language, the cipher language does not satisfy this need to the point of isolating it from its connection to the historistic selfhood characterizing myths as such.

The combination of the existential element anchored in the processes of elucidating selfhood and of the more structured and communicative facet that developed in the framework of the explication of Being in the cipher language realizes what Jaspers saw as a condition for the constitution of the consciousness of Being: maintaining the tension between objectivity and subjectivity.[178] He walks "on the double ground" that consciousness of Being has "both in objectivity and in subjectivity."[179] So the cipher's viewpoint represents the process in which the development of the person's selfhood gradually becomes a reflection of transcendence,[180] without losing the connection with the concrete reality of

Existenz.[181] Jaspers described the new situation created by the symbolic observation of reality as follows:

> In the cipher, what is connected to the root of my Being and yet does not unite with me faces me as a Being. I am real in that I exist in the cipher as myself without chasing a [certain] end or serving some interest of existence.[182]

Finally, the concept of cipher becomes a crossroads where the meeting of different aspects of Jaspers's philosophy led to the maturation of metaphysical consciousness—a maturity expressed in its ability to acquire a new philosophical language that does not involve losing the connection with its constituent elements. The ability of the cipher language to speak also the language of the philosophizing that characterized the elucidation of selfhood not only revealed the metaphysical depth contained in the Being of Existenz, but also demonstrated the thematic continuity from the elucidation of selfhood to the explication of Being. At this point we can find grounds for a comparison between Jaspers and Ricoeur, who argued that understanding the symbolic aspects is a moment of self-comprehension.[183] In this respect, the concept of cipher expressed a meeting between two potencies: the one existing in immanence, whose roots are in transcendence, and the one typical of Existenz, described in this context as experiencing reality as "the pure self-presence of transcendence in immanence."[184] The same experience that in the perception of the encompassing was held in the duality between "the encompassing that is us" and "the encompassing that is Being itself" led in the framework of the cipher's viewpoint to the integration of Existenz and immanence with transcendence. As Jaspers put it: "in the cipher text *the separation between the symbol and what it symbolizes* [is] *impossible*,"[185] since "the cipher is a parable that is Being or Being that is a parable."[186]

Eleven

BETWEEN BEING AND TRANSCENDENCE

1. "Being" and "Transcendence"

Karl Jaspers's unsystematic usage throughout his different writings of the concepts "Being" (*Sein*) and "transcendence" (*Transzendenz*) creates difficulties in elucidating the boundaries of the framework of the explication of Being. As we have seen, in the early works where Jaspers dealt with the elucidation of selfhood, the concepts "Being" and "transcendence" hardly appeared at all. With the constitution of the Being of Existenz in *Philosophy*, where these concepts appeared for the first time, their discussion was subjugated to the elucidation of Existenz's selfhood. The word "Being" was usually attributed to Existenz's Being, while the discussion of transcendence was derived from the ways Existenz related to it.[1] The relation of Existenz toward transcendence expressed the particular ability of selfhood to expand the boundaries of its awareness and its capability to experience. We can state that from the viewpoint of Existenz, characterized by a drive to transcend itself and not to be satisfied with the boundaries of existence alone, the discussion of the difference between the concepts of Being and transcendence was not crucial. In general, within the framework of the explication of selfhood the discussion regarding reality was not directed to the elucidation of Being or transcendence, but focused on Existenz itself. Even when, within this framework, there appeared a discussion of transcendence, it was intended for the functional needs of Existenz, whose resources were mostly devoted to explicating its selfhood. The framework of clarifying Existenz was characterized by a large degree of similarity, if not actual identity, between the practice of transcending (*transzendieren*) and the very Being of transcendence (*Transzendenz*). In principle, the centrality of selfhood in the philosophical discussion did not require or even enable a real distinction between Being and transcendence, and their meaning as independent entities remained beyond the horizon of the discussion, which dealt primarily with elucidating the character of Existenz.

The awareness of the boundaries of the Being of Existenz first started to form in the context of Jaspers's discussion of the philosophical ideas included in what I have termed the transition mechanisms. Only at this stage did Jaspers turn to discuss "Being" and "transcendence" as entities existing outside or beyond the boundaries of existence and Existenz. Despite this, even within the context of the transition mechanisms we can not yet indicate a basis that would enable a distinction between the concept of Being and the concept of transcendence. A discussion whose subject was transcendence and Being only appeared with the transition to the philosophizing framework of the explication of Being, and it appears that only at this stage did the basis for a significant distinction between these two concepts start to be formulated. Jaspers himself marked the boundary line between the discussion of Being from Existenz's perspective and the one conducted from viewpoint of the explication of Being, when he argued that he "want[ed] to reach [the place] where there was no longer any possibility, but where there was only the decided real, existing only because it is Being as such."[2] In these words, Jaspers linked the removal of "possibility"—a central facet of the Being of Existenz—with the elucidation of the reality of Being. The framework of the explication of Being also presented the aim to elucidate it as a central characteristic of Existenz, but once Being had become the central target of the explication, dealing with it no longer had to meet the self-understanding needs of Existenz. In any case, within the framework of the explication of Being, neither the character of Being nor that of transcendence was determined according to the boundaries of the existential viewpoint.

The attempt to overcome the centrality of the existential viewpoint without removing Existenz itself from the arena of philosophizing was apparent in the elucidation of the concept of the encompassing, where Jaspers presented its seven modes, including transcendence, as a scheme of Being.[3] From the way these things were presented, transcendence is apparently not separate from Being, but is one of its aspects. However, Jaspers argued that "transcendence has nothing of its own… but it speaks from the other [modes of the encompassing] that include it within themselves and are penetrated by it."[4] However, in precisely the same context, Jaspers stated that "one should distinguish between the transcendence of all the modes of the encompassing and real transcendence. We transcend to each of the modes of the encompassing … but transcendence in its real meaning is only the encompassing as such, the encompassing of all the encompassings."[5] This second statement may serve as a basis for understanding transcendence not as part of Being or an aspect of Being, but as another Being existing beyond the boundaries of the encompassing. This duality also arises from Jaspers's discussion of the question of the relation between the unity of Being and its expressions in the multiple ways of the encompassing.[6]

The difficulty in distinguishing between the concepts of Being and transcendence also arises from the perception of ciphers. The ciphers of transcendence reflect, on the one hand, a viewpoint of immanence and not another reality. In the concept of "immanent transcendence," placed at the center of the elucidation of the concept of cipher, Jaspers presented a perception of immanence whereby this reality is not identical to its understanding as mere empiricism, but contains metaphysical depth that makes it into a symbol of transcendence.[7] On the other hand, already during his discussion of the concept of cipher Jaspers indicated the urgent need for the "*separation of the description of transcendence from transcendence* [itself]."[8] The distinction between the perception of transcendence achieved through the interpretation of immanent reality and transcendence itself is also apparent in several other statements in this context of the discussion. Jaspers argued that "there is no simple parallel between the fullness of the tangible and the fullness of the content of Being"[9]; that "*the reality of transcendence* does not enter metaphysical thought in any way"[10]; that the cipher is not an expression of a person's mental reality, but is an objectivity that can be compared only to itself, and "through which transcendence speaks"[11]; and that "the observable *symbolism* does not know *anything absolute*."[12] In this respect, we can also state that even if the cipher's viewpoint constitutes an interpretative stance toward immanence without proving the existence of a transcendent reality, at least it does not disprove it. However, other statements, primarily the argument that "the presence of Being turns to us only in itself and through itself,"[13] support the understanding whereby Jaspers saw transcendence as a reality existing outside the boundaries of the immanence he included in the concept of Being.

As with the perception of the encompassing, so in the framework of the concept of cipher Jaspers's words can be considered the basis for two perceptions: one including transcendence within the framework of immanent reality and making it part of the concept of Being, and the other presenting it as a different reality exceeding the boundaries of immanence and distinct from the reality of Being. These two different perceptions are also reflected in the interpretations of the concept of transcendence in the secondary literature.

2. The Concept of Transcendence as Reflected in Research

The secondary literature dealing with Jaspers's philosophy devoted special attention to the concept of transcendence. There are three main interpretative directions: immanent, theological-religious, and ethical.

A. The Immanent Interpretation

The image of the "missing God" is a central motif in Jeanne Hersch's immanent interpretation of Jaspers's concept of transcendence. In her opinion, this concept denotes the hidden God who does not achieve self-expression, but appears as lacking absolute essence. Since this entity is only felt by Existenz, in Hersch's opinion there is no point asking about its reality, its time, and its place. Hersch argues that transcendence never denotes a different world than the one existing in the empirical reality where the ciphers exist.[14] She believes that their main significance is in their constituting a barrier against the confusion of transcendence with the meaning people give it.[15] In her later article, "Existenz in empirical reality," Hersch argues that transcendence is not evidence of something, but it means that by being there, in the place and time where Existenz reaches its decision, it arrives at an awareness that it did not create itself, and that its essence is not exhausted solely by itself. When it deals with transcendence, Existenz "transposes" and "bisects" time, as Hersch puts it, but at the same time is not detached from it. The discussion of transcendence is mainly important, in Hersch's view, as a means for stressing the weight of empiricism in Jaspers's thought, which is unique in "not disarming reality."[16]

Hans Kunz derived the basis for his immanent viewpoint of the concept of transcendence from people's experiences of the boundaries of their existence, and especially from dealing with death as the certain destiny of their actual existence. His argument in principle is that human beings' transition from mere existence to authentic existence is not based on Existenz's relation to transcendence as an extra-worldly Being, but is enabled by the very dealing with death as a potential element revealed to people in existence as an immanent possibility of their cessation.[17] From this point of view, because death entails the end of life and portends the atemporality that has an identical meaning to the perception of the end of life, this is perceived as eternality and permanence. So Kunz believes that Jaspers's movement between the world and what is outside it does not reflect experience in the direct meaning of the word, but expresses a confrontation with the possibility of the loss of immanent existence through death.[18] In the end, immanent death as an absolute element of human existence enables, in Kunz's opinion, interpreting the existential relation to transcendence and even transcendence itself as immanent.[19]

The immanent interpretation of Jaspers's concept of transcendence led some scholars, such as Joseph Lenz and Arnold Gehlen, to define Jaspers's perception of Being as an idealistic world view. The premise behind Lenz's interpretation was that since Immanuel Kant there has been no possibility of proposing a metaphysics that could pass a rational test.[20] In his opinion, "the basic motif of Jaspers's philosophy is constant tension between radical doubt of objective order and blind faith in the Being of the self, between realizing the drive to know and its doubtedness."[21] Despite this tension, Lenz believes that Jaspers's metaphysical philosophy reflects an attempt to unify Being with thought. In his opinion, this attempt makes it irrational, impossible except as a sort of faith combining a process of people's return to themselves with a pantheistic position lacking "any view to what is beyond."[22] Like Lenz, Gehlen, too, tried to examine Jaspers's concept of transcendence through clarifying the relations between Being and thought in his philosophy. He argued that Jaspers's renunciation of general validity and objectivity led him to create a "negative dogmatism" relying on what he termed "the undeniable subjectivity of the whole."[23] Eventually even the idealistic interpretations of Lenz and Gehlen located Jaspers's concept of transcendence within the immanent boundaries of the explication of selfhood. For further discussion, see also the idealistic interpretation of Erich Frank.[24] The influence of the idealistic tradition on the concept of transcendence and Jaspers's method of transcending on the one hand, and Jaspers's studies in the history of philosophy (*The Great Philosophers*,[25] *Nicolaus Causanus*, *Schelling*,[26] and others) on the other hand, is extensively discussed in Alan M. Olson's study. Olson's main argument is that Jaspers's connection to the idealist tradition does not express an adoption of it with small changes, but that Jasper offers a reading of idealism in light of the philosophy of Existenz, which enables him to understand idealism itself as a mystical appeal for transcendence.[27]

B. The Theological-Religious Interpretation

The combination appearing in Jaspers's thought—between the inability to objectivize the absolute basis of the existence with which the cipher's viewpoint deals on the one hand, and the aim, despite this, to constitute a significant relation to Being as a wholeness that exceeds the boundaries of human existence on the other hand—led some interpreters to present his concept of transcendence as a religious concept and to grant his philosophy a theological nature. One of the extreme conclusions arising from the attempt to examine the religious aspects of Jaspers's philosophy is portrayed in Claus Uwe Hommel's interpretation, stating that the perception of Being eventually denies the reality of the world. Hommel argued that just as for Kant the world remained an idea and did not become an object, so for Jaspers everything that is known is always within the world but never reflects the world itself.[28] The constant doubt regarding the world's reality inevitably becomes a datum that does not enable Existenz to experience the world as its "fatherland." Instead of accepting this situation that indicates the predicted realization of the possibility of Existenz's cessation as such, in Hommel's opinion it must "drop its anchor in transcendence"—which eventually leads to its self-actualization through a mystical union.[29] It transpires, according to this interpretation, that the experience of the world as full of the presence of transcendence depends on a person's ability to abandon the perception of the world as "earthly," or this experience would lead to "the world getting lost between Existenz and transcendence."[30] Karl Löwith expressed a similar criticism of Jaspers's metaphysical philosophy. In his opinion, Jaspers, like other existentialists, expressed in his thought excessive esteem for the a-worldly internality and preference for general humanity—which in his opinion returns Jaspers's philosophy to the realm of German idealism.[31]

The perception of Jaspers's concept of transcendence as having theological implications is also reflected in the interpretation of Fritz-Joachim Von Rinteln, who distinguished between two concepts of transcendence: "non-actual transcendence," with no restriction on the contexts where it applies, and "actual transcendence," which becomes the reality at the center of Jaspers's philosophy.[32] These two concepts express, in his opinion, two basic meanings of transcendence:

as absolute emptiness or fullness.[33] One is aimed at fulfilling the requirement that transcendence lack contents, be non-objective, avoid any satisfaction or "solidifying" (*Verfestigung*), and stress the value of searching and the desire to remain uncertain.[34] The other, in contrast, is aimed at providing us with the perfect satisfaction embodied in God's love. Eventually Von Rinteln argues that everything in reality becomes transcendence according to Jaspers, while immanence itself becomes absurd, which in his opinion brings Jaspers's philosophy close to mystical approaches.[35]

A religious viewpoint, although much more moderate than that of Hommel and Rinteln's interpretations, also appears in F. Imle, who defined Jaspers's philosophy as "apology" that could denote for modern people the way back to the religion of revelation.[36] In his opinion, the centrality of Existenz in Jaspers's thought does not detract from this understanding, since any positive faith starts with the yearning accompanying people's search for self.[37] In any case, in his opinion, the search for God in Jaspers is characterized by vacillating between pantheism and vague theism.[38] A similar position is presented by Robert Winkler, who argued that the separation between "the religious basis and the religious subject" reflects a misunderstanding of theology.[39] In his opinion, although God remains hidden in Jaspers's thought, this should not remove his philosophy from the realm of theology.[40] Similarly, Wolfgang Stegmüller states that the idea of people's givenness to themselves is equivalent, to a great extent, to the Christian concept of grace (*Gnade*).[41] In this context, Stegmüller also indicated the basic similarity between Jaspers's philosophy and that of Plotinus.[42] A similar argument appears in Ludwig Armbruster.[43]

In addition to these interpretations, we could note several other approaches, which while perceiving Jaspers's philosophy as religious thought, still do not identify it with a particular historical religion. Schmuel Hugo Bergman argued that the criticism of modernity arising from Jaspers's entire work expresses his philosophical position toward religion. In his opinion, Jaspers "would like to see the renewal of the philosophical faith entailed in religious faith or the turning of religion into philosophy."[44] In this spirit, Leo Gabriel states that Jaspers's concept of transcendence does not reflect by any means a particular religious form, since in his opinion transcendence is "essentially the encompassing (*Umgreifende*) and not the perceived (*Eingreifende*)."[45] Johannes Ell argued that while Jaspers has a "meeting point" with God, this is not accompanied by any aspect of regularity or permanence.[46] Werner Schneiders well expressed the difference between the interpretations that saw Jaspers's philosophy as expressing a religious position related to a particular religion and those that characterized this philosophy by the general term "religious thought," when he stated that "while Jaspers is religious (*religiös*), he is not Christian (*Christ*)."[47]

C. The Ethical Interpretation

Hanoch Tennen defines transcendence as the highest and most encompassing metaphysical introduction to Jaspers's perception of ethics. It is a concept or category that on the one hand enables and on the other hand requires ethics.[48] The ethical approach Tennen stresses in his interpretation of Jaspers's philosophy led him to define "transcendence [as] existing for man only immanently within existence, meaning as immanent transcendence," since immanence is the arena of ethical activity.[49] Tennen stresses that the presence of transcendence in existential existence does not exhaust its Being, which in itself is not dependent upon the relation human beings constitute toward it.[50] Although the very definition of transcendence as a metaphysical introduction indicates its relation to an extra-immanent world, it is not examined except through the ethical activity of existence that represents its immanence in practice. The understanding of transcendence as a depth aspect of Existenz, arising from Tennen's interpretation, also appears in Winkler[51] and Wilhelm Andersen.[52] Tennen himself noted the similarity of his interpretation to that of Andersen.[53] However, Andersen's interpretation also refers to the religious aspects typical of Jaspers's idea of Existenz. In his opinion, Jasper made the transition from pure immanent philosophy to a religious understanding of Existenz.[54] Winkler, too, argued that Jaspers refers to transcendence as "the other in itself."[55]

Like Tennen, Johannes Reis also understood Jaspers's concept of transcendence as serving the individual's self-realization.[56] In his opinion, the expression of transcendence in the world of Existenz as awareness and as moral life does not lead to the exposure of transcendence, which in any case remains in Jaspers's philosophy in a state of constant undefinedness and concealment.[57] However, in his opinion, the real life of Existenz reveals a certain facet of the reality of transcendence that could not be expressed without Existenz.[58]

The gap between the substantial Being of transcendence, which is not accessible to people's forms of experience and consciousness on the one hand, and the ability to identify its presence in human existence and its influence upon it, as Reis and Tennen understood on the other hand, is presented by Fritz Kaufmann as the relation between two concepts of transcendence: "pure transcendence" and "the God of the Covenant." To the extent that the ethical viewpoint is perceived as being focused on the human attempt to rise above existence and to determine for human beings ideals that they can realize in their lives, Kaufmann's interpretation expresses the ethical viewpoint of Jaspers's concept of transcendence. Kaufmann argues that transcendence reflects Jaspers's opposition to the dynamics of life itself and his search for signs that could give people meaning. Transcendence, as guidance and power for human beings, prevents them from identifying themselves with their global tasks.[59] In this respect, Kaufmann argues that transcendence is a correlative of existential existence, and even depends on the Existenz for which it exists. The use of the term correlation, which is central in neo-Kantian thought, is a conscious usage by Kaufmann, who also argued for an influence of the neo-Kantian style, to which Jaspers had been exposed while in Heidelberg.[60] Transcendence is the ally of Existenz. Its second meaning as "pure transcendence," in contrast, maintains the superiority of transcendence over Existenz and its detachment from human existence—both as incomprehensible to people and as lacking influence over people's lives.[61]

In the three interpretative directions to the concept of transcendence in Jaspers's philosophy presented above we can note the presence of two approaches: one seeing transcendence as part of immanent reality and of Jaspers's perception of Being, and the other seeing it as separate from immanence and so as beyond the boundary of Being. The criticism presented below will not attempt to disprove the interpretations reviewed above, but to show them as different expressions of the way Jaspers's complex philosophy was received.

The hidden God, the limitations of time and place within which human existence as such is structured, and the subjective unity between Being and thought, which are central motifs in the immanent interpretation of the concept of transcendence, make the possibility of the existence of a transcendent Being separate from immanence irrelevant to the philosophical discussion, and perhaps even remove it altogether. Kunz's disputing the very connection between the concept of Existenz and the concept of transcendence, arguing that the concept of Existenz can be clarified without requiring the concept of transcendence, makes him the most radical proponent of this group.[62] Compared with Kunz, who completely rejected a philosophical concept so central to Jaspers's thought, the criticism of other scholars regarding the concept of transcendence was limited. Hersch focuses on what can be learned from Jaspers's philosophy regarding immanence, while Lenz and Gehlen express a rational criticism of the concept of transcendence. However, all those who understood the concept of transcendence as immanent eventually return the discussion of transcendence to the boundaries of the explication of selfhood. The assimilation of the discussion of transcendence within the framework of the explication of selfhood accords with the basic understanding presented at the beginning of this discussion, whereby the centrality of selfhood in the philosophical discussion did not necessitate or even enable a real distinction between Being and transcendence. In this respect, the immanent interpretative direction can be seen as supporting the understanding that the distinction between the concepts of Being and transcendence is not essential for the explication of selfhood.

The theological-religious interpretations of the concept of transcendence, unlike those defined as immanent, show an attempt to distinguish between the concept of Being and the concept of transcendence. The perception of transcendence as separate from immanence is prominent in Hommel's interpretation, connecting the concept of transcendence with the denial of the reality of the world. Unlike Hommel's interpretation, that of Von Rinteln, presenting two concepts of transcendence, does not distinguish unambiguously between Being and transcendence. However, his argument that the mystical meaning of transcendence makes immanence absurd can be seen as a basis for the perception of transcendence as a Being separate from immanent reality. The position of the other interpreters in this interpretative direction stresses the principle of the relation toward God, and does not discuss the apparently factual aspects connected to it. These scholars viewed Jaspers's philosophy as an attempt to establish a new type of religiosity, which would give real weight to the critical consciousness typical of modern people.[63] We can state that they do not find it crucial to distinguish between the concept of Being and the concept of transcendence. The main importance of these interpreters to our discussion of the ability to distinguish between these two concepts is in their not perceiving the elucidation of the treatment of transcendence as part of the explication of selfhood. The mode of Existenz's existence behind these interpretations—existence as Existenz in the face of transcendence—is typical of the framework of the explication of Being as presented at the beginning of the discussion in this section of the study. In this respect, their interpretations can be seen as supporting the understanding that the distinction between these two terms is relevant mainly to the context of the explication of Being instead of to that of selfhood. We should expect the distinction between the concept of Being and the concept of transcendence to be based in particular on the concepts of the encompassing and the cipher, on which, as we have seen, the explication of Being is founded, instead of on the concepts typical of the explication of selfhood.

The ethical interpretation illuminates the question of the distinction between the concept of Being and the concept of transcendence from a unique angle. On the one hand, the focus on Existenz's self-realization through ethical existence and the hiddenness of transcendence that are typical of this interpretative direction do not necessitate the distinction between the concept of Being and the concept of transcendence. In addition, the emphasis granted to the search for Existenz's possibilities of realization, and these interpretations not dealing with defining the legitimate forms of this realization, unlike the religious approaches, may indicate the connection between the ethical interpretation of the concept of transcendence and the discussion framework aimed at the explication of selfhood. On the other hand, the general perception of ethical activity as expressing an attempt to go beyond existence and the understanding of the moral act as anchored in an extra-immanent Being may indicate once more how essential it is to distinguish between these two concepts. In the end, we can state that even if the ethical interpretations do not reject the existence of a transcendent Being, as the immanent interpretations of the concept of transcendence did, their focus of interest is on elucidating the ethical activity that takes place mainly within the boundaries of

Being, which, according to the perception of the encompassing, contain immanence.

Apart from these three interpretative directions that entail, as we have seen, a position regarding the distinction between the concept of Being and the concept of transcendence, one can indicate another position. This position reflects handling the problem of distinguishing between these two concepts, but it does not find in Jaspers's thought a real basis enabling the distinguishing of the two perceptions presented regarding transcendence. Johannes Thyssen asks whether the multiplicity of ciphers breaches the unity of Being of transcendence. Thyssen replies that the unity of transcendence is clarified through the different and even contradictory existential experiences in the ciphers.[64] In his opinion, in addition to the definition of the ciphers as a semi-objective form explaining how Existenz is able to experience transcendence,[65] it also grants tangible expression to the particular presence of transcendence: a Being present both in the different forms of experience of the person searching for it, and at the same time hidden from him in the same experiences. Thyssen criticized Jaspers for not enabling the distinction between the two forms of presence of transcendence, arguing that this was an irrational element in his philosophy.[66] While rationality expressed a clearer distinction between the concept of Being and the concept of transcendence, the irrationality Thyssen found in Jaspers's approach enables the establishment of two simultaneous perceptions of transcendence: a perception incorporating it along with immanence in the wider framework of Being, and a perception separating it from Being and placing it beyond immanent reality. Some the awareness of the lack of distinction between Being and transcendence also appears in the interpretations of Olson and Stephen A. Erickson. Olson argues that the inability to mediate between anthropology and ontology served as a basis for the approach viewing metaphors and symbols as an expression of the "divided referentiality" reflecting a dialectic at both the level of reality and the level of Existenz. At this point, in his opinion, a basic difference exists between Jaspers and Martin Heidegger.[67] Erickson, too, compares Jaspers's and Heidegger's concepts of transcendence. He believes that in terms of the location in the world, Jaspers has a more Aristotelian position, while Heidegger tended toward a more Platonic approach. The image of God as the "unmoved mover," the duality of matter and form, and the tension of yearning between them, typical of Aristotelian thought, can serve as a fertile basis for a thesis seeing Jaspers's perception of Being as an expression of undecidedness.[68] Olson, too, discussed the Platonic influences reflected in Jaspers's thought.[69]

3. Facing the Contradiction

Inevitably, the question arises whether these difficulties raised by dealing with Jaspers's ideas expresses a contradiction between different aspects of his thought, or whether the vagueness and ambiguity was deliberate on his part. According to the interpretation offered here, this basic fact, reflected also in the perceptions Jaspers expressed regarding other issues, should not be viewed as representing a contradiction. This is because along with Jaspers's prominent effort to offer a conceptual framework for discussing Being, he himself referred to the problematic entailed in his attempt, a problematic he defined as the "*impermanence of the metaphysical objects*" revealed in a "circle, as a tautology, or as an internal contradiction"[70] and as stemming from the particular nature of Existenz and transcendence as such.[71] These words undoubtedly rule out the possibility of seeing these difficulties as expressing Jaspers's lack of awareness of the contradictions entailed in his words, or of seeing them as the result of deliberate vagueness on his part.

So the question may be asked, what is the value of the philosophical effort presented above to distinguish the concept of Being and the concept of transcendence? Jaspers partially answered this question when he argued that as awareness of the possibilities where selfhood can be clarified increases, and as it finds clearer the "boundaries where it is denied," and recognizes is insufficiency for itself, so it becomes more real and more ready for the otherness of transcendence.[72] Emphasizing the connection between transcendence and the self-perception of Existenz makes tangible the possibility that the experience of foundering would not lead to breaching the framework of the explication of selfhood. In any case, we cannot find in Jaspers's arguments evidence of direct handling of the question of the relation between Being and transcendence from the viewpoint of the framework of the explication of Being.

The simultaneous presence of two concepts of transcendence—the perception including it with immanence in the framework of the concept of Being, and the perception seeing it as a reality separate from immanence—reveals a fundamental contradiction in Jaspers's thought. Apparently, the interpretations presented above, each of which finding support in Jaspers's words, reflect different ways of dealing with a philosophical text characterized by obvious vagueness. Whether consciously or not, we can argue that no scholar can avoid taking decisions in a situation where the text is unclear, and in this respect room exists for the three interpretative approaches that expressed a decision and also for the approach that avoided presenting such a decision. However, understanding the complexity of Jaspers's explication of Being necessitates dealing with the way he perceived the meaning of the contradictions in philosophy.

Jaspers the philosopher did not discuss the issue of contradiction, and its discovery requires deliberate interpretation, but when he faced this problem as a scholar and interpreter, he was able to clarify this position in principle regarding the role of contradictions in philosophical thought. In his extensive study of Friedrich Nietzsche's philosophy, he pointed to the problematic approach to the Being based on the "mind," meaning the attempt to use logical tools to elucidate Being,[73] whose use leads, in his opinion, to erroneous simplifications of Being.[74] Jaspers argued there that the contradictions arising in the study of Being are *inevitable and necessary*, and that they originate in the "thing" from which they stem, meaning from Being itself. The task of the interpreters aiming to expose the wholeness of thought is not to settle the contradictions forming before their eyes, but instead "to be forever dissatisfied where we cannot find also contradictions, and then perhaps experience these contradictions in their essentialness. Instead of pushing the contradictions randomly, we should search for the source of the contradictoriness."[75]

Jaspers's basic approach, seeing the contradictions arising from Nietzsche's thought as an essential part of the process of elucidating the philosophy of Being and a final criterion for the truth of the philosophy,[76] may help us explain the basic contradiction arising from his perception of Being.[77] Walter Kaufmann argues that "Jaspers's position depends on his own Existenzphilosophie."[78] This approach, granting philosophical value to the exposure of contradictions by interpreters, is aimed at shaping their stance in relation to complex questions such as the one discussed in this chapter. The very inability to settle the contradictions that the interpreters can expose may help them overcome the consciousness of control typical of modern people's stance toward the tasks they set themselves. Perhaps this overcoming will open horizons hidden from people when they were determined to grant maximal meaning and clarity to everything they encountered. Facing an insoluble contradiction ends the explication of Being, and this has decisive significance in more precisely clarifying Jaspers's approach in principle to dealing with the presence of contradictions. We learn that the philosophical position, characterized by the ability to contain contradictions, should appear only after the interpreters tried to settle the contradictions and not to accept them as a predetermined decree. However, once these attempts have been exhausted and some of them remain standing, only then are they entitled and even obligated to face them as the final datum of the philosophical experience.

In the end, the boundaries of metaphysical consciousness in whose philosophical constitution Jaspers would have wanted to see himself involved are not determined according to the ontological or epistemological distinctions in which the discussion of philosophical concepts is often anchored, but on the basis of his stance toward philosophical problems. The character of the philosophizer Jaspers envisaged was characterized by the constant aim of removing philosophical "barriers"—the barriers without which new horizons would open to the philosophizing that would lead people to the "boundary" beyond which we cannot progress even one step further.[79]

CONCLUSION

Karl Jaspers's philosophical search for Being was based on the search for comprehensive existential wholeness. Unlike systematic wholeness, where the role of its system is merely the element that directs the process of philosophizing, the comprehensive wholeness does not function as a "guiding principle" but instead as a "fundamental drive," a deep motivation that cannot be silenced.[1] In this study, which aimed to make contact with the primary elements on which Jaspers's philosophy was based, as they developed over the long years of his work, I tried to find the element connecting the varied philosophical themes with which he dealt. These issues transpired during the study as combining into a unity that goes beyond the sum of all its components. I have called this unity "metaphysical consciousness." Since philosophizing was, for Jaspers, a drive rather than just a way of observing reality, the interpretation I have proposed to his philosophy sought to express the internal tension apparent in the process of the development of metaphysical consciousness and to avoid as much as possible eroding it through an interpretation that would devote itself to illuminating this philosophy as a harmonious whole.

The effort to reveal the wholeness at the basis of Jaspers's thought relied on two viewpoints, genealogical and thematic, on which the research methodology of this study was based. The *genealogical viewpoint* was intended to clarify the development dynamic of Jaspers's work, from his psychiatric period up to the peak of the philosophical period, while the *thematic viewpoint* was aimed at elucidating the various issues presented in the different chapters. However, with hindsight it seems that the fuller understanding of the metaphysical consciousness in Jaspers's thought did not rely mainly on the implementation of these two viewpoints, each of which illuminated Jaspers's work from a different angle, but instead on the fact that it was not actually possible to separate them.

It was not possible to present the stages of the development of Jaspers's philosophy from the genealogical viewpoint without being aware of the various issues discussed in the framework of the thematic study. In this respect, the thematic viewpoint served as an infrastructure enabling the genealogical study. Only thanks to the existence of this understanding in the background of the genealogical study was it possible to determine what would be considered as a milestone in the development of Jaspers's ideas, and to distinguish between the primary and secondary stages. The genealogical study of Jaspers's philosophy could not be structured as a descriptive spread, a sort of "narrative of the development of Jaspers's ideas" from the "starting point" to the "end," since the "narrative" itself was only enabled on the basis of acquaintance with its end. Against the background of these ideas we can characterize the genealogical viewpoint as a "progressive method" in the sense that it always aimed to advance from the early to the late point. The awareness whereby in the background of this viewpoint there must exist a thematic understanding of the subject enables us to understand more precisely the nature of the genealogical study, and to see it as a detracting progress, meaning progress achieved from extricating the aspects relevant to the subject and abandoning those the thematic understanding already knows are not essential for elucidating the topic.

At the same time, the formulation of the discussion of the different issues in Jaspers's philosophy, the focus of the study from the thematic viewpoint, would not have been possible without understanding the philosophical moves that led to the constitution of the issues included in the wider topic of the metaphysical consciousness. The thematic viewpoint, relying on the background genealogical study, can thus be defined as a "regressive method." But since this method is eventually aimed at revealing the connection between the issues in the studied philosophy, we can make the definition of the thematic viewpoint more precise, and see it as cumulative regression, meaning a method that requires acquaintance with the early stages of the development of the philosophy in order to formulate the topic on which the study is focused.

In the end, it transpired that not only is there no way of separating the two viewpoints on which the research methodology in this book was based—they actually simultaneously present the existence of both continuous phenomena and non-continuous phenomena in Jaspers's philosophy. We can call the non-continuous phenomena "tears" (*Zerrissenheit*) in the sense Jaspers gave this term in the context of the perception of Being.[2] As the genealogical study reflected the different stages of the philosophy's development and served as a basis for its division into periods, so this study showed the continuity unifying all the various stages of development. But as the thematic study aimed at reaching a coherent understanding of central topics and concepts in Jaspers's thought referring to their appearances throughout the years of his work, so it also revealed the processes of alteration and meaning-change these topics and concepts underwent during the development of his thought.

This book exposed two philosophizing axes along which Jaspers's philosophy developed: one aimed at achieving what I have called the "explication of selfhood," the other aimed at what I have defined as the "explication of Being." The structure of the book apparently reflects the understanding that the first axis of philosophizing led to the second, but against the background of the renewed discussion of the nature of the two viewpoints on which the research methodology was based, we can state that these two axes were actually simultaneously present throughout the stages of the development of this philosophy, and only the mode of their presence is what changed. Our study of the explication of selfhood, relying on the publications where Jaspers discussed this issue directly, showed that the perception of Being was also present implicitly in the background of insights that were apparently not related to it, but to selfhood. In contrast, in the explication of Being his arguments were aimed directly at Being, and apparently they had nothing to add to the character of selfhood that had been elucidated earlier. Subjectivity or Existenz, which were focused only on elucidating their selfhoods, were revealed as different from those perceiving themselves as existing in the face of transcendence.

The change in the mode of presence of Being and selfhood in the two axes of the explication can also be understood as Jaspers's attempt to exhaust his discussion of these two objects of philosophizing on two levels: as a possibility (*Möglichkeit*) and as a reality (*Sein*). Within the explication of selfhood, selfhood portrayed the reality to which the philosophizing was directed, while Being itself was placed in the background of this framework of explication as a possibility that had yet to find its realization within the philosophizing. In the second explication, in contrast, Being or transcendence constituted the reality the philosophical discussion was intended to elucidate, while selfhood was delegated to the background. In this respect, the category of reality expresses the central object of the philosophizing that is given overtly and directly, while the category of possibility has two different meanings. In the explication of selfhood it refers to the Being portraying the horizons beyond the boundaries of the philosophical discussion, which still lacked the tools to explicate it. In the explication of Being this category represents selfhood, which had served in Jaspers's philosophy as an a-priori infrastructure on which the discussion was based, and which actually enabled it.

Illuminating the changing mode of presence of the two main objects of Jaspers's philosophy has great significance for understanding it as one whole. It prevents the option of seeing selfhood or Being as a decisive issue in this thought, and implies that in fact there is no significance to Jaspers's perception of selfhood without his perception of Being, and *vice versa*. Just as the explication of selfhood was unable to fulfill all the needs of selfhood, which required the explication of Being to complement it, so it is impossible to understand the explication of Being without knowing the existential infrastructure that led to it and remains implicit within it. The completion of the two frameworks of explication can only be achieved outside them. In this respect, the "turning point" in Jaspers's thought reflected primarily the context in which it was revealed. From the perspective of the entire philosophy, however, the transition from the explication of selfhood to the one aimed at Being is perceived as the exposure and realization of philosophical potentials that had existed in this thought from the very beginning. In this sense, the three parts composing this book reflect the essential limitations of the philosophical explication, which by its very nature was unable to illuminate the wholeness of the philosophy all at once without spreading it out over several stages.

The illumination of each of the two objects of explication, both as a possible element and as a real element, reveals the depth of meaning of the metaphysical consciousness being constituted in Jaspers's philosophy. On the one hand, it is presented as the realization of a possibility that selfhood had chosen, and thus it should be seen as having significance only for selfhood rather than as an expression of a deterministic process. On the other hand, the very existence of the possibility as background and even as an a-priori condition for the constitution of metaphysical consciousness contains the basis for the realization of this possibility—a reality that is not tested by its actual realization, but that has value even without this realization. Jaspers's philosophy does not lay down "the road to the constitution of metaphysical consciousness," but only entails one of the possibilities for constituting such a consciousness.

Finally, just as the method guiding this study was not prior to the very act of research, but was formulated during it, so also the metaphysical consciousness typical of Jaspers's thought was not a teleological object to which the philosophizing consciously aimed itself, but became tangible only after it had actually been achieved. The secret of the authenticity of Jaspers's philosophy stems from the constant dialog he conducted with the basic intuitions that had guided him at the beginning, intuitions that at various stages along the way were put to the test, but that survived despite the criticism of them as part of the framework of philosophizing, which constantly expanded. Metaphysical consciousness, portraying at the early stages of the development of his thought the self-consciousness of Existenz, and seeking at the later stages to meet not only the "searchlight" illuminating Being, but also "this light itself,"[3] apparently always found its way to the selfhood in which its starting point was anchored.

NOTES

Introduction

1 Henri Bergson. *The Creative Mind*. Translated by Mabelle L. Andison. New Jersey: Littlefield, Adams & Co.,1965, pp. 108–109.

2 Berthold P. Reisterer, "Existenz and Transcendence. Karl Jaspers and the Crisis of Contemporary Liberalism." In Leonard Ehrlich and Richard Wisser (eds.) *Karl Jaspers: Philosoph unter Philosophen*. Würzburg: Konigshausen & Neumann, 1993, pp.228–234; Michael Ignatieff, *The Need of Strangers: An Essay on Privacy and the Politics of Being Human*, New York: Penguin, 1988, pp. 181 ff.; Fritz K. Ringer, *The Decline of The German Mandarins, The German Academic Community, 1890–1933*. Cambridge, Mass.: Harvard University Press, 1969; Herbert Schnändelbach, *Philosophy in Germany, 1831–1933*. Cambridge: Cambridge University Press, 1984; Michael Harrington, *The Politics at God's Funeral: The Spiritual Crisis of Western Civilization*. New York: Henry Holt, 1983.

3 Karl Jaspers, *Philosophy* 3, Heidelberg: Springer, 1994 [1932], p. 24 [26].

4 *Ibid*., p. 27.

5 *Ibid*., p. 27.

6 *Ibid*., p. 26.

7 Karl Jaspers, *Philosophy* 1, Heidelberg: Springer, 1994 [1932], p. 32.

8 *Ibid*., p. 33.

9 Sebastian Samay, *Reason Revisited: The Philosophy of Karl Jaspers*. Dublin: Gill and Macmillan,1971, p. 167.

10 Karl Jaspers, *Psychologie der Weltanschauungen*. Berlin: Springer, 1985 [1919], p. ix (from the Introduction written in 1954).

11 Martina Plümacher, *Philosophie nach 1945 in der Bundesrepublik Deutschland*. Hamburg: Rowohlt Taschenbuch Verlag, 1996, pp. 20 ff.; Kurt Wuchterl, *Streitgespräche und Kontroversen in der Philosopie des 20. Jahrhunderts*. Stuttgart: UTB, 1982.

12 Karl Jaspers, *Vernunft und Freiheit*, Ausgewählte Schriften. Stuttgart-Zürich-Salzburg: Europäischer Buchklub, 1959, pp. 49–50; Karl Jaspers, *Vernunft und Widervernunft in unserer Zeit*, Drei Gastvorlesungen. Munich: Piper, 1950, p. 63; Fritz Heinemann, *Existenzphilosophie–lebendig oder tot?* Stuttgart: PUB, 1954, pp. 80 ff.

13 Karl Jaspers, *Vernunft und Widervernunft in unserer Zeit*; *Was ist Erziehung?* Munich: Piper, 1981; *Die Idee der Universität*. 1. Berlin: Schriften der Universität Heidelberg, 1946; *Die Schuldfrage*. Heidelberg: L. Schneider, 1946; *Über Bedingungen und Möglichkeiten eines neuen Humanismus*. Munich: P. Reclam jun, 1951; *Die Atombombe und die Zukunft des Menschen*. Munich: Piper, 1961; *Philosophie und Welt*, Reden und Aufsätze. Munich: Piper, 1958; *Vernunft und Freiheit*.

14 Plümacher, *Philosophie nach 1945 in der Bundesrepublik Deutschland*, pp. 20 ff.; Rudolf Mense, "Der Anspruch der Philosophie," *Zeitschrift für philosophische Forschung*, 1, (1946), pp. 173–189; Ludwig Landgrebe, *Was bedeutet uns Philosophie? Eine*

Einführung. Hamburg: Marion von Schroder, 1948; Hans-Georg Gadamer, "Das Verhältnis der Philosophie zu Kunst und Wissenschaft." In Gadamer (ed.), *Über die Ursprünglichkeit der Philosophie*. Berlin: Chronos, 1948; Alexander Von Pechmann, "Die Philosophie der Nachkriegszeit in München (1945–1960) Eine Dokumentation, *Widerspruch, Münchener Zeitschrift für Philosophie* (1990); Hermann Krings, "Die Philosophie zwischen Anpassung und Selbstbehauptung," Gespräch mit Prof. Hermann Krings, *Widerspruch*, Münchener Zeitschrift für Philosophie (1987), pp. 15–26.

15 Karl Jaspers, *Die Wandlung* 1, 5, (1945), cited from Plümacher, *Philosophie nach 1945 in der Bundesrepublik Deutschland*, p. 20; Jürgen von Kempski, *Archiv für Philosophie*, 1, (1947), (Geleitwort), pp. 5–8; von Kempski, "Kant und der Geist der Europäischen Philosophie," *Archiv für Philosophie*, 1, (1947), pp. 9–38.

16 Jeanne Hersch, Jan Milic Lochman, and Reiner Wiehl (eds.), *Karl Jaspers—Philosoph, Arzt, politischer Denker*. Munich and Zürich: Piper, 1986; Kurt Salamun, *Karl Jaspers, Zur Aktualität seines Denkens*. Munich and Zürich: Piper,1991; Elisabeth Salamun-Hybasek and Kurt Salamun, (eds.). *Jahrbuch der österreichischen Karl Jaspers Gesellschaft*, 9, (1996); Donatella Di Cesare, *Die Sprache in der Philosophie von Karl Jaspers*, Tübingen and Basel: Francke, 1996; Dietrich Harth (ed.), *Karl Jaspers*, Denken zwischen Wissenschaft, Politik und Philosophie. Stuttgart: Metzler, J.B., 1989; Alan M. Olson (ed.), *Heidegger & Jaspers*. Philadelphia: Temple University Press, 1994; Kay Ganahl, *Sphären des Zersetzenden, Ein Beitrag zur Jaspers Forschung*. Berlin: Verlag für Wissenschaft und Bildung, 1994; Yusuf Örnek, *Karl Jaspers, Philosophie der Freiheit*. Freiburg and Munich: K. Alber, 1986; Rudolf Lengert (ed.) *Philosophie der Freiheit*. Oldenburg: Holzberg, 1983; Leonard Ehrlich & Richard Wisser (eds.), *Karl Jaspers Today, Philosophy at the Threshold of the Future*. Washington, D.C.: University Press of America, 1988.

17 Jaspers, *Philosophy* 1, p. 1.

18 Bernhard Bollen, *Existential Thinking, A Philosophical Orientation*, Pittsburgh: University Duquesne, 1968, pp. 1–35.

19 Jaspers, *Philosophy* 1, p. 28.

20 *Ibid.*, Epilogue to the 1955 edition, p. xv.

21 *Ibid.*, pp. 4–6.

22 Immanuel Kant, *Critique of Pure Reason*. Translated and edited by Paul Guyer and Allen W. Wood. New York: Cambridge University Press, 1977, p. 406, 407 n.

23 Samay, *Reason Revisited: The Philosophy of Karl Jaspers*, pp. 15–18, 33, 276 n. 37; Heinemann, *Existenzphilosophie—lebendig oder tot?*, p. 72; Elisabeth Young-Bruehl, *Freedom and Karl Jaspers' Philosophy*. New Haven: Yale University Press, 1981, pp. 19–20.

24 Kant, *Critique of Pure Reason*, pp. 399–404.

25 Gerhard Kwiatkowski (ed.), *Die Philosophie, Ein Sachlexikon der Philosophie*. Mannheim: Dudenverlag, 1985, pp. 463–367.

26 Jaspers, *Philosophy* 1, pp. 45, 210–236.

27 *Ibid.*, p. 45.

28 *Ibid.*, p. 46.

29 *Ibid.*, p. 26.

30 *Ibid.*, pp. 46–48.
31 *Ibid.*, p. 49.
32 *Ibid.*, p. 50.
33 *Ibid.*, p. 53.
34 Kant, *Critique of Pure Reason*, p. 407.
35 Jaspers, *Philosophy* 1, p. 39.
36 *Ibid.*, p. 52.
37 *Ibid.*, p. 52.
38 *Ibid.*, pp. 322 ff.
39 Karl Jaspers, *Allgemeine Psychopathologie, Ein Leitfaden für Studierende, Ärzte und Psychologen*. Berlin: Springer, 1st ed., 1913, p.1.
40 Jaspers, *Psychologie der Weltanschauungen*, p. 6.
41 Jaspers, *Philosophy* 1, p. 45.
42 Kant, "Prolegomena to any future metaphysics that will be able to come forward as a science." Translated by Gary Hatfield. In *Immanuel Kant: Theoretical Philosophy after 1781*. Henry Allison and Peter Heath (eds.). New York: Cambridge University Press, 2002, p. 142.
43 Kant, *Critique of Pure Reason*, p. 215.
44 Kant, "Prolegomena to any future metaphysics that will be able to come forward as a science," p. 157, 142.
45 *Ibid.*, pp. 142–143; Jaspers, *Philosophy* 1, pp. 92–93.
46 Urs Richli, *Transzendental Reflexion und sittliche Entscheidung, Zum Problem der Selbsterkenntnis der Metaphysik bei Jaspers und Kant*. Bonn: H. Bouvier, 1967; Rudolf J. Gerber, "Karl Jaspers and Kantian Reason," *New Scholasticism*, 43, (1969), pp. 400–423; Erich P. Grünert, "Der Einfluss Kants auf Karl Jaspers: Zugang zur Transzendenz bei Kant und Karl Jaspers," *Freiburger Zeitschrift für Philosophie und Theologie*, III, (1956), pp. 21–28; Ronny Miron,"Was Jaspers Really Kantian?" *Yearbook of the Austrian Karl Jaspers Society*, 19, (2006), pp. 73–106.
47 Jaspers, *Rechenschaft und Ausblick*, Tübingen: Reden und Aufsätze, 1958, p. 341; *Rechenschaft und Ausblick*: "Mein Weg zur Philosophie" (1951), pp. 323–332; "Uber meine Philosophie" (1941), pp. 333–365.
48 Jaspers, *Philosophy* 1, p. ix; Karl Jaspers, *Nietzsche*, Einführung in das Verständnis seines Philosophierens, Berlin: Walter De Gruyter, 1950, p. 9.
49 Leonard Ehrlich, *Karl Jaspers: Philosophy as Faith*. Amherst: University of Massachusetts Press, 1975; Aloys Klein, *Glaube und Mythos, Eine kritische, religionsphilosophisch-theologische Untersuchung des Mythos-Begriffs bei Karl Jaspers*. Munich: F. Schöningh, 1973; Samay, *Reason Revisited: The Philosophy of Karl Jaspers*; Hans Kunz, "Critique of Jaspers' Concept of Transcendence." In *The Philosophy of Karl Jaspers*. Paul Arthur Schlipp, (ed.). New York: Tudor, 1957, pp. 115–140; Alan M. Olson, *Transcendence and Hermeneutics, An Interpretation of the Philosophy of Karl Jaspers*. The Hague and Boston: M. Nijhoff, 1979; Salamun, *Karl Jaspers*. Munich: Beck, 1985; Otto Friedrich Bollnow, *Existenzphilosophie*. Stuttgart: W. Kohlhammer, [1942] 1960; Heinrich Knittermeyer, *Die Philosophie der Existenz von der Renaissance bis zur Gegenwart*. Vienna and Stuttgart: Humboldt, 1961.

50 Chris Walker, "Karl Jaspers and Edmund Husserl—I: The Perceived Convergence," *Philosophy, Psychiatry and Psychology*, 1:2, (1994), pp. 117–134; Walker, "Karl Jaspers and Edmund Husserl—II: The Divergence," *Philosophy, Psychiatry and Psychology*, 1:4, (1994), pp. 245–266; Walker, "Karl Jaspers and Edmund Husserl—III: Jaspers as a Kantian Phenomenologist," *Philosophy, Psychiatry and Psychology*, 2:1, (1995), pp. 65–82; Walker, "Karl Jaspers and Edmund Husserl—IV: Phenomenology as Empathic Understanding," *Philosophy, Psychiatry and Psychology*, 2:3, (1995), pp. 247–266; Walker, "Karl Jaspers as a Kantian Psychopathologist, I: The Philosophical Origins of the Concept of Form and Content," *History of Psychiatry*, 4, (1993a), pp.209–238; Walker, "Karl Jaspers as a Kantian Psychopathologist, II: The Concept of Form and Content in Jaspers' Psychopathology," *History of Psychiatry*, 4, (1993b), pp. 321–348; Walker, "Karl Jaspers as a Kantian Psychopathologist, III: "The Concept of Form in Georg Simmel's Social Theory: a Comparison with Jaspers," *History of Psychiatry*, 5, (1994), pp. 37–70.

51 Fritz-Joachim Von Rinteln, *Beyond Existentialism*. London: Allen and Unwin, 1961, p. 204; Charles F. Wallraff, "Jaspers in English: A Failure in Communication," *Philosophy and Phenomenological Research*, 37, (1977), pp. 537–548; Heinemann, *Existenz-philosophie—lebendig oder tot?*, pp. 65, 71; Hans Mader, "Das Seindenken bei Karl Jaspers," *Wissenschaft und Weltbild*, 10, (1957), p. 58.

52 Kurt Hoffman, "The Basic Concept of Jaspers' Philosophy." In *The Philosophy of Karl Jaspers*. Paul Arthur Schilpp, (ed.). New York: Tudor, 1957, pp. 95 ff.; Adolph Lichtigfeld, *Jaspers' Metaphysics*. London: Colibri Press, 1954.

53 Avi Sagi, *Kierkegaard, Religion, and Existence: The Voyage of the Self*. Translated by Batya Stein. Amsterdam: Rodopi, 2000, pp. 45–46, 67–74.

54 Heinemann, *Existenzphilosophie—lebendig oder tot?* pp. 11–32.

Chapter One

1 Karl Jaspers, "Heimweh und Verbrechen" (Dissertation). In *Archiv für Kriminal-Anthropologie und Kriminalistik*, 35, (1909); Jaspers, "Ein Beitrag zur Frage: 'Entwicklung einer Persönlichkeit' oder 'Prozess'?" *Zeitschrift für die gesamte Neurologie und Psychiatrie*. 1, (1910), pp. 567–637; Jaspers, "Die Methode der Intelligenzprüfung und der Begriff der Dimenz," *Zeitschrift für die gesamte Neurologie und Psychiatrie*, (referatential), (1910) pp. 402–452; (1912), pp. 289–354; Jaspers, "Zur Analyse der Trugwahrnehmungen (Leibhaftigkeit und Realitätsurteil)," *Zeitschrift für die gesamte Neurologie und Psychiatrie*, 6, (1911) pp. 460–535; Jaspers, "Die phänomenologische Forschungsrichtung in Psychopathologie," *Zeitschrift für die gesamte Neurologie und Psychiatrie*, 9, (1912) pp. 391–408; Jaspers, "Die Trug-wahrnehmungen," *Zeitschrift für die gesamte Neurologie und Psychiatrie*, 4, (referatential); Jaspers, "Kausale und 'verständliche' Zusammenhange zwischen Schicksal und Psychose bei der Dementia praecox (Schizophrenie)," *Zeitschrift für die gesamte Neurologie und Psychiatrie*, 14, (1913) pp. 158–263; Jaspers, *Allgemeine Psychopathologie, Ein Leitfaden für Studierende, Ärzte und Psychologen*. Berlin: Springer, 1st ed., 1913; Jaspers, *Allgemeine Psychopathologie*, Berlin and Heidelberg: Springer, 8th ed., 1965.

2 Hans Saner, *Jaspers*. Rowohlt, Hamburg, 1991 [1970], p. 31; Herbert Spiegelberg, *Phenomenology in Psychology and Psychiatry*. Evanston: Northwestern University Press, 1972, pp. 173–193; Manfred Spitzer, *Phenomenology, Language & Schizophrenia*. In Manfred Spitzer, Friedrich Uehlein, and Michael A. Schwarts (eds.). New York and Berlin: Springer 1992, pp. 35–69; Chris Walker, "Karl Jaspers and Edmund Husserl—I: The Perceived Convergence," *Philosophy, Psychiatry and Psychology*, 1:2, (1994), pp. 117–134; Walker, "Karl Jaspers and Edmund Husserl—II: The Divergence," *Philosophy, Psychiatry and Psychology*, 1:4, (1994), pp. 245–266; Walker, "Karl Jaspers and Edmund Husserl—IV: Phenomenology as Empathic Understanding," *Philosophy, Psychiatry and Psychology*, 2:3, (1995), pp. 247–266; Fritz Heinemann, *Existenzphilosophie—lebendig oder tot?* Stuttgart: Kohlhammer, 1954, pp. 61–66; Ernst Moritz Manasse, "Max Weber's Influence on Jaspers." In *The Philosophy of Karl Jaspers*. Paul Arthur Schlipp, (ed.). New York: Tudor, 1957, pp. 369–393; Walker, "Karl Jaspers and Edmund Husserl—III: Jaspers as a Kantian Phenomenologist," *Philosophy, Psychiatry and Psychology*, 2:1, (1995), pp. 65–82; Walker, "Karl Jaspers as a Kantian Psychopathologist, II: The Concept of Form and Content in Jaspers' Psychopathology," *History of Psychiatry*, 4, (1993b), pp. 321–348; Walker, "Karl Jaspers as a Kantian Psychopathologist, III: The Concept of Form in Georg Simmel's Social Theory: a Comparison with Jaspers," *History of Psychiatry*, 5, (1994), pp. 37–70; Hans Peter Rickman, "The Philosophic Basis of Psychiatry: Jaspers and Dilthey," *Philosophy of the Social Science*, 17, (1987), pp. 180–181.

3 Jaspers, *Allgemeine Psychopathologie*, p. 1.

4 Max Weber, *The Protestant Ethic and the Spirit of Capitalism*. New York: C. Scribner's Sons, 1958, pp. 79–92; Weber, *Gesammelte Aufsätze zur Wissen-schaftslehre*, Tübingen: J.C.B. Mohr, 1922, pp. 524–555.

5 Jaspers, *Allgemeine Psychopathologie*, p. 2.

6 *Ibid*., p. 2.

7 *Ibid*., pp. 1–2.

8 Jaspers, "Die phänomenologische Forschungsrichtung in Psychopathologie," *Zeitschrift für die gesamte Neurologie und Psychiatrie*, 9, (1912), p. 408.

9 Jaspers, *Allgemeine Psychopathologie*, p. 2.

10 Wilhelm Dilthey, *Der Aufbau der geschichtlichen Welt in den Geisteswissenschaften*, Stuttgart and Goettingen: Teubner and Vandenhoeck, 1927, pp. 79–88; Fritz K. Ringer, *The Decline of The German Mandarins, The German Academic Community, 1890–1933*. Cambridge: Harvard University Press, 1969, p. 315 ff.; Herbert Schnädelbach, *Philosophy in Germany, 1831–1933*. Cambridge: Cambridge University Press, 1984, p. 54 ff.; Walker, "Karl Jaspers and Edmund Husserl—IV: Phenomenology as Empathic Understanding," *Philosophy, Psychiatry and Psychology*, 2:3, (1995), pp. 247–266.

11 Jaspers, *Allgemeine Psychopathologie*, p. 1

12 Joachim-Felix Leonard, (ed.), *Karl Jaspers in seiner Heidelberger Zeit*. Heidelberg: Heidelberger Verlagsanstalt und Druckerei, 1983; Heinz Häfner, "Einleitung in den psychiatrischen Teil." In *Karl Jaspers—Philosoph, Arzt, politischer Denker*. Jeanne Hersch, Jan Milic Lochman and Reiner Wiehl (eds.). Munich and Zurich: Piper, 1986, pp. 83–87; Werner Janzarik, "Jaspers, Kurt Schneider und die Heidelberger Psycho-

pathologie." In *Karl Jaspers—Philosoph, Arzt, politischer Denker*. Jeanne Hersch, Jan Milic Lochman, and Reiner Wiehl (eds.). Munich and Zurich: Piper, 1986, pp. 112–126.

13 Jaspers, *Allgemeine Psychopathologie*, pp. 94–144.

14 *Ibid.*, p. 22.

15 Aleida Assmann, *Arbeit am nationalen Gedächtnis, Eine kurze Geschichte der deutschen Bildungsidee*. Frankfurt and New York: Campus, 1993; Assmann, "Jaspers' Achsenzeit, oder: Vom Glück und Elend der Zentralperspektive in der Geschichte." In *Karl Jaspers, Denken zwischen Wissen-schaft, Politik und Philosophie*. Dietrich Harth (ed.). Stuttgart: Metzler, 1989, pp. 187–205.

16 Jaspers, *Allgemeine Psychopathologie,* p. 2.

17 *Ibid.*, p. 9.

18 Jaspers, *Allgemeine Psychopathologie,* p. 5.

19 Jaspers, *Allgemeine Psychopathologie,* (1965), pp. 651–661; Spiegelberg, *Phenomenology in Psychology and Psychiatry*, pp. xxxiv–xxxv.

20 Jaspers, *Allgemeine Psychopathologie,* p. 3.

21 *Ibid.*, p. 4; 4, n. 1.

22 *Ibid.*, p. 3.

23 Jaspers, *Psychologie der Weltanschauungen*, Berlin: Springer, 1985 [1919], p. 1.

24 Jaspers, *Philosophie*. Berlin: Springer, 1994 [1932], 1, pp. 26–27, 19.

25 Kurt Schneider, "Die phänomenologische Richtung in den Psychiatrie," *Philosophischer Anzeiger*, IV, (1926), pp. 382–404; Arthur Kronfeld, "Über neuere pathologisch-phänomenologische Arbeiten", *Zentralblatt für die gesamte Neurologie und Psychiatrie*, XXVIII, (1922), pp. 441–459; Spiegelberg, "The Relevance of Phenomenological Philosophy for Psychology." In *Phenomenology and Existentialism.* Edward N. Lee and Maurice Mandelbaum, (eds.). Baltimore: Johns Hopkins Press, 1967, xxvi–xlv; Ulrich Sonnemann, *Existence and Therapy: An Introduction to Phenomenological Psychology and Existential Analysis*. New York: Grune & Stratton, 1954; Anna-Teresa Tymieniecka, *Phenomenology and Science in Contemporary Thought*, New York: Farrar, Straus and Cudahy, 1962; Adrian Van Kaam, "The Impact of Existential Phenomenology on Psychological Literature of Western Europe," *Review of Existential Psychology and Psychiatry*, I, (1961), pp. 63–92.

26 Jaspers, "Die phänomenologische Forschungsrichtung in Psychopathologie," *Zeitschrift für die gesamte Neurologie und Psychiatrie*, 9, (1912), pp. 391–408.

27 *Ibid.*, pp. 400–402.

28 *Ibid.*, p. 391.

29 Jaspers, *Allgemeine Psychopathologie,* p. 13.

30 Jaspers, "Die phänomenologische Forschungsrichtung in Psychopathologie," p. 393.

31 Jaspers, *Allgemeine Psychopathologie,* p. 13.

32 Jaspers, "Die phänomenologische Forschungsrichtung in Psychopathologie," p. 402.

33 *Ibid.*, pp. 404–405.

34 *Ibid.*, p. 404.

35 Jaspers, *Allgemeine Psychopathologie,* p. 12.

36 *Ibid.*, p. 12.
37 *Ibid.*, p. 14.
38 *Ibid.*, pp. 147–148; Jaspers, *Allgemeine Psychopathologie,* (1965), pp. 296; Dilthey, *Der Aufbau der geschichtlichen Welt in den Geisteswissenschaften*, pp. 94 ff.
39 Jaspers, *Allgemeine Psychopathologie,* pp. 14–15.
40 *Ibid.*, p. 8; Wilhelm Griesinger, *Pathologie und Therapie der psychischen Krankheiten*, Braunschweig: Wreden, 4th ed., 1786.
41 Jaspers, *Allgemeine Psychopathologie,* p. 8.
42 *Ibid.*, p. 8; 12; 15; 20; Jaspers, "Die phänomenologische Forschungsrichtung in Psycho-pathologie," p. 396.
43 Dilthey, *Selected Writings*. Cambridge: Cambridge University Press, 1976, p. 93.
44 Jaspers, *Allgemeine Psychopathologie,* (1965), p. 460, 6.
45 Jaspers, *Allgemeine Psychopathologie,* pp. 12–13.
46 Jaspers, "Die phänomenologische Forschungsrichtung in Psychopathologie," p. 391; Spiegelberg, *Phenomenology in Psychology and Psychiatry*. Evanston: Northwestern University Press, 1972, p. 186; Walker, "Karl Jaspers and Edmund Husserl—IV: Phenomenology as Empathic Understanding;" Osborne Wiggins, Michael Schwartz and Manfred Spitzer, "Phenomenological / Descriptive Psychiatry: The Methods of Edmund Husserl and Karl Jaspers." In *Phenomenology, Language and Schizophrenia*. Manfred Spitzer, Friedrich Uehlein and Michael Schwartz (eds.).New York: Springer, 1992, pp. 56 ff.
47 Jaspers, *Allgemeine Psychopathologie,* (1965), p. 254.
48 Jaspers, "Die phänomenologische Forschungsrichtung in Psychopathologie," p. 397; Jaspers, *Allgemeine Psychopathologie,* (1965), pp. 7–8; Dilthey, *Selected Writings*, p. 94.
49 Jaspers, "Die phänomenologische Forschungsrichtung in Psychopathologie," pp. 394–395.
50 *Ibid.*, p. 396.
51 *Ibid.*, p. 392.
52 *Ibid.*, p. 396.
53 *Ibid.*, p. 404.
54 *Ibid.*, p. 405.
55 Jaspers, "Ein Beitrag zur Frage: 'Entwicklung einer Persönlichkeit' oder 'Prozess'?" *Zeitschrift für die gesamte Neurologie und Psychiatrie*, 1, (1910), pp. 567–602, 637.
56 Jaspers, *Allgemeine Psychopathologie,* p. 3.
57 *Ibid.*, pp. 6–7.
58 *Ibid.*, pp. 6–7.
59 *Ibid.*, p. 2.
60 *Ibid.*, p. 12.
61 Jaspers, *Vernunft und Widervernunft in unserer Zeit, Drei Gastvorlesungen*. Munich: Piper, 1950, pp. 9–29; Jaspers, *Die geistige Situation der Zeit*. Berlin: Walter de Gruyter, 1931, pp. 137–139; Jaspers, "Zur Kritik de Psychoanalyse," *Rechenschaft und Ausblick, Reden und Aufsätze*. Munich: Piper, 1958, pp. 260–271; Kurt Kolle, "Jaspers as

Psychopathologist." In *The Philosophy of Karl Jaspers*. Paul Arthur Schlipp (ed.). New York: Tudor, 1957, pp. 459–461.

62 Jaspers, *Allgemeine Psychopathologie,* (1965), p. 40.

63 *Ibid.*, p. 6.

64 *Ibid.*, p. 644.

65 Jaspers, *Allgemeine Psychopathologie,* p. 13.

66 Jaspers, *Allgemeine Psychopathologie,* (1965), pp. 624–686.

67 *Ibid.*, p. 464.

68 *Ibid.*, p. 464; Jaspers, *Philosophie*, 1, pp. 212–239.

69 Jaspers, *Allgemeine Psychopathologie,* (1965), pp. 20–21.

70 *Ibid.*, pp. 26–27.

71 Jaspers, *Vernunft und Existenz*. Munich: Piper, [1935] 1987, pp. 35–58; Jaspers, *Von der Wahrheit*, Munich: Piper, [1947] 1991.

72 Jaspers, *Von der Wahrheit*, p. 109.

73 Jaspers, *Allgemeine Psychopathologie,* (1965), p. 634.

74 *Ibid.*, p. 627.

75 Georg Wilhelm Friedrich Hegel, *The Phenomenology of Spirit*. Oxford: Oxford University Press, 1961, pp. 86–87; Jon Stewart, *The Unity of Hegel's Phenomenology of Spirit, a Systematic Interpretation*. Evanston: Northwestern University Press, 2000, p. 32 ff.

76 Jaspers, *Allgemeine Psychopathologie,* (1965), p. 627.

77 *Ibid.*, p. 8.

78 *Ibid.*, p. 464.

79 *Ibid.*, p. 627.

80 Jaspers, *Allgemeine Psychopathologie,* (1965), p. 634, 637.

81 Heinrich Schipperges, "Medizin als konkrete Philosophie." In *Karl Jaspers—Philosoph, Arzt, politischer Denker*. Jeanne Hersch, Jan Milic Lochman and Reiner Wiehl (eds.). Munich and Zurich: Piper, 1986, p. 88; Jaspers, "*Die Idee des Arztes*" and "*Arzt und Patient*." In Jaspers, *Philosophie und Welt, Reden und Aufsätze*, Munich: Piper, 1958, pp. 169–207.

Chapter Two

1 Ronny Miron, "Transcendence and Dissatisfaction in Jaspers's Idea of the Self," *Phaenomenologische Forschungen*, NS 10, (2005), pp. 221–241.

2 Karl Jaspers, *Psychologie der Weltanschauungen*. Berlin: Springer, [1919] 1985.

3 *Ibid.*, pp. 52–216.

4 *Ibid.*, p. ix; Hans Saner, *Jaspers*. Hamburg: Rowohlt, [1970] 1991, pp. 31–37.

5 Wilhelm Dilthey, *Weltanschauungslehre, Abhandlung zur Philosophie der Philosophie, Gesammelte Schriften*, VIII. Stuttgart and Goettingen: Teubner and Vandenhoeck, 1962; Max Scheler, *Philosophische Weltanschauung*. Munich: Lehnen Verlag, 1954; Sigmund Freud, *New Introductory Lectures on Psycho-Analysis and Other Works*. Translated by James Starchey. London: Hogarth Press and the Institute of Psycho–Analysis, 1964, pp. 158–182.

6 Jaspers, *Psychologie der Weltanschauungen*, p. 1.
7 *Ibid.*, pp. 1–2.
8 *Ibid.*, p. 4.
9 *Ibid.*, p. 7.
10 *Ibid.*, p. 4.
11 *Ibid.*, pp. 465–486.
12 *Ibid.*, p. iiix.
13 *Ibid.*, p. iiix.
14 *Ibid.*, p. 5.
15 *Ibid.*, p. 21.
16 *Ibid.*, p. 22.
17 *Ibid.*, pp. 22–23.
18 *Ibid.*, p. 25.
19 *Ibid.*, p. 24.
20 *Ibid.*, p. 10.
21 *Ibid.*, pp. 4 ff.
22 *Ibid.*, p. 97.
23 Saner, *Karl Jaspers in der Diskussion*. Munich: Piper, 1973, pp. 70–100; Martin Heidegger, *Pathmarks*. Cambridge: Cambridge University Press, 1998, p. 6.
24 Jaspers, *Psychologie der Weltanschauungen*, p. 6.
25 *Ibid.*, pp. 13–14.
26 *Ibid.*, p. xi.
27 *Ibid.*, p. 16, 6.
28 *Ibid.*, pp. 10–11.
29 *Ibid.*, p. 5.
30 *Ibid.*, p. 14.
31 *Ibid.*, p. 8.
32 *Ibid.*, pp. 14–15.
33 *Ibid.*, pp.19–20.
34 *Ibid.*, p.19.
35 *Ibid.*, p. 18.
36 *Ibid.*, p. x.
37 *Ibid.*, pp.2–3.
38 *Ibid.*, p. 6.
39 *Ibid.*, p.14.
40 *Ibid.*, pp.16–17.
41 *Ibid.*, p. 18.
42 Jaspers, *Allgemeine Psychopathologie, Ein Leitfaden für Studierende, Ärzte und Psychologen*. Berlin: Springer, 1st ed., 1913, p. 12.
43 Rollo May, et al. (eds.). *Existence: A New Dimension in Psychology and Psychiatry*. New York: Basic Books, 1958.
44 Jaspers, *Psychologie der Weltanschauungen*, p. 18.
45 *Ibid.*, p. 57.
46 *Ibid.*, p. x–xi. These words appear in the preface to the book, written in 1954.

47 *Ibid.*, p. vii.
48 *Ibid.*, p. 5.
49 *Ibid.*, p. 5.
50 *Ibid.*, pp. 65–66.
51 *Ibid.*, pp. 65–66.
52 *Ibid.*, p. 66.
53 *Ibid.*, p. 64.
54 *Ibid.*, p. xii.
55 *Ibid.*, p. 231.
56 Jaspers, *Philosophie*, 1. Berlin: Springer, [1932] 1994.
57 Heidegger, *Pathmarks*, p. 24.
58 *Ibid.*, p. 25.
59 Heidegger, *Sein und Zeit*. Tübingen: M. Niemeyer, [1927] 1993.
60 Jaspers, *Philosophie*, 1, p. 1.
61 Jaspers, *Psychologie der Weltanschauungen*, p. 21.
62 Jaspers, *Allgemeine Psychopathologie, Ein Leitfaden für Studierende, Ärzte und Psychologen*. Berlin: Springer, 1st ed., 1913.
63 Jaspers, *Allgemeine Psychopathologie*. Berlin and Heidelberg: Springer, 8th ed., 1965.
64 Heidegger, *Pathmarks*, p. 10, pp. 17–18.
65 *Ibid.*, p. 32.
66 *Ibid.*, p. 17.
67 *Ibid.*, p. 20.
68 Jaspers, *Psychologie der Weltanschauungen*, p. 69 ff.
69 *Ibid.*, p. 231.
70 *Ibid.*, p. 231.
71 *Ibid.*, p. 6.
72 *Ibid.*, p. 6.
73 *Ibid.*, p. 6.
74 Heidegger, *Pathmarks*, p. 2.
75 Jaspers, *Psychologie der Weltanschauungen*, p. 6.
76 *Ibid.*, p. 51.
77 *Ibid.*, p. 6.
78 *Ibid.*, p. 6.
79 *Ibid.*, p. 6.

Chapter Three

1 Karl Jaspers, *Psychologie der Weltanschauungen*. Berlin: Springer, [1919] 1985.
2 Jaspers, *Philosophie* (1–3). Berlin: Springer, [1932] 1994.
3 Jaspers, *Rechenschaft und Ausblick, Reden und Aufsätze*. Munich: Piper, 1958, pp. 392 ff.
4 Jaspers, *Philosophie 1*, p. 12.
5 Jaspers, *Die geistige Situation der Zeit*, Berlin: Walter de Gruyter, 1931, p. 23 ff.

6 Jaspers, *Philosophie*, 1, p. 1; Elisabeth Young-Bruehl, *Freedom and Karl Jaspers's Philosophy*. New Haven: Yale University Press, 1981, pp. 64–65; pp. 105–106.

7 Jaspers, *Philosophie*, 2, p. 9, 18, 134 ff.

8 Jaspers, *Von der Wahrheit*. Munich: Piper, [1947] 1991.

9 Jaspers, *Philosophie*, 1, p. 69.

10 *Ibid*., p. 63.

11 *Ibid*., p. 63.

12 Thomas Räber, *Das Dasein in der "Philosophie" von Karl Jaspers, Eine Untersuchung im Hinblick auf die Einheit und die Realität der Welt im existentiallen Denken*. Bern: Francke, 1955, p. 30 ff., 33 ff., 133 ff., 135 ff.

13 *Ibid*., p. 69.

14 *Ibid*., pp. 74–75.

15 *Ibid*., pp. 84 ff.

16 Alan M. Olson, *Transcendence and Hermeneutics, An Interpretation of the Philosophy of Karl Jaspers*. The Hague and Boston: M. Nijhoff, 1979, p. 10.

17 *Ibid*., pp. 11–12.

18 Werner Schneiders, *Karl Jaspers in der Kritik*. Bonn: Bouvier, 1965, p. 167, 167, n. 38(a); Wilhelm Andersen, *Der Existenzbegriff und das existenzielle Denken in der neueren Philosophie und Theologie* (Diss). Tübingen: Bertelsmann, 1940.

19 Jaspers, *Von der Wahrheit*, p. 62.

20 Jaspers, *Philosophie*, 1, p. 67.

21 Jaspers, *Allgemeine Psychopathologie, Ein Leitfaden für Studierende, Ärzte und Psychologen*. 1. Aufl. Berlin: Springer, 1913, pp. 98 ff.; Jaspers, "Zur Analyse der Trugwahrnehmungen (Leibhaftigkeit und Realitätsurteil)," *Zeitschrift für die gesamte Neurologie und Psychiatrie*, 6, (1911), pp. 460–535; Jaspers, "Die Trugwahrnehmungen," *Zeitschrift für die gesamte Neurologie und Psychiatrie*, 4, (referatential) (1912), pp. 289–354.

22 Jaspers, *Psychologie der Weltanschauungen*, p. 21.

23 Jaspers, *Psychologie der Weltanschauungen*, pp. 228–229.

24 *Ibid*., pp. 231–247.

25 Ronny Miron, "From Opposition to Reciprocity: Karl Jaspers on Science, Philosophy and What Lies Between Them," *International Philosophical Quarterly*, 44, (2004), pp. 147–163; Bernhard Bollen, *Existential Thinking, A Philosophical Orientation*. Pittsburgh: Duquesne University Press, 1968, pp. 1–12; Fritz K. Ringer, *The Decline of The German Mandarins, The German Academic Community, 1890–1933*. Cambridge, Mass.: Harvard University Press, 1969, pp. 367–434; Franz Clemens Brentano, "Genuine and Fictitious Objects." In *Realism and the Background of Phenomenology*. Chisholm, Roderick Milton (ed.). Glencoe: The Free Press, 3, 1960, pp.71–75; Herbert Spiegelberg, "Der Begriff der Intentionalität in der Scholastik bei Brentano und Husserl," *Philosophische Hefte*, 5, (1936), pp. 75–91; Gottlob Frege, "On Concept and Object." In *Translations from Philosophical Writings of Gottlob Frege*. Peter Greach and Max Black (eds.). Oxford: Basil Blackwell and Mott, 1970, pp. 42–55; Alexius Meinung, "The Theory of Objects." In *Realism and the Background of Phenomenology*. Chisholm, Roderick Milton (ed.). Glencoe: Free Press, 1960, pp. 76–117; Henry Leonard,

"Interrogative, Imperatives, Truth, Falsity, and Lies," *Philosophy of Science*, 26, (1959), pp. 176–186; John E. Llewelyn, "What is a Question?" *The Australian Journal of Philosophy*, 42, (1964), pp. 69–85; Emerich S. G. Coreth, *Metaphysik: Eine methodisch-systematische Grundlegung*. Innsbruck: Tyrolia, 1961, pp. 95–98; Wolfgang Stegmüller, *Probleme und Resultate der Wissenschaftstheorie und analytischen Philosophie*, I. Berlin–Heidelberg–New York: Springer, 1969.

26 Jaspers, *Philosophie*, 1, p. 14.

27 *Ibid.*, p. 10.

28 *Ibid.*, pp. 11–12.

29 *Ibid.*, pp. 17–18.

30 Gabriel Marcel, "Grundsituation und Grenzsituationen." In *Karl Jaspers in der Diskussion*, Hans Saner (ed.). Munich: Piper, 1973, p. 160.

31 Jaspers, *Philosophie*, 1, pp. 14–15.

32 Søren Kierkegaard, *Concluding Unscientific Postscript*. Princeton: Princeton University, 1974, p. 545.

33 Young-Bruehl, *Freedom and Karl Jaspers's Philosophy*, pp. 5–9; Fritz Heinemann, *Existenzphilosophie—lebendig oder tot?* Stuttgart: Kohlhammer, 1954, pp. 61–83.

34 Jaspers, *Philosophie*, 1, p. 17.

35 Jaspers, *Von der Wahrheit*, pp. 225–449.

36 Sebastian Samay, *Reason Revisited: The Philosophy of Karl Jaspers*. Dublin: Gill and Macmillan, 1971, pp. 146 ff.; Olson, *Transcendence and Hermeneutics, An Interpretation of the Philosophy of Karl Jaspers*, p. 20; Young-Bruehl, *Freedom and Karl Jaspers's Philosophy*, p. 2.

37 Jaspers, *Philosophie*, 1, p. 30.

38 Samay, *Reason Revisited: The Philosophy of Karl Jaspers*, pp. 71–73.

Chapter Four

1 Karl Jaspers, *Philosophie*, 2, Berlin: Springer, [1932] 1994, p. 3.

2 Otto Friedrich Bollnow, *Existenzphilosophie*. Stuttgart: W. Kohlhammer, [1942] 1960, pp. 11–26; Bollnow, "Existenzerhellung und philosophische Anthropologie," *Bulletin für deutsche Philosophie*, 12:2, (1938–1939), pp. 136–139, 157; Joseph Lenz, *Der moderne deutsche und französische Existentialismus*. Trier: Paulinus Verlag, 1951, p. 14, 32; F. Imle "Jaspers als Existenz-philosoph," *Philosophisches Jahrbuch der Görres-gesellschaft*, 50, (1937), pp. 86 ff.; Imle, "Jaspers als Existenzphilosoph," *Philosophisches Jahrbuch der Görresgesellschaft*, 49, (1936), p. 503; Jürgen von Kempski, "Philosophie als Anruf." In *Brechungen, Kritischer Versuch zur Philosophie der Gegenwart*. Jürgen von Kempski (ed.). Hamburg: Rowohlt, 1964, pp. 235–250; Jeanne Hersch, *Die Illusion, Der Weg der Philosophie*. Bern: Francke, 1965, pp. 120 ff.; Hans-Rudolf Müller-Schwefe, *Existenzphilosophie, Das Verständnis von Existenz in Philosophie und christlichem Glauben*. Gottingen: Vandenhoeck & Ruprecht, 1961, pp. 39 ff.; Johannes Reis, "Menschliche Existenz bei Jaspers," *Die Neue Ordnung*, 4, (1950), pp. 418–426, 527–531.

3 Jaspers, *Psychologie der Weltanschauungen*. Berlin: Springer, [1919] 1985, pp. 51–216.

4 Jaspers, *Philosophie*, 2, p. 6.

5 Ronny Miron, "Transcendence and Dissatisfaction in Jaspers's idea of the Self," *Phaenomenologische Forschungen*, NS 10, (2005), pp. 221–241.

6 Alan M. Olson, *Transcendence and Hermeneutics, An Interpretation of the Philosophy of Karl Jaspers*. The Hague and Boston: M. Nijhoff, 1979, p.20, 20, n. 6.

7 Jaspers, *Philosophie*, 2, p. 6.

8 *Ibid.*, p. 6.

9 *Ibid.*, p. 6.

10 *Ibid.*, p. 8.

11 Bollnow, *Existenzphilosophie*, p. 24.

12 Bollnow, "Existenzerhellung und philosophische Anthropologie," pp. 136–139.

13 Bollnow, *Existenzphilosophie*, p. 11.

14 *Ibid.*, p. 27.

15 *Ibid.*, p. 16; Bollnow, "Existenzerhellung und philosophische Anthropologie," p. 157.

16 Kurt Salamun, *Karl Jaspers*. Munich: Beck, 1985, p. 46; Fritz Heinemann, *Existenzphilosophie—lebendig oder tot?* Stuttgart: Kohlhammer, 1954, pp. 30 ff.; Fritz-Joachim Von Rinteln, *Beyond Existentialism*. London: Allen and Unwin, 1961, p. 204; William Barrett, *Irrational Man: A Study in Existential Philosophy*. London: Anchor Books, 1964.

17 Joseph Lenz, *Der moderne deutsche und französische Existentialismus*. Trier: Paulinus–Verlag, 1951, p. 32, 14 ff.

18 F. Imle, "Jaspers als Existenzphilosoph," *Philosophisches Jahrbuch der Görresgesellschaft*, 50, (1937), p. 86.

19 Imle, "Jaspers als Existenzphilosoph," *Philosophisches Jahrbuch der Görresgesellschaft*, 49, (1936), p. 503.

20 Imle, "Jaspers als Existenzphilosoph," (1937), pp. 246 ff., 251 ff.

21 Lenz, *Der moderne deutsche und französische Existentialismus*, p. 54.

22 Leo Gabriel, *Existenzphilosophie von Kierkegaard bis Sartre*. Vienna: Verlag Herold, 1951, pp. 17 ff., 20.

23 *Ibid.*, p. 174.

24 *Ibid.*, p. 170.

25 *Ibid.*, p. 193.

26 *Ibid.*, pp. 221–222.

27 Wolfgang Stegmueller, *Hauptströmungen der Gegenwartsphilosophie*. Stuttgart: Alfred Kroner, 1960, pp. 233 ff.; Heinemann *Existenzphilosophie—lebendig oder tot?*, p. 61, 72 ff.

28 Stegmüller, *Hauptströmungen der Gegenwartsphilosophie*, pp. 240 ff.; Marcel Reding, *Die Existenzphilosophie, Heidegger, Sartre, Gabriel Marcel und Jaspers in kritischer-systematischer Sicht*. Düsseldorf: Schwann 1949, pp. 69–109.

29 Von Kempski, "Philosophie als Anruf," p. 250.

30 *Ibid.*, p. 243, 250; Werner Schneiders, *Karl Jaspers in der Kritik*. Bonn: Bouvier, 1965, pp. 70 ff.

31 Jeanne Hersch, *Die Illusion, Der Weg der Philosophie.* Bern: Francke, 1965, p. 120, 128.

32 *Ibid.*, p. 101; Hans-Rudolf Müller-Schwefe, *Existenzphilosophie, Das Verständnis von Existenz in Philosophie und christlichem Glauben.* Gottingen: Vandenhoeck & Ruprecht, 1961, p. 39; Heinrich Knittermeyer, *Die Philosophie der Existenz von der Renaissance bis zur Gegenwart.* Vienna: Humboldt, 1961, pp. 48–49; Johannes Reis, "Menschliche Existenz bei Jaspers," *Die Neue Ordnung*, 4, (1950), pp. 418–426, 527–531.

33 Schneiders, *Karl Jaspers in der Kritik*, p. 169.

34 Jaspers, *Philosophie*, 2, p. 4.

35 *Ibid.*, p. 12.

36 *Ibid.*, p. 9.

37 *Ibid.*, p. 11.

38 *Ibid.*, p. 9.

39 *Ibid.*, p. 12.

40 *Ibid.*, p. 32.

41 *Ibid.*, pp. 175 ff;

42 *Ibid.*, p. 21.

43 *Ibid.*, p. 149.

44 *Ibid.*, p. 149.

45 *Ibid.*, p. 158.

46 *Ibid.*, p. 150.

47 *Ibid.*, p. 151.

48 *Ibid.*, p. 156.

49 *Ibid.*, p. 166.

50 *Ibid.*, p. 27.

51 *Ibid.*, p. 151.

52 C. D. Rollins, "Solipsism." In *The Encyclopedia of Philosophy*, 7. Paul Edwards (ed.). New York: MacMillan, 1967, p. 487.

53 Jaspers, *Philosophie*, 2, p. 151.

54 *Ibid.*, p. 152.

55 *Ibid.*, p. 153.

56 *Ibid.*, p. 150.

57 *Ibid.*, p. 162.

58 James Collins, *The Existentialists.* Chicago: H. Regnery, 1968, pp. 77–87; Austin Marsden Farrer, *The Freedom of the Will.* New York: Charles Scribner's Sons, 1960; Hazel Estella Barnes, *An Existentialist Ethics.* New York: Alfred Knopf, 1967; Reymond Diane Barsoum, *Existentialism and the Philosophical Tradition.* New Jersey: Prentice Hall, 1991, pp. 440–504; Robert Goodwin Olson, *An Introduction to Existentialism.* New York: Dover, 1962, pp. 100–161.

59 Jaspers, *Philosophie*, 2, pp. 336–337.

60 Jaspers, *Psychologie der Weltanschauungen*, p. 21.

61 *Ibid.*, p. 22.

62 Jaspers, *Philosophie* 2, p. 336.

63 *Ibid.*, p. 339.

64 Sebastian Samay, *Reason Revisited: The Philosophy of Karl Jaspers*. Dublin: Gill and Macmillan, 1971, p. 24, 27, 21–22; Ludwig Armbruster, *Objekt und Transzendenz bei Karl Jaspers, Sein Gegenstandsbegriff und die Möglichkeit der Metaphysik*. Innsbruck: F. Rauch, 1957, pp. 11 ff.

65 Jaspers, *Psychologie der Weltanschauungen*, pp. 20–21; Samay, *Reason Revisited: The Philosophy of Karl Jaspers*, pp. 21–35; Maximilian Beck, "Kritik der Schelling-Jaspers-Heidegger'schen Ontologie," *Philosophische Hefte*, IV, (1934), p. 103.

66 Jaspers, *Psychologie der Weltanschauungen*, p. xiii.

67 Jaspers, *Philosophie*, 1, p. 8, p. 4; Jaspers, *Philosophie*, 2, p. 338.

68 Jaspers, *Philosophie*, 2, pp. 339–340.

69 *Ibid*., pp. 339–340; Samay, *Reason Revisited: The Philosophy of Karl Jaspers*, pp. 37–46

70 Jaspers, *Philosophie*, 2, p. 346.

71 *Ibid*., p. 346.

72 *Ibid*., p. 347.

73 Jaspers, *Psychologie der Weltanschauungen*, pp. 232 ff., 411.

74 *Ibid*., pp. 284 ff.

75 Jaspers, *Philosophie*, 2, p. 337.

76 *Ibid*., p. 342, 337–338, 349, 392.

77 *Ibid*., pp. 342–343.

Introduction to Transition Mechanisms

1 Karl Jaspers, *Philosophie*, 2. Berlin: Springer, [1932] 1994.

2 Jaspers, *Psychologie der Weltanschauungen*. Berlin: Springer, [1919] 1985, pp. 229–280.

3 Jaspers, *Vernunft und Existenz*. Munich: Piper, [1935] 1987.

4 Jaspers, *Von der Wahrheit*. Munich: Piper, [1947] 1991.

5 Jaspers, *Philosophie*, 3. Berlin: Springer, [1932] 1994.

6 Jaspers, *Philosophie*, 2, p. 5.

7 *Ibid*., p. 4.

8 *Ibid*., p. 9.

9 *Ibid*., p. 5.

Chapter Five

1 Karl Jaspers, *Psychologie der Weltanschauungen*. Berlin: Springer, [1919] 1985.

2 Jaspers, *Philosophie*, 1. Berlin: Springer, [1932] 1994.

3 Jaspers, *Psychologie der Weltanschauungen*, pp. 124–125, 276–375, p. 379.

4 Jaspers, *Philosophie*, 2, pp. 60–61.

5 *Ibid*., p. 51.

6 *Ibid.*, pp. 60–61; Günter Junghänel, "Über den Begriff der Kommunikation bei Karl Jaspers," *Deutsche Zeitschrift für Philosophie*, 9:4, 1961, pp. 481–483.

7 Jaspers, *Philosophie*, 2, p. 55.

8 *Ibid*, p. 56.

9 Jaspers, *Vernunft und Existenz*. Munich: Piper, [1935] 1987.

10 Hanna Arendt, "Jaspers as Citizen of the World." In *The Philosophy of Karl Jaspers*, Paul Arthur Schilpp (ed.). New York: Tudor, 1957, pp. 539–549; Arendt, "Karl Jaspers," *Reden zur Verleihung des Friedenspreises, des deutschen Buchhandels*. Munich: Piper, 1958, pp. 27–40; Jeanne Hersch, *Karl Jaspers, Eine Einführung in sein Werk*. Bern: Francke, 1978, pp. 97 ff.; Jürgen Habermas, *Philosophisch-politische Profile*. Frankfurt: Suhrkamp, 1981, pp. 87 ff.; Kurt Salamun, *Karl Jaspers*. Munich: Beck, 1985, pp. 72 ff.; Hans Saner, *Karl Jaspers in Selbstzeugnissen und Bilddokumenten*. Hamburg: Rowohlt, [1979] 1991, pp. 100 ff.; Jürgen Schultheiss, *Philosophieren als Kommunikation, Versuch zu Karl Jaspers's Apologie des kritischen Philosophierens*. Meisenheim: Forum Academicum, 1981, pp. 97 ff.; Franz Josef Fuchs, "Seinverhältnis, Karl Jaspers's Existenzphilosophie," *Existenz und Kommunikation*, Frankfurt, Bern, New York, Nancy: Peter Lang, 1984; Donatella Di Cesare, *Die Sprache in der Philosophie von Karl Jaspers*. Tübingen and Basel: Francke, 1996, pp. 11–23.

11 Erich Fromm, *Escape from Freedom*. New York: Rinehart and Company, 1941, pp. 3–39.

12 Herbert Marcuse, *One Dimensional Man: Studies in the Ideology of Advanced Industrial Society*. Boston: Beacon Press, 1964; Jürgen Habermas, "Psychic Thermidor and the Rebirth of Rebellious Subjectivity," *Berkeley Journal of Sociology* 24–25, (1980), pp. 1–12; Salamun, *Karl Jaspers*, pp. 78 ff.

13 Jaspers, *Philosophie*, 2, p. 61.

14 *Ibid.*, p. 61.

15 Jaspers, "Einsamkeit," *Revue Internationale de Philosophie*, 37, (1983), pp. 390–409.

16 *Ibid.*, pp. 393 ff.

17 Di Cesare, *Die Sprache in der Philosophie von Karl Jaspers*, pp. 11–23; Arendt, "Karl Jaspers," pp. 27–40.

18 Jaspers, "Einsamkeit," p. 407.

19 Fritz Kaufmann, "Karl Jaspers and a Philosophy of Communication." In *The Philosophy of Karl Jaspers*. Paul Arthur Schilpp (ed.). New York: Tudor, 1957, p. 214.

20 *Ibid.*, pp. 232–240.

21 *Ibid.*, pp. 255 ff.

22 *Ibid.*, pp. 259 ff.

23 Werner Schneiders, *Karl Jaspers in der Kritik*. Bonn: Bouvier, 1965, pp. 150–151.

24 Jaspers, *Philosophie*, 2, p. 56.

25 *Ibid.*, p. 4.

26 Martin Heidegger, *Sein und Zeit*. Tübingen: M. Niemeyer, [1927] 1993, pp. 117–125.

27 Jean Marie Paul. "Der Weg des Menschen oder Kommunikation und Liebe bei Jaspers." In *Karl Jaspers, Denken zwischen Wissenschaft, Politik und Philosophie*, Dietrich Harth (ed.). Stuttgart: Metzler, J.B., 1989, p. 49.

28 Junghänel, "Über den Begriff der Kommunikation bei Karl Jaspers," pp. 477–479.

29 Schneiders, *Karl Jaspers in der Kritik*, p. 152.

30 Georg Lukács, *Die Zerstörung der Vernunft: Der Weg des Irrationalismus von Schelling zu Hitler*. Berlin: Aufbau-Verlag, 1955.

31 Jaspers, "Reply to my critics." In *The Philosophy of Karl Jaspers*. Paul Arthur Schilpp (ed.). New York: Tudor, 1957, p. 847.

32 Saner, *Jaspers*. Hamburg: Rowohlt, [1970] 1991, pp. 32 ff., 142–143.

33 Manfred Gangl, "Karl Jaspers und Georg Lukács, Rechte und linke Kulturkritik in der Weimar-Republik." In *Karl Jaspers, Denken zwischen Wissenschaft, Politik und Philosophie*, Dietrich Harth (ed.). Stuttgart: Metzler, J.B., 1989, pp. 87–110.

34 Jaspers, *Philosophie*, 2, p. 50.

35 *Ibid*., p. 53.

36 Di Cesare, *Die Sprache in der Philosophie von Karl Jaspers*, p. 13.

37 Jaspers, *Philosophie*, 2, p. 56.

38 *Ibid*., p. 88.

39 *Ibid*., p. 56.

40 *Ibid*., p. 57.

41 *Ibid*., p. 56.

42 *Ibid*., p. 67.

43 *Ibid*., p. 56.

44 Alan M. Olson, *Transcendence and Hermeneutics: An Interpretation of the Philosophy of Karl Jaspers*. The Hague and Boston: M. Nijhoff, 1979, pp. 45 ff., 76 ff.; Olson, "Hegel and Jaspers on the Comparative Philosophy of Religion." In *Karl Jaspers: Philosoph unter Philosophen*. Leonard Ehrlich and Richard Wisser (eds.). Würzburg: Konigshausen & Neumann, 1993, pp. 41–64.

45 Jaspers, *Philosophie*, 2, p. 2.

46 *Ibid*., p. 56.

47 Johannes Reis, "Menschliche Existenz bei Jaspers," *Die Neue Ordnung*, 4, (1950), pp. 528–530; Hans-Rudolf Müller-Schwefe, *Existenzphilosophie: Das Verständnis von Existenz in Philosophie und christlichem Glauben*. Gottingen: Vandenhoeck & Ruprecht, 1961, p. 48; Heinrich Knittermeyer, *Die Philosophie der Existenz von der Renaissance bis zur Gegenwart*. Vienna: Humboldt, 1961, pp. 48–49; Junghänel, "Über den Begriff der Kommunikation bei Karl Jaspers," pp. 477 ff.

48 Hans Urs Von Balthasar, *Einsame Zwiesprache, Martin Buber und Christentum*. Cologne: Johannes, 1958.

49 Heinz Horst Schrey, *Dialogisches Denken*. Darmstadt: Wissenschaftliche Buchgesellschaft, 1970, p. 35.

50 Elisabeth Young-Bruehl, *Freedom and Karl Jaspers's Philosophy*. New Haven: Yale University Press, 1981, pp. 10 ff., 184, n. 49; Balthasar, *Einsame Zwiesprache: Martin Buber und Christentum*, p. 35.

51 Michael Theunissen, *Der Andere, Studien zur Sozialontologie der Gegenwart*. Berlin: W. de Gruyter, 1981, pp. 476 ff.

52 Harry Wardlaw, "Jaspers's Account of Truth as a Way into the Discussion of Theological Truth–Claims." *Sophia*, 44:1, (2005), pp. 77–90.

53 Jaspers, *Philosophie*, 2, p. 64.

54 *Ibid.*, p. 64.

55 Salamun, *Karl Jaspers*, pp. 79–80; Theodor Litt, *Mensch und Welt, Grundlinien einer Philosophie des Geistes*. Munich–Heidelberg: Quelle & Meyer, 1961; Romano Guardini and Otto Friedrich Bollnow (eds.), *Begegnung und Bildung*. Würzburg: Werkbund, 1960, p. 20; Bollnow, *Existenzphilosophie und Pädagogik*. Stuttgart: W. Kohlhammer, 1959, p. 130; Karl Löwith, *Das Individuum in der Rolle des Mitmenschen*. Darmstadt: Wissenschaftliche Buchgesellschaft, 1969, p. 56.

56 Jaspers, *Philosophie*, 2, p. 61.

57 *Ibid.*, p. 56.

58 Jaspers, *Psychologie der Weltanschauungen*, pp. 117–138.

59 Steffen Graefe, "Von der 'Zugkraft des Seins,' Existentielle Kommunikation und der platonische Eros." In *Karl Jaspers: Philosoph unter Philosophen,* Leonard Ehrlich and Richard Wisser (eds.). Würzburg: Konigshausen and Neumann, 1993, pp. 272–278

60 Jaspers, *Philosophie*, 2, p. 73.

61 *Ibid.*, p. 73.

62 *Ibid.*, p. 65.

63 *Ibid.*, p. 64.

64 *Ibid.*, p. 65.

65 *Ibid.*, p. 64.

66 Salamun, *Karl Jaspers*, p. 83, 77.

67 Schneiders, *Karl Jaspers in der Kritik*, pp. 135–136.

68 *Ibid.*, pp. 136–144.

69 Heinrich End, Existentiale Handlungen im Strafrecht, Die Pflichtenkollision im Lichte der Philosophie von Karl Jaspers. Munich: Beck, 1959; Ulrich Hommes, *Die Existenzerhellung und das Recht*. Frankfurt am Main: Klostermann, 1962; Erich P. Grunert, *Objektiv Norm, Situation und Entscheidung, Ein Vergleich zwischen Thomas von Aquino und Karl Jaspers*. Dissertation. Bonn, 1953.

70 Jaspers, *Psychologie der Weltanschauungen*, p. xii [1954].

71 See *Philosophy*, 2, p. 107.

72 Heidegger, *Sein und Zeit*, pp. 12–14.

73 William Earle, "Anthropology in the Philosophy." In: *The Philosophy of Karl Jaspers*. Paul Arthur Schilpp (ed.). New York: Tudor, 1957, pp. 530–531.

74 Urs Richli, *Transzendental Reflexion und sittliche Entscheidung, Zum Problem der Selbsterkenntnis der Metaphysik bei Jaspers und Kant*. Bonn: H. Bouvier, 1967, p. 174.

Chapter Six

1 Karl Jaspers, *Philosophie*, 1. Berlin: Springer, [1932] 1994.

2 Georg Wilhelm Friedrich Hegel. *Vorlesungen über die Philosophie der Geschichte*. Leipzig: P. Reclamjun, 1974, pp. 142 ff.; Nathan Rotenstreich. *Between Past and Present*. New Haven: Yale University Press, 1958, pp. 1–25.

3 Jaspers, *Philosophie*, 2, pp. 118–119.

4 *Ibid.*, p. 119.

5 Jaspers, *Psychologie der Weltanschauungen*. Berlin: Springer, [1919] 1985.

6 Elisabeth Young-Bruehl. *Freedom and Karl Jaspers's Philosophy*. New Haven: Yale University Press, 1981, pp. 19–20.

7 Jaspers, *Philosophie*, 2, pp. 119–120.

8 *Ibid.*, p. 120.

9 *Ibid.*, p. 130.

10 *Ibid.*, p. 121.

11 *Ibid.*, p. 123.

12 *Ibid.*, p. 123.

13 Alan M. Olson. *Transcendence and Hermeneutics: An Interpretation of the Philosophy of Karl Jaspers*. The Hague and Boston: M. Nijhoff, 1979, pp. 24–26.

14 Jaspers, *Philosophie*, 2, p. 123.

15 *Ibid.*, p. 123.

16 *Ibid.*, p. 122.

17 *Ibid.*, p. 122.

18 *Ibid.*, p. 123.

19 *Ibid.*, p. 129.

20 *Ibid.*, p. 126.

21 Jaspers, *Psychologie der Weltanschauungen*, pp. 109–117; Walter Schweidler, "Die Ethik des Augenblicks. Jaspers, Kierkegaard, Wittgenstein." In *Karl Jaspers: Philosoph unter Philosophen*. Leonard Ehrlich and Richard Wisser (eds.). Würzburg: Konigshausen & Neumann, 1993, pp. 202–214.

22 Jaspers, *Philosophie*, 2, p. 129.

23 Jaspers, *Philosophie*, 1, p. 3.

24 Jaspers, *Philosophie 2*, p. 138 ff.

25 *Ibid.*, p. 123.

26 *Ibid.*, pp. 124–125.

27 *Ibid.*, pp. 121–122.

Chapter Seven

1 Martin Heidegger, *Pathmarks*. Cambridge: Cambridge University Press, 1998, p. 10; German original: Hans Saner (ed.). *Karl Jaspers in der Diskussion*. Munich: Piper, 1973, p. 77; Edwin Latzel, "The Concept of 'Ultimate Situation' in Jaspers's Philosophy." In *The Philosophy of Karl Jaspers*. Paul Arthur Schilpp (ed.). New York: Tudor, 1957, pp. 169–170; Otto Friedrich Bollnow, *Existenzphilosophie*. Stuttgart: W. Kohlhammer, 1964, p. 61.

2 Karl Jaspers, *Psychologie der Weltanschauungen*. Berlin: Springer, [1919] 1985, p. 231; Jaspers, *Philosophie*, 2. Berlin: Springer, [1932] 1994, p. 204.

3 Latzel, "The Concept of 'Ultimate Situation' in Jaspers's Philosophy," pp. 194 ff.; Latzel, "Bemerkungen zum Umgang mit Existenzphilosophie," *Zeitschrift für philosophische Forschung*, VI, (1951/1952), pp. 399–410.

4 Jaspers, *Psychologie der Weltanschauungen*, p. 1.

5 *Ibid.*, p. 229.

6 *Ibid.*, p. 231.

7 *Ibid.*, p. 232.

8 Latzel, "The Concept of 'Ultimate Situation' in Jaspers's Philosophy," p. 195.

9 Jaspers, *Psychologie der Weltanschauungen*, p. 281.

10 Kurt Salamun, *Karl Jaspers*. Munich: Beck, 1985, pp. 66–67.

11 J. Rudolf Gerber, "Karl Jaspers and Kantian Reason," *New Scholasticism*, 43, (1969), p. 412.

12 *Ibid.*, p. 411.

13 Erich P. Grünert, *Objektiv Norm, Situation und Entscheidung, Ein Vergleich zwischen Thomas von Aquino und Karl Jaspers*. Dissertation. Bonn, 1953; Grünert, "Der Einfluss Kants auf Karl Jaspers: Zugang zur Transzendenz bei Kant und Karl Jaspers," *Freiburger Zeitschrift für Philosophie und Theologie*, III, (1956), pp. 21–28.

14 Immanuel Kant, *Critique of Pure Reason*. Translated and edited by Paul Guyer and Allen W. Wood. New York: Cambridge University Press, 1977, pp. 459–460.

15 Jaspers, *Psychologie der Weltanschauungen*, p. 232.

16 Chris Walker, "Karl Jaspers as a Kantian Psychopathologist, I: The Philosophical Origins of the Concept of Form and Content," *History of Psychiatry*, 4, (1993a), pp. 209–238; Walker, "Karl Jaspers as a Kantian Psychopathologist, II: The Concept of Form and Content in Jaspers's Psychopathology," *History of Psychiatry*, 4, (1993b), pp. 321–348; Walker, "Karl Jaspers as a Kantian Psychopathologist, III: "The Concept of Form in Georg Simmel's Social Theory: a Comparison with Jaspers," *History of Psychiatry*, 5, (1994), pp. 37–70.

17 Jaspers, *Psychologie der Weltanschauungen*, pp. 240 ff.

18 *Ibid.*, p. 240.

19 *Ibid.*, pp. 240–241.

20 *Ibid.*, p. 241.

21 *Ibid.*, p. 1.

22 Jaspers, *Allgemeine Psychopathologie*. 8th edition. Berlin–Heidelberg: Springer, 1965, 1, p. 4, n.

23 Leo Gabriel, *Existenzphilosophie von Kierkegaard bis Sartre*. Vienna: Verlag Herold, 1951, p. 170; Werner Schneiders, *Karl Jaspers in der Kritik*. Bonn: Bouvier, 1965, p. 57.

24 Jaspers, *Psychologie der Weltanschauungen*, p. 229.

25 *Ibid.*, p. 219.

26 *Ibid.*, p. 220, 284, 285 ff.

27 *Ibid.*, p. 284.

28 William D. Blattner, "Heidegger's Debt to Jaspers's Concept of Limit-Situation." In *Heidegger and Jaspers*. Alan. M. Olson (ed.). Philadelphia: Temple University Press, 1994, p. 157.

29 Jaspers, *Philosophie*, 2, p. 203.
30 *Ibid.*, p. 216.
31 *Ibid.*, p. 203.
32 *Ibid.*, p. 209.
33 *Ibid.*, p. 211.
34 *Ibid.*, p. 203.
35 *Ibid.*, p. 204.
36 *Ibid.*, p. 204.
37 Gabriel Marcel, "Grundsituation und Grenzsituationen." In *Karl Jaspers in der Diskussion*, Hans Saner (ed.). Munich: Piper, 1973, p. 166; Latzel, "The Concept of 'Ultimate Situation' in Jaspers's Philosophy," p. 189.
38 Jaspers, *Philosophie*, 2, pp. 216–217.
39 *Ibid.*, p. 252.
40 *Ibid.*, p. 253.
41 Salamun, *Karl Jaspers*, pp. 68 ff.
42 Latzel, "The Concept of 'Ultimate Situation' in Jaspers's Philosophy," p. 189.
43 *Ibid.*, pp. 192–193.
44 *Ibid.*, p. 183.
45 Salamun, *Karl Jaspers*, pp. 71–71; Schneiders, *Karl Jaspers in der Kritik*, p. 152, 149.
46 Latzel, "The Concept of 'Ultimate Situation' in Jaspers's Philosophy," pp. 186 ff.
47 Jaspers, *Philosophie*, 2, pp. 220 ff.; Jaspers, *Psychologie der Weltanschauungen*, p. 261.
48 *Ibid.*, p. 253.
49 *Ibid.*, p. 208.
50 *Ibid.*, p. 209.
51 *Ibid.*, p. 204.

Transition Mechanisms: A Concluding Overview

1 Karl Jaspers, *Philosophie*, 2. Berlin: Springer, [1932] 1994, pp. 50 ff.
2 Georg Wilhelm Friedrich Hegel, *The Phenomenology of Spirit*. Oxford: Oxford University Press, 1961, pp. 229 ff.
3 Jaspers, *Philosophie*, 2, pp. 260–261.
4 Jaspers, *Philosophie*, *1*, pp. 24 ff., 56 ff., 266 ff.; *Philosophie*, 2, p. 70, 137.
5 Jaspers, *Philosophie*, 2, pp. 261–263.
6 *Ibid.*, p. 291, 267.
7 *Ibid.*, p. 266.
8 *Ibid.*, p. 266.
9 *Ibid.*, p. 260.
10 *Ibid.*, p. 257.
11 *Ibid.*, p. 268.
12 *Ibid.*, p. 272.

13 Martin Heidegger, *Sein und Zeit*. Tübingen: M. Niemeyer, [1927] 1993, pp. 270–301; Paul Tillich, "Heidegger and Jaspers." In *Heidegger and Jaspers*. Alan M. Olson (ed.). Philadelphia: Temple University Press, 1994, p. 23; Karsten Harris, "Shame, Guilt, Responsibility." In *Heidegger & Jaspers*, Olson, Alan M. (ed.). Philadelphia: Temple University Press, 1994, pp. 49–64; Jean Paul Sartre, *Being and Nothingness: An Essay on Phenomenological Ontology*. London: Methuen, 1957, pp. 73–218;

14 Sartre, *The Transcendental Ego: An Existentialist Theory of the Consciousness*. New York: Noonday Press, 1957; Simon Gzynn (ed.). *Sartre: An Investigation of Some Major Themes*. Aldershot: Avebury, 1987, pp. 1–21.

15 Jaspers, *Philosophie*, 2, pp. 281–282.

16 *Ibid*., p. 279.

17 *Ibid*., p. 280.

18 Jaspers, *Der philosophische Glaube angesichts der Offenbarung*. Munich: Piper, 1962; *Der philosophische Glaube*. Munich: Piper, [1948] 1960, pp. 148 ff.; Claus Uwe Hommel, *Chiffer und Dogma, vom Verhältnis der Philosophie zur Religion bei Karl Jaspers*. Zurich: EVZ Verlag, Abt. Editio Academica, 1968; Wolf Hertel, *Existentieller Glaube, Eine Studie über den Glaubensbegriff von Karl Jaspers und Paul Tillich*. Meisenheim am Glan: Verlag Anton Hain, 1971; Elisabeth Young-Bruehl, *Freedom and Karl Jaspers's Philosophy*. New Haven: Yale University Press, 1981, pp. 150–161; Leonard Ehrlich, *Karl Jaspers: Philosophy as Faith*. Amherst: University of Massachusetts Press, 1975; Gregory J. Walters, "Jaspers's Philosophical Faith and Revelational Faith Today: Can the Two Faiths Meet in the Struggle for Human Liberation?" In *Karl Jaspers: Philosoph unter Philosophen*. Leonard Ehrlich and Richard Wisser (eds.). Würzburg: Konigshausen & Neumann, 1993, pp. 217–227; Richard Wisser, *Karl Jaspers: Philosophy in der Bewährung, Vorträge und Aufsätze*. Würzburg: Königshausen & Neumann, 1995, pp. 3–28; Johannes Baptist Lotz, *Sein und Existenz*. Freiburg: Herder, 1965, pp. 296–306; Oskar Hammelsbeck, "Die Theologische Bestreitung des Philosophischen Glaubens." In *Offener Horizont, Festschrift für Karl Jaspers, zum 70*., Klaus Piper (ed.). Munich: Piper, 1953, pp. 27–35; John F. Kane, *Pluralism and Truth in Religion*. Chico, CA: Scholars Press, 1981, pp. 45–75; Albrecht Kiel, "Der 'Philosophische Glaube' (Jaspers) und die Logik." In *Glauben und Wissen, Dritter Teil (Hegel-Jahrbuch 2005)*. Andreas Arndt (ed.). Berlin: Akademie Verlag, 2005, pp. 291–297; Istvan Czako, "Das Problem des Glaubens und der Geschichte in der Philosophie Kierkegaards und Karl Jaspers." *Kierkegaard Studies*, Yearbook, 2000, pp. 373–382.

19 Jaspers, *Philosophie*, 2, p. 282.

20 *Ibid*., p. 282.

21 *Ibid*., p. 282.

22 *Ibid*., p. 283.

23 Jaspers, *Psychologie der Weltanschauungen*. Berlin: Springer, [1919] 1985, p. xii.

Chapter Eight

1 Karl Jaspers, *Philosophie*, 3. Berlin: Springer, [1932] 1994, p. 2.

2 *Ibid*., p. 4.

3 *Ibid*., p. 4.
4 Jaspers, *Philosophie*, 2, p. 56.
5 Jaspers, *Philosophie*, 3, p. 3.
6 Hans Kunz, "Critique of Jaspers's Concept of Transcendence." In *The Philosophy of Karl Jaspers*. Paul Arthur Schilpp (ed.). New York: Tudor, 1957, pp. 507–509.
7 Jaspers, *Philosophie*, 3, p. 3.
8 Jaspers, *Philosophie*, 1, p. 27.
9 Jaspers, *Philosophie*, 3, p. 5.
10 *Ibid*., p. 9.
11 *Ibid*., p. 40.
12 *Ibid*., p. 67.
13 *Ibid*., p. 43.
14 *Ibid*., p. 45.
15 *Ibid*., p. 4.
16 Martin Heidegger, "What is Metaphysics?" In *Basic Writings*. David Farrell Krell (ed.). London: Routledge and Kegan Paul, 1993, pp. 109–110; Gabriel Gideon Motzkin, *The Problem of Transcendence in the Secular World: From Kant to Heidegger*. Dissertation. Ann Arbor: University Microfilms International, 1982, 2, pp. 831–977.
17 Jaspers, *Philosophie*, 3, p. 44.
18 *Ibid*., p. 43.
19 *Ibid*., p. 6.
20 *Ibid*., p. 47.
21 *Ibid*., p. 48.
22 *Ibid*., p. 47.
23 *Ibid*., p. 51.
24 *Ibid*., p. 9.
25 Heidegger, *The End of Philosophy*. Translated by Joan Stambaugh. London: Souvenir Press, 1973, pp. 95–110; Heidegger, "What is Metaphysics?", pp. 307–342; Heidegger, *Gelassenheit*. Pfullingen: Neske, 1959; Richard Wisser, *Karl Jaspers: Philosophy in der Bewährung, Vorträge und Aufsätze*. Würzburg: Königshausen & Neumann, 1995, pp. 51–222; Julius I. Löwenstein, "Das Bleibende von Jaspers und Heidegger." In *Karl Jaspers Today, Philosophy at the Threshold of the Future*. Leonard Ehrlich and Richard Wisser (eds.). Washington. D.C.: University Press of America, 1988, pp. 317–340; Wisser, "Aneignung und Unterscheidung: Existenzphilosophie im Kampf um die Existenz der Philosophie." In *Karl Jaspers Today, Philosophy at the Threshold of the Future*. Leonard Ehrlich and Richard Wisser (eds.). Washington, D.C.: University Press of America, 1988, pp. 341–361; Franz Josef Brecht, *Heidegger und Jaspers, Die beiden Grundformen der Existenzphilosophie*. Wuppertal: Marées, 1948; Jennifer Anna Gosetti, "Tragedy and Truth in Heidegger and Jaspers." *International Philosophical Quarterly*. S 02; 42:3, (2002), pp. 301–314; Robert Denoon Cumming, *Phenomenology and Deconstruction 4: Solitude*. Chicago: University of Chicago Press, 2001.
26 Jaspers, *Philosophie*, 3, p. 220.
27 Jaspers, *Psychologie der Weltanschauungen*. Berlin: Springer, [1919] 1985, pp. 51–216.

28 Jaspers, *Philosophie*, 1, pp. 58 ff.; *Philosophie*, 2, pp. 4 ff.

29 Johannes Thyssen, "The Concept of 'Foundering' in Jaspers's Philosophy." In *The Philosophy of Karl Jaspers*. Paul Arthur Schilpp (ed.). New York: Tudor, 1957, p. 314.

30 *Ibid*., p. 317.

31 *Ibid*., p. 319.

32 *Ibid*., p. 319.

33 Fritz-Joachim Von Rinteln, *Beyond Existentialism*. London: Allen and Unwin, 1961, p. 204.

34 Jaspers, *Philosophie*, 3, p. 221.

35 Johannes Pfeiffer, *Existenzphilosophie, Eine Einführung in Heidegger und Jaspers*. Leipzig: Felix Meiner, 1952, p. 41.

36 Kurt Salamun, *Karl Jaspers*. Munich: Beck, 1985, pp. 64 ff.

37 Thyssen, "The Concept of 'Foundering' in Jaspers's Philosophy," p. 297.

38 Von Rinteln, *Beyond Existentialism*, p. 204.

39 William Barrett, *Irrational Man: a Study in Existential Philosophy*. London: Anchor Books, 1964.

40 Avi Sagi, *Albert Camus and the Philosophy of the Absurd*. Translated by Batya Stein. Amsterdam: Rodopi, 2002, pp. 59–66.

41 Jaspers, *Philosophie*, 3, pp. 68–127.

42 *Ibid*., p. 3.

43 *Ibid*., p. 225.

44 *Ibid*., p. 227.

45 *Ibid*., p. 227.

46 *Ibid*., p. 228.

47 Jaspers *Philosophie*, 1, p.165, 186, 189, 193, 203, 225, 234; *Philosophie*, 2, p. 296.

48 Jaspers, *Philosophie*, 3, pp. 173–174.

49 *Ibid*., p. 228.

50 *Ibid*., p. 228.

51 *Ibid*., p. 228.

52 Jaspers, *Philosophie*, 2, pp. 65 ff., 230–246.

53 Jaspers, *Philosophie*, 3, p. 229.

54 *Ibid*., p. 223.

55 *Ibid*., p. 229.

56 *Ibid*., p. 229.

57 *Ibid*., p. 230.

58 *Ibid*., p. 230.

59 Jaspers, *Philosophie*, 2, pp. 246–254, 332 ff.; *Philosophie*, 3, pp.102 ff., 225 ff.

60 Jaspers, *Philosophie*, 3, pp. 217–219, 226.

61 *Ibid*., p. 233.

62 *Ibid*., p. 336.

Chapter Nine

1 Karl Jaspers, *Philosophie*, 3. Berlin: Springer, [1932] 1994, p. 236.

2 Jaspers, *Vernunft und Existenz*. Munich: Piper, [1935] 1987; *Existenzphilosophie*. 3rd edition. Berlin: Walter de Gruyter, [1937] 1964; *Von der Wahrheit*. Munich: Piper, [1947] 1991.

3 Ernst Mayer, "Philosophie und philosophische Logik bei Karl Jaspers." In *Offener Horizont, Festschrift für Karl Jaspers, zum 70*. Klaus Piper (ed.). Munich: Geburtstag, Piper, 1953, p. 64.

4 Jaspers, *Psychologie der Weltanschauungen*. Berlin: Springer, [1919] 1985. pp. 465–486.

5 Kurt Salamun, *Karl Jaspers*. Munich: Beck, 1985, p. 88; Gerhard Knauss, "The Concept of the 'Encompassing' in Jaspers's Philosophy." In *The Philosophy of Karl Jaspers*. Paul Arthur Schilpp (ed.). New York: Tudor, 1957, pp. 142 ff.; Knauss, *Gegenstand und Umgreifendes*. Dissertation. Basel: Verlag fur Recht und Gesellschaft, 1954.

6 Urs Richli, *Transzendental Reflexion und sittliche Entscheidung, Zum Problem der Selbsterkenntnis der Metaphysik bei Jaspers und Kant*. Bonn: H. Bouvier, 1967, pp. 119 ff., 199, n. 37.

7 Jaspers, *Vernunft und Existenz*, p. 35.

8 Salamun, *Karl Jaspers*, p. 88.

9 Jaspers, *Vernunft und Existenz*, p. 36.

10 Jaspers, *Von der Wahrheit*, p. 3.

11 Jaspers, *Philosophie*, 1, p. 327.

12 Jaspers, *Von der Wahrheit*, p. 39.

13 Jaspers, *Existenzphilosophie*, p. 13.

14 *Ibid*., p. 15.

15 Jaspers, *Vernunft und Existenz*, pp. 58–83.

16 Jaspers, *Psychologie der Weltanschauungen*, p. vii.

17 Jaspers, *Von der Wahrheit*, p. 221.

18 *Ibid*., p. 221.

19 Knauss, "The Concept of the 'Encompassing' in Jaspers's Philosophy," pp. 171 ff; Fritz Heinemann, *Existenzphilosophie—lebendig oder tot?* Stuttgart: Kohlhammer, 1954, pp. 77–78.

20 Jaspers, *Allgemeine Psychopathologie, Ein Leitfaden für Studierende, Ärzte und Psychologen*. 1st Edition. Berlin: Springer, 1913, p. 36; Jaspers, *Philosophie*, 1, p. 54; Jaspers, *Max Weber, Politiker-Forscher-Philosoph*. Munich: Piper, 1958, p. 50.

21 Jaspers, *Philosophie*, 1, p. 19.

22 *Ibid*., p. 49.

23 *Ibid*., pp. 35–36.

24 Jaspers, *Von der Wahrheit*, p. 41.

25 Jaspers, *Philosophie*, 1, p. 134.

26 Sebastian Samay, *Reason Revisited: The Philosophy of Karl Jaspers*. Dublin: Gill and Macmillan, 1971, pp. 48–49.

27 *Ibid*., p. 277 n. 54.

28 *Ibid*., p. 58, 49.

29 *Ibid*., p. 66.

30 Hans Mader, "Das Seindenken bei Karl Jaspers," *Wissenschaft und Weltbild*, 10, (1957), pp. 55–56.

31 Mader, "Das Seindenken bei Karl Jaspers," *Wissenschaft und Weltbild*, 10, (1957), pp. 55–56; Mader, *Problemgeschichtliche Studie zur Periechontologie Karl Jaspers*. Dissertation. Vienna, 1952.

32 Mader, "Das Seindenken bei Karl Jaspers," p. 58; Heinemann, *Existenzphilosophie—lebendig oder tot?*, p. 78.

33 Heinemann, *Existenzphilosophie—lebendig oder tot?*, p. 72.

34 Jaspers, *Philosophie*, 3, p. 1.

35 *Ibid.*, p. 3.

36 *Ibid.*, p. 3.

37 Jaspers, *Von der Wahrheit*, p. 3.

38 *Ibid.*, p. 1.

39 *Ibid.*, pp. 30–31.

40 Jaspers, *Von der Wahrheit*, pp. 223–499.

41 *Ibid.*, pp. 391 ff.

42 *Ibid.*, p. 31.

43 *Ibid.*, p. 36.

44 *Ibid.*, p. 703.

45 *Ibid.*, p. 706, 261, 873, 956.

46 Jaspers, *Philosophie*, 1, pp. 64 ff., 78 ff., 104 ff., 218 ff.

47 Jaspers, *Philosophie*, 2, pp. 249 ff.

48 Richli, *Transzendental Reflexion und sittliche Entscheidung*, pp. 134 ff.

49 Jaspers, *Von der Wahrheit*, pp. 3–6.

50 *Ibid.*, pp. 2–3.

51 *Ibid.*, p. 6.

52 *Ibid.*, p.185.

53 *Ibid.*, p.120.

54 *Ibid.*, p. 50.

55 *Ibid.*, pp. 114–115.

56 *Ibid.*, p. 11.

57 Jaspers, *Vernunft und Existenz*, pp. 53–54.

58 Jaspers, *Von der Wahrheit*, p. 119.

59 James Collins, "Karl Jaspers's Philosophical Logic," *The New Scholasticism*, 23, (1959), p. 416.

60 Jaspers, *Von der Wahrheit*, p. 26; Samay, *Reason Revisited: The Philosophy of Karl Jaspers*, p. 218.

61 Heinemann, *Existenzphilosophie—lebendig oder tot?*, pp. 74–75.

62 *Ibid.*, p. 73.

63 *Ibid.*, p. 71.

64 Werner Schneiders, *Karl Jaspers in der Kritik*. Bonn: Bouvier, 1965, p. 68.

65 Heinemann, *Existenzphilosophie—lebendig oder tot?*, p. 81.

66 Martina Plümacher, *Philosophie nach 1945 in der Bundesrepublik Deutschland*. Hamburg: Rowohlt Taschenbuch Verlag, 1996, pp.20 ff.

67 Jaspers, *Von der Wahrheit*, p. 8.
68 *Ibid.*, p. 8.
69 *Ibid.*, p. 7.
70 *Ibid.*, p. 6.
71 *Ibid.*, p. 41.
72 Jaspers, *Philosophie*, 1, p. 36.
73 Jaspers, *Vernunft und Existenz*, pp. 54–55.
74 Jaspers, *Philosophie*, 3, p. 38.
75 Jaspers, *Von der Wahrheit*, pp. 49–50.
76 Jaspers, *Existenzphilosophie*, p. 24.
77 Jaspers, *Von der Wahrheit*, pp. 50–51.
78 Jaspers, *Existenzphilosophie*, p. 12; Ronny Miron, "Toward Reality: The Development of the Philosophical Attitude to Reality in Karl Jaspers's Thought," *Journal of the British Society for Phenomenology*, 37:2, (2006), pp. 152–172.
79 Jaspers, *Existenzphilosophie*, p. 56.
80 *Ibid.*, p. 57.
81 *Ibid.*, p. 58.
82 Ernst Mayer, "Philosophie und philosophische Logik bei Karl Jaspers." In *Offener Horizont, Festschrift für Karl Jaspers, zum 70.* Klaus Piper (ed.). Munich: Geburtstag, Piper, 1953, p. 63.
83 Jaspers, *Existenzphilosophie*, pp. 59–60.
84 *Ibid.*, p. 12.
85 Jaspers, *Von der Wahrheit*, pp. 41–42.
86 *Ibid.*, p. 2.
87 *Ibid.*, p. 36.
88 *Ibid.*, p. 357.
89 *Ibid.*, p. 50, 307, 390, 344, 487.
90 *Ibid.*, pp. 357–358.
91 Kurt Hoffman, "The Basic Concept of Jaspers's Philosophy." In *The Philosophy of Karl Jaspers.* Paul Arthur Schilpp (ed.). New York: Tudor, 1957, pp. 104–106.
92 Herbert Schnädelbach, *Philosophy in Germany, 1831–1933*. Cambridge: Cambridge University Press, 1984, p. 193.
93 *Ibid.*, pp. 192–218.
94 Nicolai Hartmann, *Kleine Schriften*. Berlin: Walter de Gruyter, 1955, p. 1; Hartmann, *Zur Grundlegung der Ontologie.* Berlin: Walter de Gruyter, [1935] 1948.
95 Jaspers, *Vernunft und Existenz*, p. 78.
96 Heinrich Rickert, *Der Gegenstand der Erkenntnis, Einführung in die Transzendentalphilosophie*. Tübingen: Mohr, 1928.
97 Edmund Husserl, "Philosophy as Rigorous Science." In *Phenomenology and the Crisis of Philosophy*. Translated by Quentin Lauer. New York: Harper and Row, 1965, pp. 71–147.
98 Jaspers, "Reply to my critics." In *The Philosophy of Karl Jaspers.* Paul Arthur Schilpp (ed.). New York: Tudor, 1957, pp. 748–869.

99 Samay, *Reason Revisited: The Philosophy of Karl Jaspers*, pp. 71–135; Elisabeth Young-Bruehl, *Freedom and Karl Jaspers's Philosophy*. New Haven: Yale University Press, 1981, pp. 7–25; Schneiders, *Karl Jaspers in der Kritik*, p. 4, 10; Heinemann, *Existenzphilosophie—lebendig oder tot?*, pp. 66 ff.; Charles F. Wallraff, *Karl Jaspers: An Introduction to His Philosophy*. Princeton: Princeton University Press, 1970, pp. 38–65; Wallraff, "Jaspers in English: A Failure in Communication," *Philosophy and Phenomenological Research*, 37, (1977), pp. 537–548; Dieter Heinrich, "Denken im Blick auf Max Weber." In *Karl Jaspers—Philosoph, Arzt, politischer Denker*, Jeanne Hersch, Jan Milic Lochman, and Reiner Wiehl (eds.). Munich and Zurich: Piper, 1986, pp. 207–231; Oswald O. Schrag, *Existence, Existenz, and Transcendence*. Pittsburg: Duquesne University Press, 1971; James Collins, "Jaspers on Science and Philosophy." In *The Philosophy of Karl Jaspers*. Paul Arthur Schilpp (ed.). New York: Tudor, 1957, pp. 115–140; James O. Bennett, "Karl Jaspers and Scientific Philosophy," *Journal of Philosophy*, 31, (1993), pp. 437–453; Hanoch Tennen, "Jaspers's Philosophie in kritischer Sicht—Das Verhältnis zwischen Philosophie und Wissenschaft," *Zeitschrift für philosophische Forschung*, 28:4, (1974), pp. 536–561; Kurt Rossmann, "Wert und Grenze der Wissenschaft." In *Offener Horizont, Festschrift für Karl Jaspers, zum 70*. Klaus Piper (ed.). Munich: Geburtstag, Piper, 1953, pp. 126–146; Dietrich Harth, "Grenzen der Wissenschaft." In *Karl Jaspers: Denken zwischen Wissenschaft, Politik und Philosophie*, Dietrich Harth (ed.). Stuttgart: Metzler, J.B., 1989, pp. 207–226; Miron, "From Opposition to Reciprocity: Karl Jaspers on Science, Philosophy, and What Lies Between Them," *International Philosophical Quarterly*, 44, (2004), pp. 147–163.

100 Jaspers, *Existenzphilosophie*, p. 22; Jaspers, *Von der Wahrheit*, pp. 187–188.

101 Jaspers, *Existenzphilosophie*, p. 21.

102 *Ibid.*, p. 58.

103 *Ibid.*, p. 24.

104 *Ibid.*, p. 1.

105 Jaspers, *Der philosophische Glaube*. Munich: Piper, [1948] 1960, pp. 148–149; Jaspers, *Descartes und die Philosophie* (1937), 4th edition. Berlin: Walter de Gruyter, 1966, pp. 63–64.

106 Stephen A. Erickson, "The Image of Socrates in the Mirror of Jaspers," *Philosophy Today*, 38, (1994), pp. 285–293.

107 Jaspers, *Von der Wahrheit*, p. 142.

108 *Ibid.*, pp. 143–151.

109 *Ibid.*, p. 36.

110 Jaspers, *Philosophie*, 1, p. 35.

111 *Ibid.*, p. 51.

112 *Ibid.*, p. 50.

113 Jaspers, *Von der Wahrheit*, p. 26.

114 Samay, *Reason Revisited: The Philosophy of Karl Jaspers*, p. 60.

115 Jaspers, *Von der Wahrheit*, p. 50.

116 *Ibid.*, pp. 53–122; Jaspers, *Vernunft und Existenz*, pp. 38–50; Jaspers, *Von der Wahrheit*, p. 143; Knauss, "The Concept of the 'Encompassing' in Jaspers's Philosophy," pp. 152–161; Samay, *Reason Revisited: The Philosophy of Karl Jaspers*, p. 50–63.

117 Jaspers, *Existenzphilosophie*, p. 17.
118 Jaspers, *Vernunft und Existenz*, p. 36.
119 *Ibid.*, p. 36.
120 Jaspers, *Von der Wahrheit*, p. 47.
121 *Ibid.*, pp. 53, 54 ff., 65 ff., 71 ff., 53–122; Jaspers, *Vernunft und Existenz*, pp. 38 ff., 39 ff., 40 ff., 35–57.
122 Jaspers, *Von der Wahrheit*, p. 65.
123 Jaspers, *Vernunft und Existenz*, p. 41.
124 Jaspers, *Von der Wahrheit*, p. 84.
125 Jaspers, *Vernunft und Existenz*, p. 43.
126 Jaspers, *Von der Wahrheit*, p. 84.
127 *Ibid.*, p. 85.
128 Jaspers, *Philosophie*, 1, p. 63, 119; Jaspers, *Von der Wahrheit*, p. 107.
129 Jaspers, *Von der Wahrheit*, p. 83.
130 *Ibid.*, p. 83.
131 *Ibid.*, p. 83.
132 Jaspers, *Philosophie*, 2, p. 5.
133 Jaspers, *Von der Wahrheit*, p. 113.
134 *Ibid.*, p. 142, 143–151.
135 *Ibid.*, p. 149.
136 Jaspers, *Der philosophische Glaube angesichts der Offenbarung*. Munich: Piper, 1962. pp. 111 ff.
137 Jaspers, *Von der Wahrheit*, p. 125, 184–185.
138 *Ibid.*, p. 124.
139 Knauss, "The Concept of the 'Encompassing' in Jaspers's Philosophy," p. 142; Samay, *Reason Revisited: The Philosophy of Karl Jaspers*, p. 61.
140 Jaspers, *Von der Wahrheit*, p. 129.
141 Jaspers, *Philosophie*, 3, p. 2.
142 Jaspers, *Von der Wahrheit*, p. 129.
143 *Ibid.*, p. 130.
144 *Ibid.*, pp. 130–137.
145 Jaspers, *Vernunft und Existenz*, p. 41.
146 Jaspers, *Von der Wahrheit*, p. 137.
147 *Ibid.*, pp. 148–149.
148 *Ibid.*, p. 130.
149 *Ibid.*, p. 155.
150 Jaspers, *Vernunft und Existenz*, p. 46.
151 Jaspers, *Von der Wahrheit*, p. 177.
152 *Ibid.*, p. 178, 720 ff.
153 *Ibid.*, p. 247.
154 Jaspers, *Vernunft und Existenz*, p. 36.
155 *Ibid.*, p. 42.

156 Walter Schweidler, "Die Ethik des Augenblicks. Jaspers, Kierkegaard, Wittgenstein." In *Karl Jaspers: Philosoph unter Philosophen.* Leonard Ehrlich and Richard Wisser (eds.). Würzburg: Konigshausen & Neumann, 1993, pp. 202–214.

157 Jaspers, *Existenzphilosophie*, p. 24; Jaspers, *Von der Wahrheit*, p. 389.

158 Jaspers, *Von der Wahrheit*, p. 179.

159 Salamun, *Karl Jaspers*, pp. 90 ff.

160 Jaspers, *Schelling, Größe und Verhängnis*. Munich: Piper, 1955, pp. 206 ff. (reference taken from Salamun, *Karl Jaspers*, p. 168 n. 2).

161 Jaspers, *Von der Wahrheit*, pp. 219–220.

162 *Ibid.*, p. 179.

163 Schneiders, *Karl Jaspers in der Kritik*, p. 176.

164 Janos Kelemen, "The 'Thing-in-itself' and the 'Encompassing'." In *Karl Jaspers: Philosoph unter Philosophen.* Leonard Ehrlich and Richard Wisser (eds.). Würzburg: Konigshausen & Neumann, 1993, p. 30.

165 *Ibid.*, pp. 20–21.

166 Jaspers, *Psychologie der Weltanschauungen*, pp. 465–486; Jaspers, *Die grossen Philosophen* (1–3). Munich: Piper, 1957, pp. 397–616; Miron, "Was Jaspers Really Kantian?" *Yearbook of the Austrian Karl Jaspers Society*, 19, (2006), pp. 73–106.

167 Jaspers, *Von der Wahrheit*, p. 50.

168 *Ibid.*, pp. 181–182.

169 *Ibid.*, p. 180; Jaspers, *Nietzsche, Einführung in das Verständnis seines Philosophierens.* Berlin: Walter De Gruyter, 1950, p. 18, 393 ff.

170 Samay, *Reason Revisited: The Philosophy of Karl Jaspers*, pp. 58 ff.

171 *Ibid.*, pp. 71–121.

172 Jaspers, *Von der Wahrheit*, pp. 158 ff.

173 *Ibid.*, p. 159; Knauss, "The Concept of the 'Encompassing' in Jaspers's Philosophy," pp. 141–142.

174 Jaspers, *Von der Wahrheit*, pp. 160–161.

175 Jaspers, *Philosophie*, 1, p. 23.

176 Jaspers, *Von der Wahrheit*, p. 160.

177 Jaspers, *Von der Wahrheit*, p. 161.

178 Heinemann, *Existenzphilosophie—lebendig oder tot?*, p. 71.

179 Mader, "Das Seindenken bei Karl Jaspers," p. 58.

180 Jaspers, *Vernunft und Existenz*, p. 36; Jaspers, *Von der Wahrheit*, p. 38.

181 Samay, *Reason Revisited: The Philosophy of Karl Jaspers*, p. 297 n. 11.

182 Heinemann, *Existenzphilosophie—lebendig oder tot?*, p. 73, 70 ff.

183 *Ibid.*, p. 65.

184 Richli, *Transzendental Reflexion und sittliche Entscheidung*, p. 119.

185 *Ibid.*, pp. 142–143.

186 *Ibid.*, p. 138.

187 Samay, *Reason Revisited: The Philosophy of Karl Jaspers*, pp. 54 ff.; Knauss "The Concept of the 'Encompassing' in Jaspers's Philosophy," pp. 146 ff.; Mader, "Das Seindenken bei Karl Jaspers," pp. 55 ff.; Ludwig Armbruster, *Objekt und Transzendenz bei*

Karl Jaspers: Sein Gegenstandsbegriff und die Möglichkeit der Metaphysik, Innsbruck: F. Rauch, 1957, pp. 61–84.

188 Jaspers, *Von der Wahrheit*, p. 184.

189 *Ibid.*, p. 227.

190 *Ibid.*, p. 167.

191 *Ibid.*, p. 388.

192 *Ibid.*, p. 109.

Chapter Ten

1 Aloys Klein, *Glaube und Mythos, Eine kritische, religionsphilosophisch-theologische Untersuchung des Mythos–Begriffs bei Karl Jaspers*. Munich: F. Schöningh, 1973, p. 88; Johannes Thyssen, "The Concept of 'Foundering' in Jaspers's Philosophy." In *The Philosophy of Karl Jaspers*. Paul Arthur Schilpp (ed.). New York: Tudor, 1957, p. 31; Kurt Hoffman, "The Basic Concept of Jaspers's Philosophy." In *The Philosophy of Karl Jaspers*. Paul Arthur Schilpp (ed.). New York: Tudor, 1957, p. 108.

2 Karl Jaspers, *Philosophie*. Berlin: Springer, [1932] 1994, 3, p. 234.

3 *Ibid.*, p. 234.

4 Thyssen, "The Concept of 'Foundering' in Jaspers's Philosophy," p. 309.

5 Xavier Tilliette, "Sinn, Wert und Grenze der Chiffernlehre: Reflexionen über die Metaphysik von Karl Jaspers." In *Karl Jaspers in der Diskussion*. Hans Saner, (ed.). Munich: Piper, 1973, pp. 390–391.

6 *Ibid.*, p. 393.

7 *Ibid.*, p 391.

8 *Ibid.*, pp. 391–393, 395.

9 Jaspers, *Philosophie*, 3, pp. 205–206.

10 Jaspers, *Von der Wahrheit*. Munich: Piper, [1947] 1991, pp. 1022 ff.

11 Jaspers, *Philosophie*, 3, p. 16.

12 Jaspers, *Psychologie der Weltanschauungen*. Berlin: Springer, [1919] 1985, p. 21.

13 *Ibid.*, p. 21; Klein, *Glaube und Mythos, Eine kritische, religions-philosophisch-theologische Untersuchung des Mythos-Begriffs bei Karl Jaspers*, pp. 5–40.

14 Jaspers, *Psychologie der Weltanschauungen*, p. 345.

15 *Ibid.*, pp. 52 ff.

16 *Ibid.*, p. 15.

17 *Ibid.*, pp. 16–17.

18 Jaspers, *Philosophie*, 2, pp. 345 ff.

19 Jaspers, *Psychologie der Weltanschauungen*, p. 4.

20 *Ibid.*, p. 16.

21 *Ibid.*, p. 14.

22 Jaspers, *Von der Wahrheit*, p. 37.

23 Jaspers, *Philosophie*, 3, p. 136.

24 Jaspers, *Philosophie*, 1, p. 35.

25 *Ibid.*, pp. 137–138.

26 Jaspers, *Philosophie*, 3, p. 197.

27 *Ibid.*, p. 138.
28 *Ibid.*, p. 137.
29 *Ibid.*, p. 140.
30 *Ibid.*, p. 39.
31 *Ibid.*, pp. 137–138.
32 *Ibid.*, p. 140.
33 Jaspers, *Von der Wahrheit*, p. 1032.
34 Jaspers, *Philosophie*, 3, pp. 129 ff.
35 Jaspers, *Chiffren der Transzendenz*. Munich: Piper, 1970.
36 Jaspers, *Philosophie*, 3, p. 137.
37 *Ibid.*, p. 146.
38 *Ibid.*, p. 139, 151.
39 *Ibid.*, p. 170.
40 Jaspers, *Von der Wahrheit*, p. 1032, 1034.
41 *Ibid.*, p. 1032.
42 *Ibid.*, pp. 256–257.
43 Jaspers, *Philosophie*, 2, p. 341.
44 Jaspers, *Philosophie*, 3, pp. 142–143.
45 *Ibid.*, p. 130.
46 *Ibid.*, pp. 178 ff.
47 *Ibid.*, pp.182 ff.
48 *Ibid.*, pp. 192 ff.
49 John Hennig, "Karl Jaspers's Attitude toward History." In *The Philosophy of Karl Jaspers*, Paul Arthur Schilpp (ed.). New York: Tudor, 1957, pp. 565–591; Jaspers, *Philosophie*, 1, pp. 330–340; Johannes Pfeiffer, "On Karl Jaspers's Interpretation of Art." In *The Philosophy of Karl Jaspers*. Paul Arthur Schilpp (ed.). New York: Tudor, 1957, pp. 703–717.
50 Jaspers, *Philosophie*, 3, p. 182; Robert Doran, "Aesthetics and the Opposites," *Thought*, 52, (1977), pp. 117–133.
51 Jaspers, *Philosophie*, 3, p. 16.
52 *Ibid.*, p. 171.
53 Jaspers, *Von der Wahrheit*, p. 1032.
54 Jaspers, *Philosophie*, 3, p. 169.
55 *Ibid.*, p. 180.
56 *Ibid.*, p. 170; Jaspers, *Philosophie*, 1, p. 134.
57 Jaspers, *Philosophie*, 1, p. 132.
58 *Ibid.*, p. 134.
59 Jaspers, *Philosophie*, 3, p. 170.
60 *Ibid.*, p. 137.
61 *Ibid.*, p. 230.
62 *Ibid.*, p. 230.
63 Jaspers, *Von der Wahrheit*, p. 1031.
64 *Ibid.*, p. 1038, 1044.
65 *Ibid.*, p. 1044.

66 Jaspers, *Philosophie*, 3, p. 146.
67 Jaspers, *Philosophie*, 1, p. 19.
68 *Ibid.*, p. 19.
69 Jaspers, *Philosophie*, 2, pp. 8 ff.
70 Jaspers, *Von der Wahrheit*, p. 1049; Jaspers, *Allgemeine Psychopathologie*. 8th edition. Berlin-Heidelberg: Springer, 1965, p. 277.
71 Jaspers, *Philosophie*, 2, p. 341.
72 Jaspers, *Von der Wahrheit*, p. 1043.
73 Jaspers, *Philosophie*, 3, p. 185.
74 *Ibid.*, p. 16.
75 Alan M. Olson, *Transcendence and Hermeneutics: An Interpretation of the Philosophy of Karl Jaspers*. The Hague and Boston: M. Nijhoff, 1979, pp. 122 ff.
76 Jaspers, *Philosophie*, 3, p. 17.
77 *Ibid.*, p. 184.
78 Jacques Waardenburg, "Symbolic Aspects of Myth." In *Myth, Symbol, and Reality*. Alan M. Olson (ed.). Notre Dame: University of Notre Dame Press, 1980, pp. 45 ff.
79 Jaspers, *Philosophie*, 3, p. 185.
80 *Ibid.*, p. 185.
81 *Ibid.*, p. 184.
82 Jaspers, *Philosophie*, 1, p. 319; Jaspers, *Von der Wahrheit*, pp. 1033–1034.
83 Jaspers, *Von der Wahrheit*, p.1034, 1046.
84 Jaspers, *Philosophie*, 3, pp. 146 ff.; Jaspers, *Von der Wahrheit*, p. 1039.
85 Jaspers, *Von der Wahrheit*, p. 1039.
86 Jaspers, *Philosophie*, 3, p. 145, 147.
87 *Ibid.*, p. 141, 147.
88 Sebastian Samay, *Reason Revisited: The Philosophy of Karl Jaspers*. Dublin: Gill and Macmillan, 1971, pp 176–177.
89 Jaspers, *Von der Wahrheit*, p.1031.
90 *Ibid.*, p. 1039.
91 *Ibid.*, p. 1031.
92 *Ibid.*, p. 1031.
93 Jaspers, *Philosophie*, 3, pp. 146–147.
94 Jaspers, *Philosophie*, 3, p. 162.
95 Jaspers, *Philosophie*, 1, p. 33.
96 Jaspers, *Philosophie*, 3, p. 153.
97 Jaspers, *Von der Wahrheit*, p. 1031.
98 *Ibid.*, p. 1048; Waardenburg, "Symbolic Aspects of Myth," pp. 53 ff.
99 Peter Wust, *Naivität und Pietät*. Tübingen: J. C. B. Mohr, 1925.
100 Wust, *Die Auferstehung der Metaphysik*. Leipzig: F. Meiner, 1921.
101 Wilhelm Vernekohl, *Peter Wust: Leben und Werk, Biographische Notizen*. Münster: Regensberg, 1967, pp. 179–219.
102 Olson (ed.). *Myth, Symbol, and Reality*. Notre Dame: University of Notre Dame Press, 1980, p. 3.

103 Kurt Salamun, *Karl Jaspers*. Munich: Beck, 1985, p. 143; Tilliette, "Sinn, Wert und Grenze der Chiffernlehre: Reflexionen über die Metaphysik von Karl Jaspers," p. 393.

104 Immanuel Kant, *Critique of the Power of Judgment*. Ed. Paul Guyer. Trans. Paul Guyer and Eric Mathews. New York: Cambridge University Press, 2000, pp. 178–182.

105 Jaspers, *Allgemeine Psychopathologie*. 8th Edition, pp. 275–276; Jaspers, *Von der Wahrheit*, p. 1042.

106 Jaspers, *Philosophie*, 1, p. 58.

107 Jaspers, *Philosophie*, 2, p. 344.

108 Jaspers, *Philosophie*, 3, pp. 31–32; Jaspers, *Von der Wahrheit*, p. 1031.

109 Jaspers, *Philosophie*, 1, p. 33.

110 *Ibid.*, p. 33.

111 Jaspers, *Von der Wahrheit*, pp. 1022–1023.

112 Jaspers, *Philosophie*, 3, p. 170.

113 *Ibid.*, p. 170.

114 *Ibid.*, p. 218.

115 Jaspers, *Philosophie*, 2, pp. 343–344.

116 Jaspers, *Philosophie*, 3, p. 142.

117 *Ibid.*, p. 143.

118 Jaspers, *Von der Wahrheit*, p. 1036.

119 *Ibid.*, p. 1037.

120 *Ibid.*, p. 1041.

121 Jaspers, *Philosophie*, 3, p. 149.

122 Olson, *Transcendence and Hermeneutics: An Interpretation of the Philosophy of Karl Jaspers*, p. 35.

123 Bernard Joseph Francis Lonergan, *Method in Theology*. New York: Herder & Herder, 1972, pp. 320–329; Lonergan, "Reality, Myth, Symbol." In Myth, *Symbol, and Reality*, Alan M. Olson (ed.), Notre Dame: University of Notre Dame Press, 1980, pp. 31–34.

124 Stephen A. Erickson, "The Space of Transcendence in Jaspers and Heidegger." In *Heidegger & Jaspers*, Alan M. Olson (ed.). Philadelphia: Temple University Press, 1994, pp. 135 ff.; Avi Sagi, *Kierkegaard, Religion, and Existence: The Voyage of the Self*. Translated by Batya Stein. Amsterdam: Rodopi, 2000, pp. 12ff. Olson, *Transcendence and Hermeneutics: An Interpretation of the Philosophy of Karl Jaspers*, p. 40; Fritz Heinemann, *Jenseits des Existentialismus*. Stuttgart: W. Kohlhammer, 1957, pp. 115–152.

125 Jaspers, *Der philosophische Glaube angesichts der Offenbarung*. Munich: Piper, 1962, pp. 45–94; Tillich, "Sinn, Wert und Grenze der Chiffernlehre: Reflexionen über die Metaphysik von Karl Jaspers," p. 67.

126 Jaspers, *Philosophie*, 3, pp. 148–149.

127 *Ibid.*, p. 150.

128 Jaspers, *Von der Wahrheit*, p. 1038.

129 Jaspers, *Philosophie*, 3, p. 215.

130 Jaspers, *Von der Wahrheit*, pp. 1036–1037.

131 Jaspers, *Philosophie*, 3, p. 217.

132 Jaspers, *Von der Wahrheit*, p. 1046.

133 Jaspers, *Philosophie*, 3, p. 150, 218.
134 Waardenburg, "Symbolic Aspects of Myth," p. 47.
135 Jaspers, *Philosophie*, 3, p. 32.
136 *Ibid.*, p. 33, 161 ff.; Jaspers, *Von der Wahrheit*, p. 1046.
137 Jaspers, *Philosophie*, 3, p. 146.
138 *Ibid.*, pp. 178–179.
139 *Ibid.*, p. 137.
140 *Ibid.*, p. 140.
141 Hermann-Josef Seideneck, "Das Wagnis der Schwebe, Der Gottesgedanke im philosophischen Werk von Karl Jaspers." In *Karl Jaspers: Philosoph unter Philosophen.* Leonard Ehrlich and Richard Wisser (eds.). Würzburg: Konigshausen and Neumann, 1993, p. 251.
142 *Ibid.*, pp. 252–253.
143 Jaspers, *Philosophie*, 2, p. 344.
144 Jaspers, *Philosophie*, 3, p. 201.
145 *Ibid.*, p. 201.
146 *Ibid.*, p. 236.
147 *Ibid.*, p. 6.
148 Jaspers, *Philosophie*, 1, p. 33.
149 Jaspers, *Philosophie*, 3, pp. 129 ff.; Jaspers, *Von der Wahrheit*, p. 1032, 1038 ff.
150 Jaspers, *Philosophie*, 3, p. 35; Jaspers, *Philosophie*, 1, pp. 32 ff., 58, 274, 340; Jaspers, *Philosophie*, 2, pp. 129 ff., 217 ff., 282 ff., 326 ff.; Jaspers, *Philosophie*, 3, pp. 31 ff., 99 ff., 128 ff., 134 ff., 141ff., 150 ff., 165 ff., 192 ff.
151 Olson, *Transcendence and Hermeneutics: An Interpretation of the Philosophy of Karl Jaspers*, pp. 139 ff.
152 Jaspers, *Philosophie*, 3, p. 130.
153 Jaspers, *Philosophie*, 2, pp. 261 ff.
154 Jaspers, *Philosophie*, 3, pp. 131–132.
155 *Ibid.*, p. 133.
156 *Ibid.*, p. 134.
157 *Ibid.*, p. 135.
158 *Ibid.*, p. 135.
159 *Ibid.*, pp. 135–136.
160 Jaspers, *Von der Wahrheit*, p. 1032.
161 *Ibid.*, p. 1034.
162 Jaspers, *Philosophie*, 3, p. 136.
163 *Ibid.*, p. 138.
164 *Ibid.*, p. 149.
165 Olson, *Transcendence and Hermeneutics: An Interpretation of the Philosophy of Karl Jaspers*; Olson, (ed.). *Myth, Symbol, and Reality*, pp. 1–12, 99–125; Olson "Jaspers's Critique of Modernity: A Postmodern Reflection." In *Karl Jaspers Today, Philosophy at the Threshold of the Future*. Leonard Ehrlich and Richard Wisser (eds.). Washington, D.C.: University Press of America, 1988, pp. 363–380; Paul Ricoeur, "Existence and Hermeneutics." In *Contemporary Hermeneutics: Hermeneutics as Method, Philosophy,*

and Critique. Josef Bleicher (ed.). London and New York: Routledge & Kegan Paul, 1980, pp. 236–256; Ricoeur, *The Rule of Metaphor: Multi-disciplinary Studies of Creation of Meaning in Language*. London: Routledge & Kegan Paul, 1986; Ricoeur, "The Relation of Jaspers's Philosophy to Religion." In *The Philosophy of Karl Jaspers*. Paul Arthur Schilpp (ed.). New York: Tudor, 1957, pp. 611–642.

166 Jaspers, *Allgemeine Psychopathologie*. 8th Edition, p. 275.

167 Olson *Transcendence and Hermeneutics: An Interpretation of the Philosophy of Karl Jaspers*, p. xiii.

168 Olson, "Myth, Symbol, and Metaphorical Truth." In *Myth, Symbol, and Reality*. Alan M. Olson (ed.). Notre Dame: University of Notre Dame Press, 1980, p. 109.

169 Thyssen, "The Concept of 'Foundering' in Jaspers's Philosophy," p. 307.

170 Samay, *Reason Revisited: The Philosophy of Karl Jaspers*, pp. 179 ff.

171 Jaspers, *Philosophie*, 3, p. 150.

172 *Ibid*., p. 129.

173 *Ibid*., p. 151.

174 *Ibid*., pp. 151–152.

175 *Ibid*., p. 141.

176 *Ibid*., p. 144.

177 *Ibid*., pp. 139–140.

178 Jaspers, *Von der Wahrheit*, p. 1031.

179 *Ibid*., p. 1023; Jaspers, *Philosophie*, 2, p. 342; Jaspers, *Von der Wahrheit*, pp. 1022–1023, 1030.

180 Jaspers, *Philosophie*, 3, p. 207.

181 *Ibid*., p. 163.

182 *Ibid*., p. 153.

183 Ricoeur, "Existence and Hermeneutics," pp. 243 ff.

184 Jaspers, *Philosophie*, 3, p.175; Waardenburg, "Symbolic Aspects of Myth," pp. 44 ff.

185 Jaspers, *Philosophie*, 3, p. 141.

186 Jaspers, *Von der Wahrheit*, p. 1033.

Chapter Eleven

1 Karl Jaspers, *Philosophie*. Berlin: Springer, [1932] 1994, 2, p. 144, 415 ff., 421 ff.; Jaspers, *Philosophie*, 1, p. 58; Jaspers, *Philosophie*, 3, pp. 68 ff.

2 Jaspers, *Philosophie*, 3, p. 131.

3 Jaspers, *Von der Wahrheit*. Munich: Piper, [1947] 1991, p. 141.

4 *Ibid*., pp. 109–110.

5 *Ibid*., pp. 108–109.

6 *Ibid*., pp. 123 ff.

7 Jaspers, *Philosophie*, 3, p. 136.

8 *Ibid*., p. 140.

9 Jaspers, *Von der Wahrheit*, p. 1034.

10 Jaspers, *Philosophie*, 3, p. 10.

11 *Ibid.*, p. 169.

12 *Ibid.*, p. 147.

13 Jaspers, *Von der Wahrheit*, p. 1040.

14 Jeanne Hersch, *Karl Jaspers, Eine Einführung in sein Werk*. Bern: Francke, 1978, pp. 36–37.

15 *Ibid.*, pp. 39–40.

16 Hersch, "Existenz in der empirischen Wirklichkeit." In *Karl Jaspers—Philosoph, Arzt, politischer Denker*, Jeanne Hersch, Jan Milic Lochman, and Reiner Wiehl (eds.). Munich and Zurich: Piper, 1986, p. 50.

17 Hans Kunz, "Critique of Jaspers's Concept of Transcendence." In *The Philosophy of Karl Jaspers*. Paul Arthur Schilpp (ed.). New York: Tudor, 1957, p. 504.

18 *Ibid.*, pp. 512–513.

19 *Ibid.*, p. 509.

20 Joseph Lenz, *Der moderne deutsche und französische Existentialismus*. Trier: Paulinus Verlag, 1951, p. 54.

21 *Ibid.*, p. 36.

22 *Ibid.*, p. 34, 51, 61.

23 Arnold Gehlen, "Jaspers's Philosophie," *Bulletin für deutsche Philosophie*, 6:3, (1932–1933), pp. 370–371.

24 Erich Frank, "Die Philosophie von Jaspers," *Theologische Rundschau*, 5:5, (1993), pp. 301–318.

25 Jaspers, *Die grossen Philosophen* (1–3). Munich: Piper, 1957.

26 Jaspers, *Schelling, Grö ße und Verhängnis*. Munich: Piper, 1955.

27 Alan M. Olson, *Transcendence and Hermeneutics: An Interpretation of the Philosophy of Karl Jaspers*. The Hague and Boston: M. Nijhoff, 1979, p. 113, 45–90; Marcel Reding, *Die Existenzphilosophie, Heidegger, Sartre, Gabriel Marcel und Jaspers in kritischer-systematischer Sicht*. Düsseldorf: Schwann, 1949, pp. 23–38.

28 Claus Uwe Hommel, *Chiffer und Dogma, vom Verhältnis der Philosophie zur Religion bei Karl Jaspers*. Zurich: EVZ Verlag, Abt. Editio Academica, 1968, p. 97.

29 *Ibid.*, pp. 98–99.

30 *Ibid.*, p. 102, 96.

31 Karl Löwith, "Existenz-Philosophie," *Zeitschrift für deutsche Bildung*, 12, (1932), pp. 602–613.

32 Fritz-Joachim Von Rinteln, *Beyond Existentialism*. London: Allen and Unwin, 1961, p. 207.

33 *Ibid.*, p. 211.

34 *Ibid.*, p. 168.

35 *Ibid.*, p. 211, 215.

36 F. Imle, "Jaspers als Existenzphilosoph," *Philosophisches Jahrbuch der Görresgesellschaft*, 49, (1936), p. 491.

37 *Ibid.*, pp. 501 ff.

38 Imle, "Jaspers als Existenzphilosoph," *Philosophisches Jahrbuch der Görresgesellschaft*, 50, (1937), pp. 246 ff.

39 Robert Winkler, "Philosophische oder theologische Anthropologie?" *Zeitschrift für Theologie und Kirche*, 14:2, (1933), pp. 133 ff.

40 *Ibid.*, p. 124.

41 Wolfgang Stegmüller, *Hauptströmungen der Gegenwartsphilosophie*. Stuttgart: Alfred Kroner, 1960, pp. 204 ff.

42 *Ibid.*, p. 240.

43 Ludwig Armbruster, *Objekt und Transzendenz bei Karl Jaspers: Sein Gegenstandsbegriff und die Möglichkeit der Metaphysik*, Innsbruck: F. Rauch, 1957, p. 133.

44 William Kluback, "Karl Jaspers and Schmuel Hugo Bergman. Believing Philosophers." In *Karl Jaspers: Philosoph unter Philosophen*. Leonard Ehrlich and Richard Wisser (eds.). Würzburg: Konigshausen & Neumann, 1993, pp. 173–185.

45 Leo Gabriel, *Existenzphilosophie von Kierkegaard bis Sartre*. Vienna: Verlag Herold, 1951, p. 278.

46 Johannes Ell, *Der Existentialismus*. Bonn: H. Bouvier, 1955, p. 33.

47 Werner Schneiders, *Karl Jaspers in der Kritik*. Bonn: Bouvier, 1965, p. 34; John F. Kane, *Pluralism and Truth in Religion*. Chico, CA: Scholars Press, 1981, pp. 77 ff.; Wolf Hertel, *Existentieller Glaube, Eine Studie über den Glaubensbegriff von Karl Jaspers und Paul Tillich*. Meisenheim am Glan: Verlag Anton Hain, 1971, pp. 17–53; Oskar Schatz, "Religionsphilosophische Aspekte bei Karl Jaspers," *Kairos*, I, (1960), pp. 25–28; Martin Werner, "Existenzphilosophie und Christentum bei Karl Jaspers." In *Karl Jaspers in der Diskussion*. Hans Saner (ed.). Munich: Piper, 1973, pp. 335–357; Paul Ricoeur, "Philosophie und Religion bei Jaspers." In *Karl Jaspers in der Diskussion*. Hans Saner (ed.). Munich: Piper, 1973, pp. 358–389.

48 Hanoch Tennen, *The Perception of Existentialist Ethics in Karl Jaspers's Philosophy*. Ramat Gan: Masada, 1977 [Hebrew], pp. 25–26.

49 *Ibid.*, p. 76.

50 *Ibid.*, pp. 77–78.

51 Winkler, "Philosopische oder theologische Anthropologie?" pp. 107–109.

52 Wilhelm Andersen, *Der Existenzbegriff und das existentielle Denken in der neueren Philosophie und Theologie*. Dissertation Gütersloh: Bertelsmann, 1940.

53 Tennen, *The Perception of Existentialist Ethics in Karl Jaspers's Philosophy*, p. 285 n. 5; Andersen, *Der Existenzbegriff und das existentielle Denken in der neueren Philosophie und Theologie*, pp. 70–71.

54 Andersen, *Der Existenzbegriff und das existentielle Denken in der neueren Philosophie und Theologie*, p. 69.

55 Winkler, "Philosophische oder theologische Anthropologie?" pp. 109 ff.

56 Johannes Reis, "Menschliche Existenz bei Jaspers," *Die Neue Ordnung*, 4, (1950), p. 529.

57 Reis, "Transzendenz bei Jaspers," in *Die Neue Ordnung*, 5, (1951), p. 327.

58 Reis, "Menschliche Existenz bei Jaspers," p. 329; Reis, "Transzendenz bei Jaspers," pp. 240 ff.

59 Fritz Kaufmann, "Karl Jaspers and a Philosophy of Communication." In *The Philosophy of Karl Jaspers*. Paul Arthur Schilpp (ed.). New York: Tudor, 1957, pp. 268–269.

60 *Ibid.*, pp. 269 ff.

61 *Ibid.*, p. 272.

62 Kunz, "Critique of Jaspers's Concept of Transcendence," pp. 504 ff.

63 John Milbank, *Theology & Social Theory: Beyond Secular Reason*. Oxford: Blackwell, 1997; Phillip Blond, *Post-Secular Philosophy: Between Philosophy and Theology*. London and New York: Routledge, 1998.

64 Johannes Thyssen, "The Concept of 'Foundering' in Jaspers's Philosophy." In *The Philosophy of Karl Jaspers*. Paul Arthur Schilpp (ed.). New York: Tudor, 1957, p. 311.

65 *Ibid.*, p. 309.

66 *Ibid.*, p. 310.

67 Alan M. Olson, "Myth, Symbol, and Metaphorical Truth." In *Myth, Symbol, and Reality*. Alan M. Olson (ed.). Notre Dame: University of Notre Dame Press, 1980, pp. 107–110.

68 Stephen A. Erickson, "The Space of Transcendence in Jaspers and Heidegger." In *Heidegger and Jaspers*, Alan M. Olson (ed.). Philadelphia: Temple University Press, 1994, pp. 131 ff.

69 Olson "Myth, Symbol and Metaphorical Truth," pp. 58–71.

70 Jaspers, *Philosophie*, 3, p. 15.

71 *Ibid.*, p. 18, 17–18, 50, 123, 146–148.

72 *Ibid.*, p 221.

73 Jaspers, *Nietzsche, Einführung in das Verständnis seines Philosophierens*. Berlin: Walter De Gruyter, 1950, p. 9.

74 *Ibid.*, p. 17.

75 *Ibid.*, p. 17.

76 *Ibid.*, p. 329.

77 *Ibid.*, pp. 119 ff.

78 Walter Kaufmann, *Nietzsche: Philosopher, Psychologist, Antichrist*. Princeton, New Jersey: Princeton University Press, 1974, p. 74 n. 2.

Conclusion

1 Karl Jaspers, *Nietzsche, Einführung in das Verständnis seines Philosophierens*. Berlin: Walter De Gruyter, 1950, p. 18.

2 Jaspers, *Von der Wahrheit*. Munich: Piper, [1947] 1991, p. 703.

3 Jaspers, *Philosophie*. Berlin: Springer, [1932] 1994, 1, p. 27.

BIBLIOGRAPHY

Andersen, Wilhelm. *Der Existenzbegriff und das existentielle Denken in der neueren Philosophie und Theologie*. Dissertation Gütersloh: Bertelsmann, 1940.

Arendt, Hanna. "Jaspers as Citizen of the World." In *The Philosophy of Karl Jaspers*, Paul Arthur Schilpp (ed.). New York: Tudor, 1957, pp. 539–549.

———. "Karl Jaspers," *Reden zur Verleihung des Friedenspreises, des deutschen Buchhandels*. Munich: Piper, 1958, pp. 27–40.

Armbruster, Ludwig. *Objekt und Transzendenz bei Karl Jaspers: Sein Gegenstandsbegriff und die Möglichkeit der Metaphysik*, Innsbruck: F. Rauch, 1957.

Assmann, Aleida. "Jaspers' Achsenzeit, oder: Vom Glück und Elend der Zentralperspektive in der Geschichte." In *Karl Jaspers: Denken zwischen Wissenschaft, Politik und Philosophie*. Dietrich Harth (ed.). Stuttgart: Metzler, 1989, pp. 187–205.

———. *Arbeit am nationalen Gedächtnis: Eine kurze Geschichte der deutschen Bildungsidee*. Frankfurt and New York: Campus, 1993.

Balthasar, Hans Urs Von. *Einsame Zwiesprache, Martin Buber und Christentum*. Cologne: Johannes, 1958.

Barnes, Hazel Estella. *An Existentialist Ethics*. New York: Alfred Knopf, 1967.

Barrett, William. *Irrational Man: a Study in Existential Philosophy*. London: Anchor Books, 1964.

Barsoum, Reymond Diane. *Existentialism and the Philosophical Tradition*. New Jersey: Prentice Hall, 1991.

Beck, Maximilian. "Kritik der Schelling-Jaspers-Heidegger'schen Ontologie," *Philosophische Hefte*, IV, (1934), pp. 97–164.

Bennett, James O. "Karl Jaspers and Scientific Philosophy," *Journal of Philosophy*, 31, (1993), pp. 437–453.

Bergson, Henri. *The Creative Mind*. Translated by Mabelle L. Andison. New Jersey: Littlefield, Adams, 1965.

Biemel, Walter, and Saner, Hans (eds.). *Martin Heideger / Karl Jaspers 1920–1963*. Frankfurt: Klostermann, 1992.

Blackham, Harold John. *Six Existentialist Thinkers*. London: Routledge, 1961.

Blattner, William D. "Heidegger's Debt to Jaspers's Concept of Limit-Situation." In *Heidegger and Jaspers*. Alan. M. Olson (ed.). Philadelphia: Temple University Press, 1994, pp. 153–165.

Blond, Phillip. *Post-Secular Philosophy: Between Philosophy and Theology*. London and New York: Routledge, 1998.

Bollen, Bernhard. *Existential Thinking: A Philosophical Orientation*. Pittsburgh: Duquesne University Press, 1968.

Bollnow, Otto Friedrich. "Existenzerhellung und philosophische Anthropologie," *Bulletin für deutsche Philosophie*, 12:2, (1938–1939), pp. 133–174.

———. *Existenzphilosophie*. Stuttgart: W. Kohlhammer, [1942] 1960.

———. "Deutsche Existenzphilosophie und französischer Existentialismus," *Zeitschrift für philosophische Forschung*, 2, (1947), pp. 231–243.
———. *Neue Geborgenheit, Das Problem einer Überwindung des Existentialismus*. Stuttgart and Cologne: W. Kohlhammer, 1955.
———. *Existenzphilosophie und Pädagogik*. Stuttgart: W. Kohlhammer, 1959.
———. "Die Objektivität der Geisteswissenschaften und die Frage nach dem Wesen der Wahrheit," *Zeitschrift für philosophische Forschung*, 16, (1962), pp. 147–167.
———. *Existenzphilosophie*. Stuttgart: W. Kohlhammer, 1964.
Brecht, Franz Josef. *Heidegger und Jaspers, Die beiden Grundformen der Existenzphilosophie*. Wuppertal: Marées, 1948.
———. *Einführung in die Philosophie der Existenz*. Heidelberg: M. Schmidt-Carstens, 1948.
Brentano, Franz Clemens. "Genuine and Fictitious Objects." In *Realism and the Background of Phenomenology*. Roderick Milton Chisholm (ed.). Glencoe: The Free Press, 3, 1960, pp.71–75.
Chadwick, Ruth F. "Commentary on 'Karl Jaspers and Edmund Husserl', *Philosophy, Psychiatry and Psychology*, 2:1, (1995), pp. 83–84.
Collins, James. *The Existentialists*. Chicago: H. Regnery, 1968.
———. "Jaspers on Science and Philosophy." In *The Philosophy of Karl Jaspers*. Paul Arthur Schilpp (ed.). New York: Tudor, 1957, pp. 115–140.
———. "Karl Jaspers' Philosophical Logic," *The New Scholasticism*, 23, (1959), pp. 414–420.
Coreth, Emerich S. G., *Metaphysik: Eine methodisch–systematische Grundlegung*. Innsbruck: Tyrolia, 1961.
Cumming, Robert Denoon. *Phenomenology and Deconstruction 4: Solitude*. Chicago: University of Chicago Press, 2001.
Czako, Istvan. "Das Problem des Glaubens und der Geschichte in der Philosophie Kierkegaards und Karl Jaspers." *Kierkegaard Studies*, Yearbook, 2000, pp. 373–382.
Di Cesare, Donatella. *Die Sprache in der Philosophie von Karl Jaspers*. Tübingen and Basel: Francke, 1996.
Dilthey, Wilhelm. "Einleitung in die Geisteswissenschaften." *Gesammelte Schriften*, 1. Leipzig and Berlin: Teubner, 1922.
———. *Der Aufbau der geschichtlichen Welt in den Geisteswissenschaften*. Stuttgart and Goettingen: Teubner and Vandenhoeck, 1927.
———. *Weltanschauungslehre, Abhandlung zur Philosophie der Philosophie, Gesammelte Schriften*, VIII. Stuttgart and Goettingen: Teubner and Vandenhoeck, 1962.
———. "Ideen über eine beschreibende und zergliedernde Psychologie," *Gesammelte Schriften*, 6. Stuttgart and Goettingen: Teubner and Vandenhoeck, 1974, pp. 139–240.
———. *Selected Writings*. Cambridge: Cambridge University Press, 1976.
Doran, Robert. "Aesthetics and the Opposites," *Thought*, 52, (1977), pp. 117–133.

Earle, William. "Anthropology in the Philosophy." In *The Philosophy of Karl Jaspers.* Paul Arthur Schilpp (ed.). New York: Tudor, 1957, pp. 523–538.

Ehrlich, Leonard. *Karl Jaspers: Philosophy as Faith.* Amherst: University of Massachusetts Press, 1975.

——— and Wisser, Richard (eds.), *Karl Jaspers Today: Philosophy at the Threshold of the Future.* Washington D.C.: University Press of America, 1988.

——— and Wisser, Richard) eds.), *Karl Jaspers: Philosoph unter Philosophen.* Würzburg: Konigshausen and Neumann, 1993.

Ell, Johannes. *Der Existentialismus.* Bonn: H. Bouvier, 1955.

End, Heinrich. *Existentiale Handlungen im Strafrecht, Die Pflichtenkollision im Lichte der Philosophie von Karl Jaspers.* Munich: Beck, 1959.

Erich, Frank. "Die Philosophie von Jaspers," *Theologische Rundschau*, 5:5, (1933), pp. 301–318.

Erickson, Stephen A. "The Image of Socrates in the Mirror of Jaspers," *Philosophy Today*, 38, (1994), pp. 285–293.

———. "The Space of Transcendence in Jaspers and Heidegger." In *Heidegger & Jaspers*, Alan M. Olson (ed.). Philadelphia: Temple University Press, 1994, pp. 126–138.

Farrer, Austin Marsden. *The Freedom of the Will.* New York: Charles Scribner's Sons, 1960.

Frank, Erich. "Die Philosophie von Jaspers," *Theologische Rundschau*, 5:5, (1993), pp. 301–318.

Frege, Gottlob. "On Concept and Object." In *Translations from Philosophical Writings of Gottlob Frege.* Peter Greach and Max Black (eds.). Oxford: Basil Blackwell and Mott, 1970. pp. 42–55.

Freud, Sigmund. *New introductory Lectures on Psycho–Analysis and Other Works.* Translated by James Starchey. London: Hogarth Press and the Institute of Psycho-Analysis, 1964, pp. 158–182.

Fromm, Erich. *Escape from Freedom.* New York: Rinehart and Company, 1941.

Fuchs, Franz Josef. "Seinverhältnis, Karl Jaspers' Existenzphilosophie," *Existenz und Kommunikation*, Frankfurt-Bern-New York-Nancy: Peter Lang, 1984.

Gabriel, Leo. *Existenzphilosophie von Kierkegaard bis Sartre.* Vienna: Verlag Herold, 1951.

Gadamer, Hans Georg. "Die Bedeutung der Philosophie für die neue Erziehung." In *Über die Ursprünglichkeit der Philosophie*, Hans Georg Gadamer (ed.). Berlin: Chronos, 1948.

———. "Das Verhältnis der Philosophie zu Kunst und Wissenschaft." In *Über die Ursprünglichkeit der Philosophie*, Hans Georg Gadamer (ed.). Berlin: Chronos, 1948.

Ganahl, Kay. *Sphären des Zersetzenden, Ein Beitrag zur Jaspers Forschung.* Berlin: VWB, 1994.

Gangl, Manfred. "Karl Jaspers und Georg Lukács: Rechte und linke Kulturkritik in der Weimar-Republik." In *Karl Jaspers: Denken zwischen Wissenschaft, Politik und Philosophie*, Dietrich Harth (ed.). Stuttgart: Metzler, J.B., 1989, pp. 87–110.

Gehlen, Arnold. "Jaspers' Philosophie," *Bulletin für deutsche Philosophie,* 6:3, (1932–1933), pp. 365–380.

Gerber, J. Rudolf. "Karl Jaspers and Kantian Reason," *New Scholasticism*, 43, (1969), pp. 400–423.

Gosetti, Jennifer Anna. "Tragedy and Truth in Heidegger and Jaspers." *International Philosophical Quarterly*. S 02; 42:3, (2002), pp. 301–314.

Graefe, Steffen, "Von der 'Zugkraft des Seins,' Existentielle Kommunikation und der platonische Eros." In *Karl Jaspers: Philosoph unter Philosophen,* Leonard Ehrlich and Richard Wisser (eds.). Würzburg: Konigshausen and Neumann, 1993, pp. 272–278.

Griesinger, Wilhelm. *Pathologie und Therapie der psychischen Krankheiten*, 4th edition. Braunschweig: Wreden, 1786.

Grunert, Erich P. *Objektiv Norm, Situation und Entscheidung, Ein Vergleich zwischen Thomas von Aquino und Karl Jaspers*. Dissertation. Bonn, 1953.

———. "Der Einfluss Kants auf Karl Jaspers: Zugang zur Transzendenz bei Kant und Karl Jaspers," *Freiburger Zeitschrift für Philosophie und Theologie*, III, (1956), pp. 21–28.

Guardini, Romano, and Bollnow, Otto Friedrich (eds.). *Begegnung und Bildung*. Würzburg: Werkbund, 1960.

Gzynn, Simon (ed.). *Sartre: An Investigation of Some Major Themes*. Aldershot: Avebury, 1987.

Habermas, Jürgen. "Psychic Thermidor and the Rebirth of Rebellious Subjectivity," *Berkeley Journal of Sociology*, 24–25, (1980), pp. 1–12.

———. *Philosophisch–politische Profile*. Frankfurt: Suhrkamp, 1981.

Häfner, Heinz. "Einleitung in den psychiatrischen Teil." In *Karl Jaspers—Philosoph, Arzt, politischer Denker*. Jeanne Hersch, Jan Milic Lochman, and Reiner Wiehl (eds.). Munich and Zurich: Piper, 1986, pp. 83–87.

Hammelsbeck, Oskar. "Die Theologische Bestreitung des Philosophischen Glaubens." In *Offener Horizont, Festschrift für Karl Jaspers, zum 70.*, Klaus Piper (ed.). Munich: Piper, 1953, pp. 27–35.

Harrington, Michael. *The Politics at God's Funeral: The Spiritual Crisis of Western Civilization*. New York: Henry Holt, 1983.

Harris, Karsten. "Shame, Guilt, Responsibility." In *Heidegger & Jaspers*, Olson, Alan M. (ed.). Philadelphia: Temple University Press, 1994, pp. 49–64.

Harth, Dietrich (ed.). *Karl Jaspers: Denken zwischen Wissenschaft, Politik und Philosophie*. Stuttgart: Metzler, J.B., 1989.

———. "Grenzen der Wissenschaft." In *Karl Jaspers: Denken zwischen Wissenschaft, Politik und Philosophie*, Dietrich Harth (ed.). Stuttgart: Metzler, J.B., 1989, pp. 207–226.

Hartmann, Nicolai. *Zur Grundlegung der Ontologie*. Berlin: Walter de Gruyter, [1935] 1948.

———. *Kleine Schriften*. Berlin: Walter de Gruyter, 1955.

Hegel, Georg Wilhelm Friedrich. *Vorlesungen über die Philosophie der Geschichte*. Leipzig: P. Reclamjun, 1974.

———. *The Phenomenology of Spirit*. Oxford: Oxford University Press, 1961.

Heidegger, Martin. *Gelassenheit*. Pfullingen: Neske, 1959.

———. *The End of Philosophy*. Translated by Joan Stambaugh. London: Souvenir Press, 1973.

———. "What is Metaphysics?" In *Basic Writings*. David Farrell Krell (ed.). London: Routledge and Kegan Paul, 1993, pp. 91–112.

———. *Pathmarks*. Cambridge: Cambridge University Press, 1998.

———. *Sein und Zeit*. Tübingen: M. Niemeyer, [1927] 1993.

Heinemann, Fritz. *Existentialism and the Modern Predicament*. London and New York: Harper and Row, 1953.

———. *Existenzphilosophie—lebendig oder tot?* Stuttgart: Kohlhammer, 1954.

———. *Jenseits des Existentialismus*. Stuttgart: W. Kohlhammer, 1957.

Heinrich, Dieter. "Denken im Blick auf Max Weber." In *Karl Jaspers—Philosoph, Arzt, politischer Denker*, Jeanne Hersch, Jan Milic Lochman, and Reiner Wiehl (eds.). Munich and Zurich: Piper, 1986, pp. 207–231.

Hennig, John. "Karl Jaspers' Attitude towards History." In *The Philosophy of Karl Jaspers*, Paul Arthur Schilpp (ed.). New York: Tudor, 1957, pp. 565–591.

Hersch, Jeanne. *Die Illusion, Der Weg der Philosophie*. Bern: Francke, 1965.

———. *Karl Jaspers, Eine Einführung in sein Werk*. Bern: Francke, 1978.

———. "Existenz in der empirischen Wirklichkeit." In *Karl Jaspers—Philosoph, Arzt, politischer Denker*, Jeanne Hersch, Jan Milic Lochman, and Reiner Wiehl (eds.). Munich and Zurich: Piper, 1986, pp. 47–58.

———, Lochman, Jan Milic & Wiehl, Reiner (eds.). *Karl Jaspers—Philosoph, Arzt, politischer Denker*. Munich and Zurich: Piper, 1986.

Hertel, Wolf. *Existentieller Glaube, Eine Studie über den Glaubensbegriff von Karl Jaspers und Paul Tillich*. Meisenheim am Glan: Verlag Anton Hain, 1971.

Hoffman, Kurt. "The Basic Concept of Jaspers' Philosophy." In *The Philosophy of Karl Jaspers*. Paul Arthur Schilpp (ed.). New York: Tudor, 1957, pp. 95–113.

Hommel, Claus Uwe. *Chiffer und Dogma, vom Verhältnis der Philosophie zur Religion bei Karl Jaspers*. Zurich: EVZ Verlag, Abt. Editio Academica, 1968.

Hommes, Ulrich. *Die Existenzerhellung und das Recht*. Frankfurt: Klostermann, 1962.

Husserl, Edmund. "Philosophy as Rigorous Science." In *Phenomenology and the Crisis of Philosophy*. Translated by Quentin Lauer. New York: Harper and Row, 1965.

Ignatieff, Michael. *The Need of Strangers: An Essay on Privacy and the Politics of Being Human*. New York: Penguin Books, 1988.

Imle, F. "Jaspers als Existenzphilosoph," *Philosophisches Jahrbuch der Görresgesellschaft*, 49, (1936), pp. 487–504.

———. "Jaspers als Existenzphilosoph," *Philosophisches Jahrbuch der Görresgesellschaft*, 50, (1937), pp.78–93.

Janzarik, Werner. "Jaspers, Kurt Schneider und die Heidelberger Psychopathologie." In *Karl Jaspers—Philosoph, Arzt, politischer Denker*, Jeanne Hersch, Jan Milic Lochman, and Reiner Wiehl (eds.). Munich and Zurich: Piper, 1986, pp. 112–126.

Jaspers, Karl. "Heimweh und Verbrechen" (Dissertation). In *Archiv für Kriminal–Anthropologie und Kriminalistik*, 35, (1909).

———. "Ein Beitrag zur Frage: 'Entwicklung einer Persönlichkeit' oder 'Prozess'?" *Zeitschrift für die gesamte Neurologie und Psychiatrie*, 1, (1910), pp. 567–637.
———. "Die Methode der Intelligenzprüfung und der Begriff der Dimenz," *Zeitschrift für die gesamte Neurologie und Psychiatrie*, (referatential) (1910), pp. 402–452.
———. "Zur Analyse der Trugwahrnehmungen" (Leibhaftigkeit und Realitätsurteil), *Zeitschrift für die gesamte Neurologie und Psychiatrie*, 6, (1911), pp. 460–535.
———. "Die Trugwahrnehmungen," *Zeitschrift für die gesamte Neurologie und Psychiatrie*, 4, (referatential) (1912), pp. 289–354.
———. "Die phänomenologische Forschungsrichtung in Psychopathologie," *Zeitschrift für die gesamte Neurologie und Psychiatrie*, 9, (1912), pp. 391–408.
———. "Kausale und 'verständliche' Zusammenhange zwischen Schicksal und Psychose bei der Dementia praecox (Schizophrenie)," *Zeitschrift für die gesamte Neurologie und Psychiatrie*, 14, (1913), pp. 158–263.
———. *Allgemeine Psychopathologie, Ein Leitfaden für Studierende, Ärzte und Psychologen*. 1st Edition. Berlin: Springer, 1913.
———. *Die geistige Situation der Zeit*. Berlin: Walter de Gruyter, 1931.
———. "Geleitwort," *Die Wandlung*, 1, (1945).
———. *Die Schuldfrage*. Heidelberg: L. Schneider, 1946.
———. *Die Idee der Universität*. 1. Berlin: Springer, Schriften der Universität Heidelberg, 1946.
———. *Nietzsche, Einführung in das Verständnis seines Philosophierens*. Berlin: Walter De Gruyter, 1950.
———. *Vernunft und Widervernunft in unserer Zeit, Drei Gastvorlesungen*. Munich: Piper, 1950.
———. *Einführung in die Philosophie, Zwölf Radiovorträge*. Zurich: Artemis, 1950.
———. *Über Bedingungen und Möglichkeiten eines neuen Humanismus*. Stuttgart: P. Reclamjun, 1951.
———. *Die Frage der Entmythologisierung*. Munich: Piper, 1954.
———. *Schelling, Grö ße und Verhängnis*. Munich: Piper, 1955.
———. *Die grossen Philosophen* (1–3). Munich: Piper, 1957.
———. "Reply to my critics." In *The Philosophy of Karl Jaspers*. Paul Arthur Schilpp (ed.). New York: Tudor, 1957, pp. 748–869.
———. *Philosophie und Welt, Reden und Aufsätze*. Munich: Piper, 1958.
———. *Rechenschaft und Ausblick, Reden und Aufsätze*. Munich: Piper, 1958.
———. *Max Weber, Politiker-Forscher-Philosoph*. Munich: Piper, 1958.
———. *Vernunft und Freiheit, Ausgewählte Schriften*. Stuttgart–Zurich–Salzburg: Europäischer Buchklub, 1959.
———. *Der philosophische Glaube*. Munich: Piper, [1948] 1960.
———. *Die Atombombe und die Zukunft des Menschen*. Munich: Piper, 1961.
———. *Der philosophische Glaube angesichts der Offenbarung*. Munich: Piper, 1962.
———. *Existenzphilosophie*. 3rd edition. Berlin: Walter de Gruyter, [1937] 1964.
———. *Allgemeine Psychopathologie*. 8th edition. Berlin–Heidelberg: Springer, 1965.
———. *Descartes und die Philosophie* (1937), 4th edition. Berlin: Walter de Gruyter, 1966.
———. *Chiffren der Transzendenz*. Munich: Piper, 1970.

———. *Was ist Erziehung?* Munich: Piper, 1981.

———. "Einsamkeit," *Revue Internationale de Philosophie*, 37, (1983), pp. 390–409.

———. *Psychologie der Weltanschauungen*. Berlin: Springer, [1919] 1985.

———. *Vernunft und Existenz*. Munich: Piper, [1935] 1987.

———. *Notizen zu Martin Heidegger*. Hans Saner, (ed.). Munich: Piper, 1989.

———. *Von der Wahrheit*. Munich: Piper, [1947] 1991.

———. *Philosophie* (1–3). Berlin: Springer, [1932] 1994.

Junghänel, Günter. "Über den Begriff der Kommunikation bei Karl Jaspers," *Deutsche Zeitschrift für Philosophie*, 9:4, (1961), pp. 472–489.

Kane, John F. *Pluralism and Truth in Religion*. Chico, CA: Scholars Press, 1981.

Kant, Immanuel. *Critique of Pure Reason*. Translated and edited by Paul Guyer and Allen W. Wood. New York: Cambridge University Press, 1977.

———. *Critique of the Power of Judgment*. Edited by Paul Guyer. Translated by Paul Guyer and Eric Mathews. New York: Cambridge University Press, 2000.

———. "Prolegomena to any future metaphysics that will be able to come forward as a science." Translated by Gary Hatfield. In *Immanuel Kant: Theoretical Philosophy after 1781*. Henry Allison and Peter Heath (eds.). New York: Cambridge University Press, 2002, pp. 29–170.

Kaufmann, Fritz. "Karl Jaspers and a Philosophy of Communication." In *The Philosophy of Karl Jaspers*. Paul Arthur Schilpp (ed.). New York: Tudor, 1957, pp. 211–295.

Kaufmann, Walter. *Nietzsche: Philosopher, Psychologist, Antichrist*. Princeton, New Jersey: Princeton University Press, 1974.

Kelemen, Janos, "The 'Thing-in-itself' and the 'Encompassing'." In *Karl Jaspers: Philosoph unter Philosophen*. Leonard Ehrlich and Richard Wisser (eds.). Würzburg: Konigshausen & Neumann, 1993, pp. 18–21.

Kiel, Albrecht. "Der 'Philosophische Glaube' (Jaspers) und die Logik." In *Glauben und Wissen, Dritter Teil (Hegel-Jahrbuch 2005)*. Andreas Arndt (ed.). Berlin: Akademie–Verlag, 2005, pp. 291–297.

Kierkegaard, Søren. *Concluding Unscientific Postscript*. Princeton: Princeton University, 1974.

Klein, Aloys. *Glaube und Mythos, Eine kritische, religionsphilosophisch–theologische Untersuchung des Mythos–Begriffs bei Karl Jaspers*. Munich: F. Schöningh, 1973.

Kluback, William. "Karl Jaspers and Schmuel Hugo Bergman. Believing Philosophers." In *Karl Jaspers: Philosoph unter Philosophen*. Leonard Ehrlich and Richard Wisser (eds.). Würzburg: Konigshausen & Neumann, 1993, pp. 173–185.

Knauss, Gerhard. *Gegenstand und Umgreifendes*. Dissertation. Basel: Verlag fur Recht und Gesellschaft, 1954.

———. "The Concept of the 'Encompassing' in Jaspers' Philosophy." In *The Philosophy of Karl Jaspers*. Paul Arthur Schilpp (ed.). New York: Tudor, 1957, pp. 141–175.

Knittermeyer, Heinrich. *Die Philosophie der Existenz von der Renaissance bis zur Gegenwart*. Vienna: Humboldt, 1961.

Kolle, Kurt, "Jaspers as Psychopathologist." In *The Philosophy of Karl Jaspers.* Paul Arthur Schilpp (ed.). New York: Tudor, 1957, pp. 437–466.

Krings, Hermann. "Die Philosophie zwischen Anpassung und Selbstbehauptung," Gespräch mit Prof. Hermann Krings, *Widerspruch, Münchener Zeitschrift für Philosophie* (1987), pp. 15–26.

Kronfeld, Arthur. "Über neuere pathologisch–phänomenologische Arbeiten," *Zentralblatt für die gesamte Neurologie und Psychiatrie*, XXVIII, (1922), pp. 441–459.

Kunz, Hans. "Critique of Jaspers' Concept of Transcendence." In *The Philosophy of Karl Jaspers.* Paul Arthur Schilpp (ed.). New York: Tudor, 1957, pp. 115–140.

Kwiatkowski, Gerhard (ed.). *Die Philosophie, Ein Sachlexikon der Philosophie.* Vienna and Zurich: Dudenverlag, Mannheim, 1985.

Landgrebe, Ludwig. *Was bedeutet uns Philosophie? Eine Einführung.* Hamburg: Marion von Schroder, 1948.

Latzel, Edwin. "Bemerkungen zum Umgang mit Existenzphilosophie," *Zeitschrift für philosophische Forschung*, VI, (1951/1952), pp. 399–410.

———. "The Concept of 'Ultimate Situation' in Jaspers' Philosophy." In *The Philosophy of Karl Jaspers.* Paul Arthur Schilpp (ed.). New York: Tudor, 1957, pp. 177–208.

Lengert, Rudolf (ed.). *Philosophie der Freiheit.* Oldenburg: Holzberg, 1983.

Lenz, Joseph. *Der moderne deutsche und französische Existentialismus.* Trier: Paulinus Verlag, 1951.

Leonard, Henry. "Interrogative, Imperatives, Truth, Falsity and Lies," *Philosophy of Science*, 26, (1959), pp. 176–186.

Leonard, Joachim-Felix (ed.). *Karl Jaspers in seiner Heidelberger Zeit.* Heidelberg: Heidelberger Verlagsanstalt und Druckerei, 1983.

Lichtigfeld, Adolph. *Jaspers' Metaphysics.* London: Colibri Press, 1954.

———. "Jaspers in English: A Failure of Communication but rather of Interpretation," *Philosophy & Phenomenological Research*, 41, (1981).

Litt, Theodor, *Mensch und Welt, Grundlinien einer Philosophie des Geistes.* Munich-Heidelberg: Quelle & Meyer, 1961.

Llewelyn, John E. "What is a Question?" *The Australian Journal of Philosophy*, 42, (1964), pp. 69–85.

Lonergan, Bernard Joseph Francis. *Method in Theology.* New York: Herder & Herder, 1972.

———. "Reality, Myth, Symbol." In Myth, *Symbol, and Reality*, Alan M. Olson (ed.), Notre Dame: University of Notre Dame Press, 1980, pp. 31–37.

Lotz, Johannes Baptist. *Sein und Existenz.* Freiburg: Herder, 1965.

Löwenstein, Julius I. "Das Bleibende von Jaspers und Heidegger." In *Karl Jaspers Today, Philosophy at the Threshold of the Future.* Leonard Ehrlich and Richard Wisser (eds.). Washington. D.C.: University Press of America, 1988, pp. 317–340.

Löwith, Karl. "Existenz-Philosophie," *Zeitschrift für deutsche Bildung*, 12, (1932), pp. 602–613.

———. *Das Individuum in der Rolle des Mitmenschen.* Darmstadt: Wissenschaftliche Buchgesellschaft, 1969.

Lukács, Georg. *Die Zerstörung der Vernunft: Der Weg des Irrationalismus von Schelling zu Hitler*. Berlin: Aufbau Verlag, 1955.

Mader, Hans. *Problemgeschichtliche Studie zur Periechontologie Karl Jaspers*. Dissertation. Vienna, 1952.

———. "Das Seindenken bei Karl Jaspers," *Wissenschaft und Weltbild*, 10, (1957), pp. 50–58.

Manasse, Ernst Moritz. "Max Weber's Influence on Jaspers." In *The Philosophy of Karl Jaspers*. Paul Arthur Schilpp (ed.). New York: Tudor, 1957, pp. 369–393.

Marcel, Gabriel. "Grundsituation und Grenzsituationen." In *Karl Jaspers in der Diskussion*, Hans Saner (ed.). Munich: Piper, 1973, pp.155–180.

Marcuse, Herbert. *One Dimensional Man: Studies in the Ideology of Advanced Industrial Society*. Boston: Beacon Press, 1964.

May, Rollo, et al. (eds.). *Existence: A New Dimension in Psychology and Psychiatry*. New York: Basic Books, 1958.

Mayer, Ernst. "Philosophie und philosophische Logik bei Karl Jaspers." In *Offener Horizont, Festschrift für Karl Jaspers, zum 70*. Klaus Piper (ed.). Munich: Geburtstag, Piper, 1953, pp. 63–73.

Meinung, Alexius. "The Theory of Objects." In *Realism and the Background of Phenomenology*. Roderick Milton Chisholm (ed.). Glencoe: Free Press, 1960, pp. 76–117.

Milbank, John. *Theology & Social Theory: Beyond Secular Reason*. Oxford: Blackwell, 1997.

Miron, Ronny. "From Opposition to Reciprocity: Karl Jaspers on Science, Philosophy, and What Lies Between Them," *International Philosophical Quarterly*, 44, (2004), pp. 147–163.

———. "Towards Reality: The Development of the Philosophical Attitude to Reality in Karl Jaspers' Thought," *Journal of the British Society for Phenomenology*, 37:2, (2006), pp. 152–172.

———. "Transcendence and Dissatisfaction in Jaspers' Idea of the Self," *Phaenomenologische Forschungen* , NS 10, (2005), pp. 221–241.

———. "Was Jaspers Really Kantian?" *Yearbook of the Austrian Karl Jaspers Society*, 19, (2006), pp. 73–106.

Motzkin, Gabriel Gideon. *The Problem of Transcendence in the Secular World: From Kant to Heidegger* (1–2). Dissertation. Ann Arbor: University Microfilms International, 1982.

Müller, Max. *Existenzphilosophie, Von der Metaphysik zur Metahistorik*. Freiburg-Munich: K. Alber, [1949] 1986.

Müller-Schwefe, Hans-Rudolf. *Existenzphilosophie, Das Verständnis von Existenz in Philosophie und christlichem Glauben*. Gottingen: Vandenhoeck & Ruprecht, 1961.

Olson, Alan M. *Transcendence and Hermeneutics: An Interpretation of the Philosophy of Karl Jaspers*. The Hague and Boston: M. Nijhoff, 1979.

——— (ed.). *Myth, Symbol, and Reality*. Notre Dame: University of Notre Dame Press, 1980.

———. "Introduction." In *Myth, Symbol, and Reality*. Alan M. Olson (ed.). Notre Dame: University of Notre Dame Press, 1980, pp.1–12.

———. "Myth, Symbol, and Metaphorical Truth." In *Myth, Symbol, and Reality*. Alan M. Olson (ed.). Notre Dame: University of Notre Dame Press, 1980, pp. 99–125.

———. "Hegel and Jaspers on the Comparative Philosophy of Religion." In *Karl Jaspers: Philosoph unter Philosophen*. Leonard Ehrlich and Richard Wisser (eds.). Würzburg: Konigshausen & Neumann, 1993, pp. 41–64.

———. "Jaspers's Critique of Modernity: A Postmodern Reflection." In *Karl Jaspers Today, Philosophy at the Threshold of the Future*. Leonard Ehrlich and Richard Wisser (eds.). Washington, D.C.: University Press of America, 1988, pp. 363–380.

——— (ed.). *Heidegger & Jaspers*. Philadelphia: Temple University Press, 1994.

Olson, Robert Goodwin. *An Introduction to Existentialism*. New York: Dover, 1962.

Örnek, Yusuf. *Karl Jaspers: Philosophie der Freiheit*. Freiburg and Munich: K. Alber, 1986.

Orozco, Teresa. *Platonische Gewalt, Gadamers politische Hermeneutik der NS-Zeit*. Berlin: Argument, 1995.

Paul, Jean Marie. "Der Weg des Menschen oder Kommunikation und Liebe bei Jaspers." In *Karl Jaspers, Denken zwischen Wissenschaft, Politik und Philosophie*. Dietrich Harth (ed.). Stuttgart: Metzler, J.B., 1989, pp. 43–64.

Pfeiffer, Johannes. *Existenzphilosophie, Eine Einführung in Heidegger und Jaspers*. Leipzig: Felix Meiner, 1952.

———. "On Karl Jaspers' Interpretation of Art." In *The Philosophy of Karl Jaspers*. Paul Arthur Schilpp (ed.). New York: Tudor, 1957, pp. 703–717.

Piper, Klaus. (ed.), *Offener Horizont, Festschrift für Karl Jaspers, zum 70*. Munich: Geburtstag, Piper, 1953.

Plümacher, Martina. *Philosophie nach 1945 in der Bundesrepublik Deutschland*. Hamburg: Rowohlt Taschenbuch Verlag, 1996.

Räber, Thomas. *Das Dasein in der "Philosophie" von Karl Jaspers: Eine Untersuchung im Hinblick auf die Einheit und die Realität der Welt im existentiallen Denken*. Bern: Francke, 1955.

Reding, Marcel. *Die Existenzphilosophie, Heidegger, Sartre, Gabriel Marcel und Jaspers in kritischer-systematischer Sicht*. Düsseldorf: Schwann, 1949.

Reis, Johannes. "Menschliche Existenz bei Jaspers," *Die Neue Ordnung*, 4, (1950), pp. 418–426, pp. 527–531.

———. "Transzendenz bei Jaspers," in *Die Neue Ordnung*, 5, (1951), pp. 230–240.

Reisterer, Berthold P. "Existenz and Transcendence. Karl Jaspers and the Crisis of Contemporary Liberalism." In *Karl Jaspers: Philosoph unter Philosophen*. Leonard Ehrlich and Richard Wisser (eds.). Würzburg: Konigshausen & Neumann, 1993, pp. 228–234.

Richli, Urs. *Transzendental Reflexion und sittliche Entscheidung, Zum Problem der Selbsterkenntnis der Metaphysik bei Jaspers und Kant*. Bonn: H. Bouvier, 1967.

Ricoeur, Paul. "The Relation of Jaspers' Philosophy to Religion." In *The Philosophy of Karl Jaspers*. Paul Arthur Schilpp (ed.). New York: Tudor, 1957, pp. 611–642.

———. "Philosophie und Religion bei Jaspers." In *Karl Jaspers in der Diskussion.* Hans Saner (ed.). Munich: Piper, 1973, pp. 358–389.

———. "Existence and Hermeneutics." In *Contemporary Hermeneutics: Hermeneutics as Method, Philosophy and Critique.* Josef Bleicher (ed.). London and New York: Routledge & Kegan Paul, 1980, pp. 236–256.

———. *The Rule of Metaphor: Multi-disciplinary Studies of Creation of Meaning in Language.* London: Routledge & Kegan Paul, 1986.

Rickert, Heinrich. "Psychologie der Weltschauungen und Philosopie der Werte," *Logos,* 9, (1920), pp. 1–42.

———. *Die Grenzen der naturwissenschaft–lischen Begriffsbildung, Eine logische Einleitung in die historischen Wissenschaften.* Tübingen: Mohr, 1921.

———. *Der Gegenstand der Erkenntnis, Einführung in die Transzendentalphilosophie.* Tübingen: Mohr, 1928.

Rickman, Hans Peter. "The Philosophic Basis of Psychiatry: Jaspers and Dilthey," *Philosophy of the Social Science,* 17, (1987), pp. 173–196.

Ringer, Fritz K. *The Decline of the German Mandarins, The German Academic Community, 1890–1933.* Cambridge, Mass.: Harvard University Press, 1969.

Rollins, C. D. "Solipsism." In *The Encyclopedia of Philosophy,* 7. Paul Edwards (ed.). New York: MacMillan, 1967, pp. 487–491.

Rossmann, Kurt. "Wert und Grenze der Wissenschaft." In *Offener Horizont, Festschrift für Karl Jaspers, zum 70.* Klaus Piper (ed.). Munich: Geburtstag, Piper, 1953, pp. 126–146.

Rotenstreich, Nathan. *Between Past and Present.* New Haven: Yale University Press, 1958.

Sagi, Avi. *Kierkegaard, Religion, and Existence: The Voyage of the Self.* Translated by Batya Stein. Amsterdam: Rodopi, 2000.

———. *Albert Camus and the Philosophy of the Absurd.* Translated by Batya Stein. Amsterdam: Rodopi, 2002.

Salamun, Kurt. *Karl Jaspers.* Munich: Beck, 1985.

——— (ed.). *Karl Jaspers, Zur Aktualität seines Denkens.* Munich: Piper, 1991.

Salamun-Hybasek, Elisabeth and Salamun, Kurt (eds.). *Jahrbuch der österreichischen Karl Jaspers Gesellschaft,* 9, (1996).

Samay, Sebastian. *Reason Revisited: The Philosophy of Karl Jaspers.* Dublin: Gill and Macmillan, 1971.

Saner, Hans. *Karl Jaspers, Werk und Wirkung, zum 80.* Munich: Geburtstag, Piper, 1963.

——— (ed.). *Karl Jaspers in der Diskussion.* Munich: Piper, 1973.

———. *Jaspers.* Hamburg: Rowohlt, [1970] 1991.

———. *Karl Jaspers in Selbstzeugnissen und Bilddokumenten.* Hamburg: Rowohlt,] 1979] 1991).

Sartre, Jean-Paul. *The Transcendental Ego: An Existentialist Theory of the Consciousness.* New York: Noonday Press, 1957.

———. *Being and Nothingness: An Essay on Phenomenological Ontology.* London: Methuen, 1957.

Schatz, Oskar. "Religionsphilosophische Aspekte bei Karl Jaspers," *Kairos*, I, (1960), pp. 23–28.

Scheler, Max. *Philosophische Weltanschauung*. Munich: Lehnen Verlag, 1954.

Schilpp, Paul Arthur (ed.). *The Philosophy of Karl Jaspers*. New York: Tudor, 1957.

Schipperges, Heinrich. "Medizin als konkrete Philosophie." In *Karl Jaspers—Philosoph, Arzt, politischer Denker*. Jeanne Hersch, Jan Milic Lochman, and Reiner Wiehl (eds.). Munich and Zurich: Piper, 1986, pp. 88–111.

Schnädelbach, Herbert. *Philosophy in Germany, 1831–1933*. Cambridge: Cambridge University Press, 1984.

Schneider, Kurt. "Die phänomenologische Richtung in den Psychiatrie." *Philosophischer Anzeiger*, IV, (1926), pp. 382–404.

Schneiders, Werner. *Karl Jaspers in der Kritik*. Bonn: Bouvier, 1965.

Schrag, Oswald O. *Existence, Existenz, and Transcendence*. Pittsburg: Duquesne University Press, 1971.

Schrey, Heinz Horst. *Dialogisches Denken*. Darmstadt: Wissenschaftliche Buchgesellschaft, 1970.

Schultheiss, Jürgen. *Philosophieren als Kommunikation, Versuch zu Karl Jaspers' Apologie des kritischen Philosophierens*. Meisenheim: Forum Academicum, 1981.

Schweidler, Walter. "Die Ethik des Augenblicks. Jaspers, Kierkegaard, Wittgenstein." In *Karl Jaspers: Philosoph unter Philosophen*. Leonard Ehrlich and Richard Wisser (eds.). Würzburg: Konigshausen & Neumann, 1993, pp. 202–214.

Seideneck, Hermann-Josef. "Das Wagnis der Schwebe, Der Gottesgedanke im philosophischen Werk von Karl Jaspers." In *Karl Jaspers: Philosoph unter Philosophen*. Leonard Ehrlich and Richard Wisser (eds.). Würzburg: Konigshausen and Neumann, 1993, pp. 250–254.

Simmel, Georg. *Die Probleme der Geschichtsphilosophie*. Leipzig: Duncker & Humblot, 1892.

———. *Hauptprobleme der Philosophie*. Leipzig: G. J. Goschen, 1911.

Solomon, Robert Charles. *From Rationalism to Existentialism: The Existentialists and their Nineteenth–Century Background*. Boston: University Press of America, 1985.

Sonnemann, Ulrich. *Existence and Therapy: An Introduction to Phenomenological Psychology and Existential Analysis*. New York: Grune & Stratton, 1954.

Spiegelberg, Herbert. "Der Begriff der Intentionalität in der Scholastik bei Brentano und Husserl," *Philosophische Hefte*, 5, (1936), pp. 75–91.

———. "The Relevance of Phenomenological Philosophy for Psychology." In *Phenomenology and Existentialism*. Edward N. Lee and Maurice Mandelbaum (eds.). Baltimore: Johns Hopkins Press, 1967.

———. *Phenomenology in Psychology and Psychiatry*. Evanston: Northwestern University Press, 1972.

Spitzer, Manfred. *Phenomenology, Language & Schizophrenia*. In Manfred Spitzer, Friedrich Uehlein, and Michael A. Schwarts (eds.). New York and Berlin: Springer 1992, pp. 35–69

Spitzer, Manfred, Uehlein, Friedrich and Schwarts, Michael A. (eds.). *Phenomenology, Language & Schizophrenia*. New York and Berlin: Springer, 1992.

Stegmueller, Wolfgang. *Hauptströmungen der Gegenwartsphilosophie*. Stuttgart: Alfred Kroner, 1960.

———. *Probleme und Resultate der Wissenschaftstheorie und analytischen Philosophie*, I. Berlin-Heidelberg-New York: Springer, 1969.

Stewart, Jon. *The Unity of Hegel's Phenomenology of Spirit: A Systematic Interpretation*. Evanston, Illinois: Northwestern University Press, 2000.

Tennen, Hanoch. *The Perception of Existentialist Ethics in Karl Jaspers' Philosophy*. Ramat Gan: Masada, 1977 [Hebrew].

———. "Jaspers' Philosophie in kritischer Sicht—Das Verhältnis zwischen Philosophie und Wissenschaft," *Zeitschrift für philosophische Forschung*, 28:4, (1974), pp. 536–561.

Theunissen, Michael. *Der Andere, Studien zur Sozialontologie der Gegenwart*. Berlin: W. de Gruyter, 1981.

Thyssen, Johannes. "The Concept of 'Foundering' in Jaspers' Philosophy." In *The Philosophy of Karl Jaspers*. Paul Arthur Schilpp (ed.). New York: Tudor, 1957, pp. 297–335.

Tillich, Paul. *A History of Christian Thought, From its Judaic and Hellenistic Origins to Existentialism*. New York: Simon & Schuster, 1967.

———. "Heidegger and Jaspers." In *Heidegger & Jaspers*. Alan M. Olson (ed.). Philadelphia: Temple University Press, 1994, pp. 16–28.

Tilliette, Xavier. "Sinn, Wert und Grenze der Chiffernlehre: Reflexionen über die Metaphysik von Karl Jaspers." In *Karl Jaspers in der Diskussion*. Hans Saner, (ed.). Munich: Piper, 1973, pp. 390–404.

Tymieniecka, Anna-Teresa. *Phenomenology and Science in Contemporary Thought*. New York: Farrar, Straus and Cudahy, 1962.

Van Kaam, Adrian. "The Impact of Existential Phenomenology on Psychological Literature of Western Europe," *Review of Existential Psychology and Psychiatry*, I, (1961), pp. 63–92.

Vernekohl, Wilhelm. *Peter Wust: Leben und Werk, Biographische Notizen*. Münster: Regensberg, 1967.

Von Kempski, Jürgen. "Geleitwort," *Archiv für Philosophie*, 1, 1947, pp. 5–8.

———. "Kant und der Geist der Europäischen Philosophie," *Archiv für Philosophie*, 1, (1947), pp. 9–38.

———. "Philosophie als Anruf." In *Brechungen, Kritischer Versuch zur Philosophie der Gegenwart*. Jürgen Von Kempski (ed.). Hamburg: Rowohlt, 1964.

Von Pechmann, Alexander. "Die Philosophie der Nachkriegszeit in München (1945–1960)—Eine Dokumentation." *Widerspruch, Münchener Zeitschrift für Philosophie*, 18, (1990), 39–62.

Von Rinteln, Fritz-Joachim. *Beyond Existentialism*. London: Allen and Unwin, 1961.

Waardenburg, Jacques. "Symbolic Aspects of Myth." In *Myth, Symbol, and Reality*. Alan M. Olson (ed.). Notre Dame: University of Notre Dame Press, 1980, pp. 41–68.

Wallraff, Charles F. *Karl Jaspers: An Introduction to His Philosophy*. Princeton: Princeton University Press, 1970.

———. "Jaspers in English: A Failure in Communication," *Philosophy and Phenomenological Research*, 37, (1977), pp. 537–548.

Walker, Chris. "Karl Jaspers as a Kantian Psychopathologist, I: The Philosophical Origins of the Concept of Form and Content," *History of Psychiatry*, 4, (1993a), pp. 209–238.

———."Karl Jaspers as a Kantian Psychopathologist, II: The Concept of Form and Content in Jaspers' Psychopathology," *History of Psychiatry*, 4, (1993b), pp. 321–348.

———."Karl Jaspers as a Kantian Psychopathologist, III: "The Concept of Form in Georg Simmel's Social Theory: a Comparison with Jaspers," *History of Psychiatry*, 5, (1994), pp. 37–70.

———. "Karl Jaspers and Edmund Husserl—I: The Perceived Convergence," *Philosophy, Psychiatry, and Psychology*, 1:2, (1994), pp. 117–134.

———. "Karl Jaspers and Edmund Husserl—II: The Divergence," *Philosophy, Psychiatry and Psychology*, 1:4, (1994), pp. 245–266.

———. "Karl Jaspers and Edmund Husserl—III: Jaspers as a Kantian Phenomenologist," *Philosophy, Psychiatry and Psychology*, 2:1, (1995), pp. 65–82.

———. "Karl Jaspers and Edmund Husserl—IV: Phenomenology as Empathic Understanding," *Philosophy, Psychiatry and Psychology*, 2:3, (1995), pp. 247–266.

Walters, Gregory J. "Jaspers's Philosophical Faith and Revelational Faith Today: Can the Two Faiths Meet in the Struggle for Human Liberation?." In *Karl Jaspers: Philosoph unter Philosophen.* Leonard Ehrlich and Richard Wisser (eds.). Würzburg: Konigshausen & Neumann, 1993, pp. 217–227.

Wardlaw, Harry. "Jaspers' Account of Truth as a Way into the Discussion of Theological Truth–Claims." *Sophia*, 44:1, (2005), pp. 77–90.

Weber, Max. *Gesammelte Aufsätze zur Wissenschaftslehre*. Tübingen: J. C. B. Mohr, 1922.

———. *The Protestant Ethic and the Spirit of Capitalism*. New York: C. Scribner's Sons, 1958.

———. *Gesammelte Aufsätze zur Religionssoziologie*. Tübingen: J. C. B. Mohr, 1963.

Werner, Martin. "Existenzphilosophie und Christentum bei Karl Jaspers." In *Karl Jaspers in der Diskussion*. Hans Saner (ed.). Munich: Piper, 1973, pp. 335–357.

Wiggins, Osborne, Schwartz, Michael and Spitzer, Manfred. "Phenomenological/descriptive psychiatry: The Methods of Edmund Husserl and Karl Jaspers." In *Phenomenology, Language and Schizophrenia*. Manfred Spitzer, Friedrich Uehlein, and Michael Schwartz (eds.). New York: Springer, 1992, pp. 46–69.

Winkler, Robert. "Philosophische oder theologische Anthropologie?" *Zeitschrift für Theologie und Kirche*, 14:2, (1933), pp. 125–140.

Wisser, Richard. "Aneignung und Unterscheidung: Existenzphilosophie im Kampf um die Existenz der Philosophie." In *Karl Jaspers Today, Philosophy at the Threshold of the Future*. Leonard Ehrlich and Richard Wisser (eds.). Washington, D.C.: University Press of America, 1988, pp. 341–361.

———. *Karl Jaspers: Philosophy in der Bewährung, Vorträge und Aufsätze*. Würzburg: Königshausen & Neumann, 1995.

———. "Karl Jaspers: The Person and his Cause, Not the Person or his Cause," *International Philosophical Quarterly*, 26, (1996), pp. 413–427.

Wuchterl, Kurt. *Streitgespräche und Kontroversen in der Philosopie des 20. Jahrhunderts*. Stuttgart: UTB, 1982.

Wust, Peter. *Die Auferstehung der Metaphysik*. Leipzig: F. Meiner, 1921.

———. *Naivität und Pietät*. Tübingen: J. C. B. Mohr, 1925.

———. *Die Dialektik des Geistes*. Münster: Regensburg, 1964.

Young-Bruehl, Elisabeth. *Freedom and Karl Jaspers' Philosophy*. New Haven: Yale University Press, 1981.

ABOUT THE AUTHOR

Dr. Ronny Miron is a senior lecturer at the Program for Hermeneutics Studies and the Philosophy Department of Bar-Ilan University. Her areas of specialization, in both teaching and research, are existentialism, phenomenology, idealism, and modern Jewish theology.

INDEX

VIBS

The **Value Inquiry Book Series** is co-sponsored by:

Adler School of Professional Psychology
American Indian Philosophy Association
American Maritain Association
American Society for Value Inquiry
Association for Process Philosophy of Education
Canadian Society for Philosophical Practice
Center for Bioethics, University of Turku
Center for Professional and Applied Ethics, University of North Carolina at Charlotte
Central European Pragmatist Forum
Centre for Applied Ethics, Hong Kong Baptist University
Centre for Cultural Research, Aarhus University
Centre for Professional Ethics, University of Central Lancashire
Centre for the Study of Philosophy and Religion, University College of Cape Breton
Centro de Estudos em Filosofia Americana, Brazil
College of Education and Allied Professions, Bowling Green State University
College of Liberal Arts, Rochester Institute of Technology
Concerned Philosophers for Peace
Conference of Philosophical Societies
Department of Moral and Social Philosophy, University of Helsinki
Gannon University
Gilson Society
Haitian Studies Association
Ikeda University
Institute of Philosophy of the High Council of Scientific Research, Spain
International Academy of Philosophy of the Principality of Liechtenstein
International Association of Bioethics
International Center for the Arts, Humanities, and Value Inquiry
International Society for Universal Dialogue
Natural Law Society
Philosophical Society of Finland
Philosophy Born of Struggle Association
Philosophy Seminar, University of Mainz
Pragmatism Archive at The Oklahoma State University
R.S. Hartman Institute for Formal and Applied Axiology
Research Institute, Lakeridge Health Corporation
Russian Philosophical Society
Society for Existential Analysis
Society for Iberian and Latin-American Thought
Society for the Philosophic Study of Genocide and the Holocaust
Unit for Research in Cognitive Neuroscience, Autonomous University of Barcelona
Whitehead Research Project
Yves R. Simon Institute

Titles Published

Volumes 1 - 214 see www.rodopi.nl

215. Anders Nordgren, *For Our Children: The Ethics of Animal Experimentation in the Age of Genetic Engineering*. A volume in **Values in Bioethics**

216. James R. Watson, Editor, *Metacide: In the Pursuit of Excellence*. A volume in **Holocaust and Genocide Studies**

217. Andrew Fitz-Gibbon, Editor, *Positive Peace: Reflections on Peace Education, Nonviolence, and Social Change*. A volume in **Philosophy of Peace**

218. Christopher Berry Gray, *The Methodology of Maurice Hauriou: Legal, Sociological, Philosophical*. A volume in **Studies in Jurisprudence**

219. Mary K. Bloodsworth-Lugo and Carmen R. Lugo-Lugo, *Containing (Un)American Bodies: Race, Sexuality, and Post-9/11 Constructions of Citizenship*. A volume in **Philosophy of Peace**

220. Roland Faber, Brian G. Henning, Clinton Combs, Editors, *Beyond Metaphysics? Explorations in Alfred North Whitehead's Late Thought*. A volume in **Contemporary Whitehead Studies**

221. John G. McGraw, *Intimacy and Isolation (Intimacy and Aloneness: A Multi-Volume Study in Philosophical Psychology, Volume One)*, A volume in **Philosophy and Psychology**

222. Janice L. Schultz-Aldrich, Introduction and Edition, *"Truth" is a Divine Name, Hitherto Unpublished Papers of Edward A. Synan, 1918-1997*. A volume in **Gilson Studies**

223. Larry A. Hickman, Matthew Caleb Flamm, Krzysztof Piotr Skowroński and Jennifer A. Rea, Editors, *The Continuing Relevance of John Dewey: Reflections on Aesthetics, Morality, Science, and Society*. A volume in **Central European Value Studies**

224. Hugh P. McDonald, *Creative Actualization: A Meliorist Theory of Values*. A volume in **Studies in Pragmatism and Values**

225. Rob Gildert and Dennis Rothermel, Editors, *Remembrance and Reconciliation*. A volume in **Philosophy of Peace**

226. Leonidas Donskis, Editor, *Niccolò Machiavelli: History, Power, and Virtue*. A volume in **Philosophy, Literature, and Politics**

227. Sanya Osha, *Postethnophilosophy*. A volume in **Social Philosophy**

228. Rosa M. Calcaterra, Editor, *New Perspectives on Pragmatism and Analytic Philosophy*. A volume in **Studies in Pragmatism and Values**

229. Danielle Poe, Editor, *Communities of Peace: Confronting Injustice and Creating Justice*. A volume in **Philosophy of Peace**

230. Thorsten Botz-Bornstein, Editor, *The Philosophy of Viagra: Bioethical Responses to the Viagrification of the Modern World*. A volume in **Philosophy of Sex and Love**

231. Carolyn Swanson, *Reburial of Nonexistents: Reconsidering the Meinong-Russell Debate*. A volume in **Central European Value Studies**

232. Adrianne Leigh McEvoy, Editor, *Sex, Love, and Friendship: Studies of the Society for the Philosophy of Sex and Love: 1993–2003*. A volume in **Histories and Addresses of Philosophical Societies**

233. Amihud Gilead, *The Privacy of the Psychical*. A volume in **Philosophy and Psychology**

234. Paul Kriese and Randall E. Osborne, Editors, *Social Justice, Poverty and Race: Normative and Empirical Points of View*. A volume in **Studies in Jurisprudence**

235. Hakam H. Al-Shawi, *Reconstructing Subjects: A Philosophical Critique of Psychotherapy*. A volume in **Philosophy and Psychology**

236. Maurice Hauriou, *Tradition in Social Science*. Translation from French with an Introduction by Christopher Berry Gray. A volume in **Studies in Jurisprudence**

237. Camila Loew, *The Memory of Pain: Women's Testimonies of the Holocaust.*. A volume in **Holocaust and Genocide Studies**

238. Stefano Franchi and Francesco Bianchini, Editors, *The Search for a Theory of Cognition: Early Mechanisms and New Ideas*. A volume in **Cognitive Science**

239. Michael H. Mitias, *Friendship: A Central Moral Value.* A volume in **Ethical Theory and Practice**

240. John Ryder and Radim Šíp, Editors, *Identity and Social Transformation, Central European Pragmatist Forum, Volume Five.* A volume in **Central European Value Studies**

241. William Sweet and Hendrik Hart, *Responses to the Enlightenment: An Exchange on Foundations, Faith, and Community.* A volume in **Philosophy and Religion**

242. Leonidas Donskis and J.D. Mininger, Editors, *Politics Otherwise: Shakespeare as Social and Political Critique.* A volume in **Philosophy, Literature, and Politics**

243. Hugh P. McDonald, *Speculative Evaluations: Essays on a Pluralistic Universe.* A volume in **Studies in Pragmatism and Values.**

244. Dorota Koczanowicz and Wojciech Małecki, Editors, *Shusterman's Pragmatism: Between Literature and Somaesthetics.* A volume in **Central European Value Studies**

245. Harry Lesser, Editor, *Justice for Older People,* A volume in **Values in Bioethics**

246. John G. McGraw, *Personality Disorders and States of Aloneness (Intimacy and Aloneness: A Multi-Volume Study in Philosophical Psychology, Volume Two),* A volume in **Philosophy and Psychology**

247. André Mineau, *SS Thinking and the Holocaust.* A volume in **Holocaust and Genocide Studies**

248. Yuval Lurie, *Wittgenstein on the Human Spirit.* A volume in **Philosophy, Literature, and Politics**

249. Andrew Fitz-Gibbon, *Love as a Guide to Morals.* A volume in **Ethical Theory and Practice**

250. Ronny Miron, *Karl Jaspers: From Selfhood to Being.* A volume in **Studies in Existentialism**

CPSIA information can be obtained at www.ICGtesting.com
Printed in the USA
BVOW021459240712

296068BV00001B/34/P

9 789042 035317